Becoming a Behavioral Science Researcher

BECOMING A BEHAVIORAL SCIENCE RESEARCHER

A GUIDE TO PRODUCING RESEARCH THAT MATTERS

Rex B. Kline

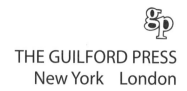

THE GUILFORD PRESS
New York   London

© 2009 The Guilford Press
A Division of Guilford Publications, Inc.
72 Spring Street, New York, NY 10012
www.guilford.com

Printed in the United States of America

This book is printed on acid-free paper.

Last digit is print number: 9 8 7 6 5 4 3

Library of Congress Cataloging-in-Publication Data

Kline, Rex B.
  Becoming a behavioral science researcher : a guide to
    producing research that matters / Rex B. Kline.
      p.   cm.
    Includes bibliographical references and indexes.
    ISBN 978-1-59385-837-7 (pbk. : alk. paper)
    ISBN 978-1-59385-838-4 (hardcover : alk. paper)
    1. Psychology—Research.   I. Title.
  BF76.5.K54   2009
  150.72—dc22
                                        2008019946

For Julia and Luke, my junior scientists

Preface and Acknowledgments

The idea for this book originated during a conversation in December 2006 with C. Deborah Laughton, Publisher, Methodology and Statistics, at The Guilford Press, about the challenges of teaching research seminars or other courses in which students conduct a thesis project. These students could be senior undergraduates in advanced programs, such as honors or specialization, or first-year graduate students. Although such students have typically taken at least two introductory courses in research methods and statistics, they are nevertheless "unfinished" in some critical ways, and thus not ready to carry out a thesis research project. For example, students' familiarity with basic concepts about design and analysis is often rather poor, despite their previous coursework. This coursework may not have introduced them to some important contemporary issues, such as statistics reform. Students' knowledge of measurement issues may be even worse still, often because they've never taken a psychometrics course. Students also need help with learning how to write cogently about their research or make formal presentations about their work. As an instructor or supervisor of thesis students, it can be difficult to specify readings that address all these needs. This is because it is often necessary to pull together works from a variety of sources, including chapters from methods or statistics books that review critical concepts, shorter or paperback books that specifically help students learn how to write better or make effective presentations, and journal articles that deal with topics just mentioned or related critical issues about how to improve behavioral science research. C. Deborah offered me this condolence: Why not write a book that addresses all these issues in one place? Well, why not indeed, especially given that doing is better than complaining. C. Deborah, thanks for getting me started.

I must also say thanks to the many psychology students in my research seminar sections over the last few years who shared with me some of their aspirations and frustrations in becoming more skilled at understanding and carrying out research. They helped me to better understand ways in which their educational backgrounds may have fallen short in preparing them to eventually become behavioral scientists. It has been rewarding for me to have played even a small role in helping them to build the foundations for later professional careers. Bruce Thompson provided invaluable commentary about several draft chapters, and many of his suggestions were incorporated into this book. This is not the first time that Bruce has given me such assistance, and I hope it is not the last. I would also like to thank the following people for their thorough reviews and thoughtful input: Theresa DiDonato, Psychology, Brown University; Larry Price, Psychometrics and Statistics, Texas State University, San Marcos; Chris L. S. Coryn, The Evaluation Center, Western Michigan University; Joseph DuCette, Educational Psychology, Temple University; and Tammy Kolbe, Educational Leadership and Policy Studies, Florida State University. It was a pleasure to work once again with the production staff at Guilford, especially Anna Nelson, Production Editor, in preparing the final version of this book. Finally, my biggest thanks go again to my family—wife, Joanna, and children, Julia and Luke—for their love and constant support.

Contents

I. PROMISE AND PROBLEMS

1. Introduction   3

Not Ready for Prime Time / 4
What Students Say They Need / 7
Plan of the Book / 7
Career Paths for Behavioral Scientists / 10
Summary / 12
Recommended Readings / 13

2. The Good, the Bad, and the (Really) Ugly   15
of Behavioral Science Research

The Good / 16
The Bad / 21
The (Really) Ugly / 27
Why? / 30
Summary / 34
Recommended Readings / 34

II. CONCEPTS

3. The Research Trinity   39
Trinity Overview / 39
Design / 41

Measurement / 46
Analysis / 47
Internal Validity / 54
Construct Validity / 62
Conclusion Validity / 64
External Validity and Sampling / 67
Summary / 70
Recommended Readings / 71
Exercises / 71

4. Design and Analysis   73
Chapter Overview / 74
From Question to Design / 74
Experimental Designs / 76
Controlled Quasi-Experimental Designs / 92
Nonequivalent-Group Designs / 94
Regression-Discontinuity Designs / 103
Other Quasi-Experimental Designs / 107
Nonexperimental Designs / 111
Resources for Learning More / 112
Summary / 112
Recommended Readings / 114
Exercises / 114

5. The Truth about Statistics   117
Study Strategy / 117
A Dozen Truths about Statistics / 118
What Statistical Significance Really Means / 121
Misinterpretations of Statistical Significance / 124
Why Are There So Many Myths? / 130
Other Drawbacks of Statistical Tests / 132
In Defense of Statistical Tests / 135
Recommendations for Changing Times / 136
Summary / 138
Recommended Readings / 138
Exercises / 139
Appendix 5.1. Review of Statistics Fundamentals / 140

6. Effect Size Estimation   153
Contexts for Estimating Effect Size / 154
Families of Parametric Effect Sizes / 155
Estimating Effect Size When Comparing Two Samples / 158
Measures of Association for More Complex Designs / 166
Effect Sizes for Dichotomous Outcomes / 169
T-Shirt Effect Sizes, Importance, and Cautions / 172

Approximate Confidence Intervals / 175
Research Examples / 178
Summary / 184
Recommended Readings / 184
Exercises / 185
Appendix 6.1. Noncentrality Interval Estimation for Effect Sizes / 186

7. Measurement   191

Chapter Scope / 191
The Critical Yet Underappreciated Role of Measurement / 193
Measurement Process Overview / 194
Resources for Finding Measures / 200
Adapting or Translating Tests / 204
Evaluation of Score Reliability and Validity / 205
Checklist for Evaluating Measures / 216
Recent Developments in Test Theory / 217
Summary / 220
Recommended Readings / 221
Exercises / 221

III. SKILLS

8. Practical Data Analysis   225

Vision First, Then Simplicity / 225
Managing Complex Analyses (Batch to the Future) / 229
Data Screening / 233
Summary / 249
Recommended Readings / 249
Exercises / 250

9. Writing   253

Plagiarism and Academic Integrity / 253
Writing as Learning / 254
Getting Started / 254
The Role of Style Guides / 255
General Principles of Good Writing / 256
Principles of Good Scientific Writing / 261
Writing Sections of Empirical Studies / 263
Effective Graphical Displays / 273
Ready for the Big Time / 276
Summary / 278
Recommended Readings / 279
Appendix 9.1. Example Results Section / 280

10. Presentations   283

Challenges of Oral Presentations / 283
Problems with PowerPoint Presentations / 286
Principles for Creating Effective PowerPoint Presentations / 289
Lessons from Multimedia Learning / 299
Other PowerPoint Issues / 300
Poster Presentations /302
Summary / 305
Recommended Readings / 305
Exercises / 306
Appendix 10.1. Example Slides, Handout, and Poster / 307

Suggested Answers to Exercises   313

References   333

Author Index   347

Subject Index   353

About the Author   367

In its encounter with Nature, science invariably elicits a sense of reverence and awe. The very act of understanding is a celebration of joining, merging, even if on a very modest scale, with the magnificence of the Cosmos.

—CARL SAGAN (1996, p. 2)

PART I

PROMISE AND PROBLEMS

CHAPTER 1

Introduction

They always say time changes things, but you
actually have to change them yourself.

—ANDY WARHOL (quoted in Honnef, 2000, p. 90)

The quote that opens this chapter speaks to the idea that it is best to be the architect of your own destiny. By taking previous courses in research methods and statistics and perhaps also by enrollment in your particular academic program, such as specialization or honors at the undergraduate level, you have already taken the first steps toward becoming a behavioral science researcher. This book is all about helping you to consolidate what you already know but in a more complete way and also to build essential skills for making the transition from

1. Reading or listening about research produced by others with some understanding to doing so with even better comprehension or conducting your own research;

2. Being a relatively passive recipient of information (a student) from authority figures (your instructors or supervisor) to someone who both takes in and disseminates knowledge through what you write and say (you become an authority figure, too); and

3. Being aware of limitations with the way research is conducted or reported in the behavioral sciences to being capable of doing

something about them (you learn to appreciate the need for reform and can act on it, too).

The last point just mentioned is a recurring theme throughout the book as we consider various issues and challenges in becoming a capable behavioral scientist.

Not Yet Ready for Prime Time

This book is intended for senior undergraduate or junior graduate students in the behavioral sciences—including psychology, education, and other disciplines where empirical studies are conducted with humans or animals—who are learning how to conduct independent (but still supervised) research. It is assumed that such students (1) have already taken at least one introductory course in both methodology and statistics and (2) are considering careers in which the ability to understand or produce research is important. The overall goal is to help such students develop the cognitive and applied skills needed in order to eventually become behavioral scientists. Specifically, this book provides information about (1) an integrative perspective on the connections among the elements of the "trinity" of research, design, analysis, and measurement; (2) structural details (including pros and cons) of many of the most widely used designs and analysis options today; (3) foundational information (what, why, how) on measurement in the behavioral sciences; (4) practical aspects of data analysis; and (5) how to write manuscript-length summaries of research results and make effective presentations about those results.

After completing basic (introductory) courses in methodology and statistics, students are usually not yet ready to carry out independent research projects. This is something that instructors of research seminar courses and supervisors of thesis projects know only too well, and students themselves often feel the same way, too. Part of the problem is that there are some critical gaps in the knowledge and skills of students who undertake thesis projects. For example, students' familiarity with basic concepts about research design and statistics is often rather poor, despite their previous coursework. Some possible reasons are outlined next.

There are some critical shortcomings in the way that methodology and statistics courses are often taught. One is that these subjects are typically dealt with in separate courses and, consequently, their integration may not be emphasized. For example, various types of research designs may be discussed in a methodology course with little attention paid to options for data analysis. Techniques for analyzing data are covered in statistics courses, but their connection with design may not be obvious. That is, both methodology and statistics may be presented outside the context of the other, but in real research projects they are integral parts of the same whole. A related problem is that too many behavioral science statistics courses are old-fashioned in that statistical tests (t, F, etc.) are the main topic. More modern approaches, including effect size estimation, the reporting of confidence intervals, and synthesis of results from replications in a meta-analysis, may not even be mentioned in a traditional statistics course (Aiken, West, Sechrest, & Reno, 1990; Frederich, Buday, & Kerr, 2000). The approaches just listed are an important part of **statistics reform**, which has been a matter of increasing importance across disciplines as diverse as psychology, wildlife management, actuarial science, and empirical economics, among many others. As a result of recent greater emphasis on reform, methods of data analysis in the behavioral sciences are changing (Kline, 2004), and students should be so informed.

A third pedagogical problem is that the instruction of measurement theory, or psychometrics, has been virtually eliminated from many undergraduate and graduate programs in psychology (Aiken et al., 1990). This is unfortunate because strong knowledge of measurement is crucial for behavioral science researchers, especially if they work with human research participants. If students have never been exposed to measurement theory, then they may lack basic skills needed in order to understand the characteristics of their scores, which are analyzed with statistical techniques. If the scores are flawed due to measurement-related problems, then the results may be tainted, too. Aiken et al. (1990) expressed the related concern that the substantial decline of measurement in the psychology curriculum opens the door to a proliferation of poorly constructed measures, the use of which would degrade the quality of psychological research.

One consequence of the problems just mentioned is that students often have difficulty when it comes time to analyze data in their own research projects. They may experience a lack of confidence in what they are doing or, worse, wind up conducting a series of statistical analyses the results of which they do not really understand. That is, students too often carry out their analyses in a relatively blind way in which they have lost sight of the connections between their hypotheses (research questions), study design and procedures, scores, and interpretation of the results. Students also tend to become overly fixated on the statistical analysis and thus pay less attention than they should to other issues, including those of methodology and measurement. The problems just described occur more often among undergraduate students, but many graduate students evidence the same difficulties, too.

Students who carry out thesis research projects need to do a lot of writing, from a proposal before starting the project to the final version of the thesis. Students in research seminar courses may also be required to make presentations about their projects. This could involve an oral presentation to the rest of the class or participation in a poster session at the end of the semester. Both of these forms of communication, written and oral, are critical skills for researchers. However, students are often unprepared to express themselves effectively in writing. This happens in part because few demands for writing may have been placed on them in earlier courses. Indeed, depending on the particular academic program and luck in course registration, it is possible to get a university degree without doing much, if any, serious writing. Thus, many students are simply unpracticed in writing before they enter a research seminar or graduate school. Even for students experienced in other types of writing, such as in the humanities, it is not easy to learn how to write research reports. This is because scientific writing has its own style and tenor, and it requires extensive practice in order to master.

Students who are obliged to make oral presentations about their research projects are often given little guidance beyond specifying a time limit (e.g., 20 minutes), asking for coverage of particular content (e.g., describe your project, hypotheses, and methods), and showing them the basic workings of Microsoft PowerPoint or similar computer tools for making and showing electronic slides (overheads). Sure, today's students see plenty of PowerPoint presentations during course lectures, some of which may be experienced as pretty awful and trivial but others as more engaging and educational. However, it is difficult for students to identify and articulate specific principles for making effective PowerPoint presentations based on hit-or-miss experiences as audience members. Consequently, it is not surprising that many students find oral presentations to be intimidating. They worry both about dealing with anxiety related to public speaking and how to organize their content in PowerPoint. A few students eventually develop by trial and error an effective presentation style, but many others do not. As you know, not all instructors are effective presenters; thus, this is not an indictment directed specifically against students. Perhaps the period of trial-and-error learning could be reduced if students (and their instructors, too) were offered more systematic instruction in how to make effective presentations, including both what to do and what not to do as a speaker and also in PowerPoint, too.

What Students Say They Need

In the last few sections of my research seminar courses in which undergraduate psychology students in specialization or honors programs conduct a thesis project, I have asked of them at the beginning of the semester the question, What do you want to learn? The students respond in writing but anonymously when I am not present. Also, they can list anything they want in response to this open-ended question. Summarized next are their most common responses:

About 75% of students indicated that they wanted to learn how to better conduct their statistical analyses and interpret the results. About the same proportion said that learning how to make effective oral presentations is a priority. A somewhat smaller proportion, but still the majority (65%), responded that they wanted to learn how to write a research paper for an empirical study. So the "big three" items on the students' wish list concern the statistical analysis and developing better communication skills. Other kinds of responses were given by a minority of the students. These include receiving information about graduate school (30%), how to manage the logistics of a research project (10%), how to make effective posters for presentation in a poster session (10%), research ethics (5%), other research areas besides their own (5%), and technical details of American Psychological Association (APA) style (5%). The latter refers to specifications for formatting manuscripts according to the *Publication Manual of the APA* (2005). I make no claim that these results are representative, but I bet that many senior undergraduate students—and junior graduate students, too—who conduct thesis projects would mention the same "big three" concerns as my own students.

Plan of the Book

The organization of this book and the contents of its three parts are intended to address the issues just discussed concerning the preparation of students for research-based careers. The starting point of this process is the discussion in the next chapter (2) about the promise and pitfalls (i.e., the good, the bad, and the ugly) of our collective research enterprise in the behavioral sciences. Many of our students could probably articulate potential benefits of a research-based education. However, the same students may be less aware of some critical problems with behavioral science research. For example, most articles published in our research literature are never cited by other authors and thus, by definition, have little or no impact on the field. There are also problems with the quality of many published studies in terms of their actual scientific contribution, how the data were analyzed, or how the results were interpreted. There is also a disconnect across many behavioral science disciplines between the conduct of research on the one hand and application of those results on the other. Many students never hear about such problems in undergraduate programs, and too many at the graduate level are also unaware of these issues. If we expect students to do a better job than those of us who now teach or supervise them, then you need to know about both the strengths and weaknesses of our research literature.

The five chapters of Part II (Chapters 3–7) concern essential concepts about design, analysis, and measurement, all presented within a framework that emphasizes their integration. In Chapter 3, this framework is laid out through description of the connections among these three pillars of research and how each is associated with a particular type of validity concerning the accuracy of inferences. Various threats to inference accuracy that involve design, analysis, measurement, and sampling, too, are also identified. Chapter 4 deals in more detail with design and analysis together. By this I mean that major types of research designs used in behavioral science research are reviewed along with options for data analysis. Emphasized in this discussion are standard statistical techniques that are more accessible to students, but I also point out a few more advanced methods. Students who go on to graduate school may later use some of these advanced methods, so it is good that you at least hear about them now.

Chapter 5 "tells the truth" about statistics in that it (1) acknowledges that many students do not have positive experiences in these courses; (2) notes that traditional statistics courses do not cover what students really need to know (they are not well prepared); and (3) points out that there are many widespread and incorrect beliefs (myths) about the outcomes of statistical tests, even among experienced researchers and university professors. The correct interpretation of outcomes of statistical tests is discussed later, and reviewed in the appendix of Chapter 5 are the fundamental statistical topics of standard errors, confidence intervals, and statistical tests. Chapter 6 deals with topics in the area of statistics reform, including the estimation and reporting of effect sizes and the construction of approximate confidence intervals for effect sizes. Described in the appendix of this chapter is an advanced method for constructing more accurate confidence intervals for effect sizes. This same method also underlies the estimation of statistical power. Some journals in psychology and education now require the reporting of effect sizes, and doing so is also called for in the APA *Publication Manual*. The basics of classical measurement theory and the estimation of score reliability and validity are the subject of Chapter 7. For too many students, the material covered in this chapter may be the only more substantial presentation about measurement they have encountered so far. Accordingly, the main goal of this chapter is to help you to make better choices about measurement in your own project, given this reality. It also briefly introduces a few more modern developments in test theory, including generalizability theory and item response theory.

Part III concerns skills that are essential for students and researchers alike. Chapter 8 deals with practical aspects of data analysis. In contrast, mainly theoretical issues are covered in statistics courses, but relatively little may be said about how to manage a real analysis. Emphasized in this chapter is the need to develop a clear analysis plan in which the simplest techniques that will get the job done are selected. That is, students are encouraged to resist the temptation to conduct too many analyses or ones that are unnecessarily complicated. Suggestions for handling more complex analyses are offered, and there is also discussion of the critical topic of data screening, or how to prepare your data for analysis. How to write a manuscript-length summary of an empirical study is the subject of Chapter 9. Also considered in this chapter are general principles of good writing and more specific requirements for good scientific writing. Examples of common writing mistakes are also given. Presented in the appendix of Chapter 9 is an example of how to write results from an actual factorial design in a way that emphasizes effect size and deemphasizes statistical significance. The last chapter (10) deals with how to make effective oral presentations using a computer tool such as PowerPoint. Tips for dealing with "stage fright" are offered in the first part of the chapter, and some common mistakes to avoid in PowerPoint presentations are identified. Next, the chapter considers specific principles for planning what to say and what to show in your presentations and compares examples of bad and better PowerPoint slides. Considered in the last part of Chapter 10 are principles for constructing effective posters when presenting your work in poster sessions. Presented in the appendix of this chapter are example slides, an audience handout, and a poster for a hypothetical 20-minute presentation based on the classical study of bystander intervention by Darley and Latané (1968).

Exercises are presented in chapters (3–8) that involve design, analysis, or measurement. These exercises are intended as opportunities for you to consolidate and apply your knowledge in each of these areas. Some of the exercises involve more theoretical matters, but others are computer exercises with small datasets. The latter are intended to give you hands-on practice with the corresponding quantitative concepts. There are also exercises for Chapter 10, but they concern preparing yourself to make a presentation about your particular research project.

Career Paths for Behavioral Scientists

At first glance it might seem that most behavioral scientists work strictly in academia—that is, as faculty members in universities. Some do, of course, but only a relatively small proportion of people with graduate degrees in psychology, education, or related areas go on to pursue academic careers. That is, the range of career possibilities for behavioral scientists is actually quite wide. Some possibilities for research-based careers are considered next.

Besides universities, behavioral scientists work in a range of government agencies or ministries, including those involved in health, education, transportation, engineering, criminal justice, statistics and standards, finance, and social services, among others. Other behavioral scientists work for nongovernmental organizations, such as those involved in human service delivery or public policy. Behavioral scientists also work in several different types of settings in the private sector, including hospitals, marketing research firms, pharmaceutical companies, software development corporations, manufacturing facilities, financial service organizations, and insurance companies, to name a few. Some also work as consultants, either as "free agents" (i.e., they work independently) or as members of consultancy firms. The main clients of such firms are governments and businesses.

Research training leaves graduates of behavioral science programs with clearly marketable skills for a wide variety of careers outside universities. And, of course, research-related work is only part of what behavioral scientists do in these positions. This could involve actually carrying out research projects from start to finish. If so, then skills other than those directly related to design, analysis, and measurement are needed, including the ability to convey study rationale to nonresearchers (i.e., write a proposal for those who control project funds) and to work out project budget and personnel needs. University faculty members deal with the same issues when they write grant proposals. Another possibility includes working to evaluate research results generated by others but then conveying your recommendations, possibly to others with no formal training in research but who count on your judgment. So, once again, the ability to communicate research results in terms that are meaningful to nonresearchers or multidisciplinary audiences is crucial for many behavioral scientists, and this is true both inside and outside universities. It helps that you really understand what your own results mean; otherwise, how can you explain them to others if you cannot first do so to yourself? This is why there is so much emphasis in this book on the correct interpretation of statistical results and on statistics reform, too.

Working as a behavioral science researcher also requires other skills that are not covered directly in this book, but they are some of the same skills needed by professionals in many other fields. One is the ability to effectively manage your work schedule. Like other busy professionals, behavioral scientists typically have too many things to do within too little time. Thus, there is often a need to prioritize among many "in-basket" tasks and deal first with the most pressing ones. The ability to work with others in a team is often critical, especially in business settings where teamwork is the norm. As mentioned, these teams may be multidisciplinary in that they are made up of people with quite different backgrounds, including those with no research credentials at all. A good sense of personal, business, and research ethics is needed, as is a general professional demeanor where others are treated with respect, honesty in communication is expected and given, and a business-like approach to tasks is taken (i.e., get the job done). Moreover, all that was just mentioned about demands on professionals must be balanced against your personal life, too. It is not easy, but few students nowadays are naïve about the challenges of a professional career. There are many rewards, too, especially for energetic, creative, and self-motivated people who want a stronger sense of making their own way than is often possible in nonprofessional positions.

As mentioned, a minority of behavioral scientists pursue academic careers. As you may know, the academic job market is highly competitive in that there are typically many more applicants than available positions, especially for tenure-track slots. In large universities with a strong emphasis on research, it is not unusual for departments to receive dozens or perhaps hundreds of applications for a single tenure-track position. The boom in academic hiring due to the retirement of senior, tenured faculty members expected in the early 1990s never materialized, in part because universities have been hiring more and more part-time, non-tenure-track (contingent) instructors instead of full-time, tenure-track professors, which reduces personnel costs. As noted by van Dalen and Klamer (2005) and others, universities now place more of a premium on relatively early manifestation of research productivity and on the ability to secure funds from granting agencies than in the past. This emphasis works against "late bloomers" who do not discover a passion for research until later in their careers. In the past, some tenured professors did not really begin their academic careers until their early 40s. This is most rare now in that the usual starting age of those with assistant-level tenure-track positions today is during the late 20s or early 30s. Indeed, it is a reality that one needs to plan for an academic position quite early in graduate school by (1) seeking out a supervisor who is a prolific researcher; (2) participating in research above and beyond one's particular thesis project; (3) presenting papers or posters at scientific conferences; and (4) publishing research articles while still a student, not just after graduation. It also does not hurt to pick up some teaching experience while in graduate school, but not at the expense of getting your research done. This is a tough business, but it is better to consider an academic position with your eyes wide open. However, the potential rewards are great for those who believe that they will thrive in academia.

Summary

The fact that many students who are about to conduct supervised research projects are not yet ready in terms of their conceptual knowledge and practical skills was discussed in this chapter. Specifically, thesis students often need help with (1) developing a more complete sense of how design, analysis, and measurement complement one another; (2) conducting their statistical analysis and correctly interpreting the results; and (3) communicating to others in written and spoken form about their findings. It was also noted that there are many career paths for those who become behavioral scientists. Some of these paths involve working in academia, but many others do not; indeed, the range of employment opportunities outside universities is wide and includes governmental, commercial, educational, and other types of settings. Do you want to see if one of these paths might be in your future? Then let us start by getting you ready. We do so in the next chapter with a review of what is right and also what is wrong with behavioral science research.

RECOMMENDED READINGS

The books by Sternberg (2006) and also by Horowitz and Walker (2005) describe various career options for students in, respectively, psychology and education, while Marek's (2004) book covers a wider range of social science career opportunities. Heiberger and Vick (2001) offer helpful suggestions for conducting an academic job search.

Heiberger, M. M., & Vick, J. M. (2001). *The academic job search handbook* (3rd ed.). Philadelphia: University of Pennsylvania Press.

Horowitz, J. A., & Walker, B. E. (2005). *What can you do with a major in education: Real people. Real jobs. Real rewards.* Hoboken, NJ: Wiley.

Marek, R. J. (2004). *Opportunities in social science careers.* New York: McGraw-Hill.

Sternberg, R. J. (Ed.). (2006). *Career paths in psychology: Where your degree can take you* (2nd ed.). Washington, DC: American Psychological Association Books.

CHAPTER 2

The Good, the Bad, and the (Really) Ugly of Behavioral Science Research

The most erroneous stories are those we think we know best—and therefore never scrutinize or question.

—STEPHEN JAY GOULD (1996, p. 57)

Considered in this chapter is the general state of psychology, education, and related areas as scientific disciplines. At first glance, it would seem that our research tradition is healthy and vibrant. This impression is supported by (1) the large and rapidly increasing number of scientific journals and articles in the behavioral sciences, and (2) requirements for research-related courses (e.g., methodology and statistics) in many behavioral science academic programs. However, there are also some serious shortcomings of our collective research enterprise—primarily in "soft" research areas where randomized designs may be difficult or impossible to use—but students rarely hear about these problems, even in graduate school. This is unfortunate because in order to truly mature as a professional in some discipline, one must learn to appreciate both its positive and negative aspects. Along similar lines, the fourth- or third-century BCE Daoist philosopher Chuang

Tzu once wrote that great knowledge sees all in one, but small knowledge breaks down into the many. I hope that the discussion in this chapter widens your knowledge about your chosen area of study. Besides, students are the future, and perhaps they will better deal with the problems described here than the current generation.

The Good

Considered next are three healthy aspects of the research tradition in the behavioral sciences.

Anchor to Reality

Sometimes students new to the behavioral sciences are surprised at the prominent role accorded to research in academic programs. For example, before taking their first psychology course, some students expect that majoring in psychology will involve learning the essence of why people are the way they are, or about fundamental truths that explain the human condition. However, they quickly discover that no such knowledge exists in psychology—or, for that matter, in any other discipline. Instead, psychology students take many content courses about specific aspects of human or animal behavior, cognition, learning, and development, all presented within a framework where research is a common thread. Results of empirical studies are summarized by instructors time and again during lectures. This perspective is further reinforced by mandatory courses in research methods and statistics. Perhaps there are similar expectations among students who contemplate majoring in education—for example, that education baccalaureate recipients know all about how people learn, or fail to learn—but such unrealistic views are probably dispatched early in university.

It makes plain sense that a research-based undergraduate program is necessary for students who aim to get a graduate degree or pursue a research-related career. However, it is true that most psychology undergraduate students do not go to graduate school and eventually work in areas outside the sciences, and thus outside psychology (Grocer & Kohout, 1997). It is also true that most education majors do not later enter the teaching profession (Henke & Perry, 2007), nor is there any formal requirement for research competency in order to be certified as a teacher. So where is the benefit of a research-based academic background for the likely majority of undergraduate students in the behavioral sciences who later pursue other lines of work or study that seem to have little to do with research?

Listed next are some potential advantages noted by Dawes (1994) to possessing the ability to think critically about how evidence is collected and evaluated that is afforded by a research-based education. These advantages may be especially important for those who work in human service fields, such as education or mental health, where there are many unsubstantiated beliefs (myths) about associations between variables or the effectiveness of certain types of practices (e.g., Dawes, 1994, Chs. 2–5; Greene, 2005):

1. Even well-intentioned efforts at intervention can produce unexpected negative consequences later on—for example, the medical literature is full of instances of treatments later found to do more harm than good—and a skeptical attitude about a proposed treatment may help to prevent such problems.

2. An empirically based, "show me" perspective may also constrain otherwise less cautious practitioners from making extreme claims without evidence. It may also prevent fads from dominating professional practice.

3. It is relatively easy for professionals to believe, based on their experience, that they have special insight about causes and mitigation of human problems. Such beliefs may not be correct, however, and it could take longer to discover so if one does not value the role of evidence.

There is a growing appreciation for the need to base practice on empirically validated methods. For example, the report of the Task Force on Promotion and Dissemination of Psychological Procedures of the Clinical Psychology division of the American Psychological Association emphasized the importance of training doctoral students in evidence-based methods of psychotherapy and assessment (Chambless, 1993). There are similar works in the education literature in which the need for research-based policy and teaching methods is stressed (Odom et al., 2005). Whether these goals are achieved in practice is a question that is considered later.

Rise of Meta-Analysis and Meta-Analytic Thinking

Although the first modern meta-analysis was published only in the late 1970s (Smith & Glass, 1977), its impact on both the behavioral science and medical research literature has been great despite its short history. Briefly, **meta-analysis** is a set of statistical techniques for summarizing results collected across different studies in the same general area. It is a type of **secondary analysis** where findings from **primary studies** (i.e., the original empirical studies) are the unit of analysis. In contrast, cases (human or animal) are the typical unit of analysis in primary studies. In the typical meta-analysis, the central tendency and variability of effect sizes are estimated across a set of primary studies, but whether results in the individual studies are statistically significant is not very relevant. This focus on effect size and not statistical significance in primary studies encourages the reader (i.e., you) to think outside the limitations of the latter.

The increasing use of meta-analysis has also encouraged **meta-analytic thinking**, which includes these perspectives (Thompson, 2002):

1. A researcher should report results so that they can be easily incorporated into a future meta-analysis. This includes the reporting of sufficient summary statistics so that effect sizes can be calculated.

2. A researcher should view his or her own individual study as making at best a modest contribution to a research literature. Hunter, Schmidt, and Jackson (1982) expressed this idea as follows: "Scientists have known for centuries that a single study will not resolve a major issue. Indeed, a small sample study will not even resolve a minor issue" (p. 10).

3. An accurate appreciation of the results of previous studies is essential, especially in terms of effect sizes.

4. Retrospective interpretation of new results, once collected, are called for via direct comparison with previous effect sizes.

There are now hundreds of published meta-analytic studies, and reviewing a good meta-analysis can be an excellent way for students to learn about the background of their research area. This assumes an established research area, though. In newer areas with few published studies, there may be no meta-analytic summary available, but thinking meta-analytically about one's own results is beneficial. Keep in mind that meta-analysis is not some magical statistical technique that automatically cuts through the clutter of results from primary studies. This is because what comes out of a meta-analysis depends much on the quality of the primary studies analyzed. This is why study quality is assessed in perhaps most meta-analyses, and results from higher-quality studies may be accorded greater weight. For a general introduction to meta-analysis, see Kline (2004, Ch. 8). Examples of introductions to meta-analysis in specific research areas include Chambers (2004) (education), Demakis (2006) (neuropsychology), and Linden and Adams (2007) (disease management).

Waxed Exceeding Mighty

The size of the research literature across all sciences has grown rapidly of late and is now truly vast. For example, there are now roughly 18,000 refereed scientific journals published by over 2,000 different commercial firms or not-for-profit organizations. Upwards of about 1½ million articles are published each year in these learned journals for a total readership of about 10–15 million persons (Mabe, 2003). In psychology alone, almost 17,000 articles were published in over 420 different research journals in the year 2002. Across all social sciences, more than 64,000 articles appeared in over 1,700 different journals in the same year (van Dalen & Klamer, 2005). These numbers will probably continue to increase, albeit perhaps at a slower rate than we have lately seen. So to judge by size, our research tradition appears to be both robust and flourishing. However, size alone is not necessarily the best indicator of survival potential in the long run—just ask the next Apatosaurus you see.

The burgeoning size of our research literature is part of the so-called **information explosion** that has been fueled by computer technology which has dramatically lowered the costs of producing printed works and also made possible electronic publication and distribution over the Internet. The same digital technology is also behind both **open-access journals** and **self-archiving research repositories**. The former are refereed electronic journals that can be accessed without cost; they are also generally free of many copyright and licensing restrictions. The latter are electronic databases where works by researchers in a common area are stored for later access by others. Perhaps most of today's electronic research archives are associated with clinical trials of medications, but archives for other research areas are sure to follow.

The flipside of information explosion is **information fatigue (burnout)**, which refers to the problem of managing an exponentially growing amount of information. For example, the total number of scientific journals is now so great that most libraries are unable to physically store the printed versions of them all, much less afford the total cost of institutional subscriptions. A related problem is that there can be dozens of different journals in the same general research area. Consequently, (1) librarians must somehow limit the total number of subscriptions, and (2) researchers need some means to decide which of many different journals offers the best information, and also where to publish their work (Dong, Loh, & Mondry, 2005).

A descriptive quantitative measure of overall journal quality that is receiving more and more attention is the **impact factor** (IF). The IF is a bibliometric index published annually by the Institute for Scientific Information (ISI),[1] which analyzes citations in over 14,000 scholarly journals. The IF reflects the number of times the typical article in a journal has been cited in the scientific literature. It is calculated as the average number of citations in 1 year by articles published in that journal during the previous 2 years (Starbuck, 2005). Given IF = 10.0, for example, we can say that the average number of times that articles in a particular journal are cited up to 2 years later is 10. The higher the value of IF, the more often articles that appear in a journal are cited in other works. Better articles are presumably cited more often than weaker articles, so the IF is generally taken as an overall index of journal quality.

Dong et al. (2005) reminded us that the IF is subject to bias by several different factors. Calculation of the IF is based mainly on English language scientific journals, and such journals consist of only about one-quarter of peer-reviewed journals worldwide. Citation patterns are different across research areas. For example, relative numbers of citations tend to be higher in new or rapidly expanding research areas compared with more traditional research areas. Articles in some research areas have short **citation half-lives**, which means that few works are cited more than a couple of years after they are published. However, if citation half-lives are longer than 2 years in a particular area, then these later citations may not contribute to the value of IF. Online availability of articles affects citation frequency: not surprisingly, articles with full-text availability are cited more often than those available on a more restricted basis. Methods for counting citations are not always accurate, so some degree of random error contributes to IF values (i.e., IF scores are not perfectly reliable). The IF is computed for a whole journal, but citations generally refer to articles, not journals. Thus, it is possible that a relatively small number of frequently cited articles are responsible for most of the value of IF for a whole journal. The tendency for authors to cite their own publications

---

[1]The ISI also publishes the *Social Sciences Citation Index* and the *Arts and Humanities Citation Index.*

can inflate IF. Indeed, upward of about 20% or more of all citations are those of authors citing their own work. Sometimes works are cited often for their notoriety, such as examples of fraud or the use of especially bad methods, not because of scientific merit. Finally, IF does not apply to other types of scholarly works, such as books, which can have great impact in a particular field.

A more controversial use of the IF is as a measure of the quality of work of individual scholars or entire academic units. For example, some funding agencies calculate IF for new applicants and track IF for currently funded investigators as measures of quality of published articles. Some academic departments place strong emphasis on IF in the evaluation of individual faculty members, and some universities allocate funds to entire departments or schools based in part on their collective IF values. Starbuck noted these limitations of such uses of IF: There is considerable randomness (error) in the editorial selection process. That is, the fate of each submission is determined by a small number of people, usually the editor and a couple of anonymous reviewers. Agreement across different reviewers is not always high, so one set of reviewers may view the same article very differently compared with another. It happens that some highly cited articles are rejected by multiple journals before finally being published. Highly prestigious, or "A-list," journals (as measured by the IF) publish quite a few articles that are not widely cited (if at all), while widely cited works are also published in less prestigious, or "B-list" (or lower), journals. That is, there is actually much overlap in articles across different levels of journal prestige. Excessive focus on publication in high-impact journals could facilitate a Matthew effect (i.e., the rich get richer, the poor poorer) that benefits the most prestigious departments or schools but penalizes those not at the very top.

The Bad

The first three of the four negative aspects of our research literature considered next are greater problems in "soft" areas of behavioral science research where experimental designs are not generally used. This includes probably most empirical studies conducted in psychology, education, political science, empirical economics, and related areas. However, these three problems are less severe in "hard" research areas, such as the behavioral neurosciences, that are closer to the natural sciences or in other areas where experimental designs are routinely used. The fourth problem discussed next may equally plague both "soft" and "hard" research areas.

Skewness and Waste

A cardinal characteristic of the research literature across all sciences is that of skewness, and this feature is present throughout the entire publication cycle. To wit: Most manuscripts submitted to peer-reviewed journals are rejected. The rejection rate for the more prestigious journals is as high as 90%, or even higher in some cases. The rejection rate is somewhat lower for less prestigious journals, but it is still about 80% overall (Starbuck, 2005). Yes, some manuscripts rejected by one journal are eventually published in another, but it is probably safe to say that most work submitted to journals is never published. Thus, the time and effort invested in preparing these unsuccessful submissions are apparently wasted.

Across all sciences, many published studies are *never* cited in a later work by a different author (Hamilton, 1990, 1991). By definition, such articles have virtually no impact and, by extension, whether they were ever published matters not. In the social sciences, it is estimated that the majority (50–75%) of all published articles are never cited (Lykken, 1991). Overall rates of uncited published works in the physical sciences and economics may be lower—about 20–25%—but it may be as high as 90% in the humanities literature (Laband & Tollison, 2003). So the situation regarding uncited publications in the behavioral sciences is not the worst example but is disquieting that so much of our research literature "disappears" into a fog of irrelevancy. van Dalen and Klamer (2005) estimated that the total direct and indirect costs to publish a typical journal article are roughly $40,000. These financial and other resources, including author, editor, and reviewer time and effort, invested into producing so many uncited articles seems all for naught. Possible reasons why so much of our research literature counts for so little are considered later.

The attribute of skewness in the scientific literature holds at the additional levels summarized next (van Dalen & Klamer, 2005). Again, these characteristics are true in the social and natural sciences alike:

1. The median article in a science journal receives few citations and has relatively few interested readers, in general about 50–200 worldwide. That is, the typical scientific article has negligible influence.

2. Only a small number of published articles are both widely read and cited. These select works correspond to about the top 5–10% of the scientific literature. A related idea is that of the so-called **80/20 rule:** About 20% of the published articles generate about 80% of the citations.

3. Likewise, a minority of journals publishes the most widely cited articles, and a minority of scientific authors write these high-impact articles and are also responsible for the bulk of the total number of publications (i.e., the 80/20 rule applies to citations, too).

The high degree of skewness in the research literature is consistent with a "superstar" model of science where an elite handful of researchers receive most of the attention and resources, but the "starlet" or rank-and-file researchers receive little or none (van Dalen & Klamer, 2005). Even if one accepts this analogy, though, it does not necessarily imply that the work of the latter is unimportant or wasteful. For example, van Dalen and Klamer estimated that the total cost of scientific publishing across all 14,000 or so journals monitored by the ISI corresponded to roughly .0006% of total world income in 2002. This level of expenditure "makes science not an entirely free lunch, but it certainly is a cheap lunch" (p. 401). Not all work of superstar researchers is widely cited; that is, probably the majority of articles published by the top researchers are not also of stellar quality.

There are some conceptual models in which the organization of beehives or termite colonies is seen as analogous to the uneven distribution of publications and citations in science (e.g., J. Cole & Cole, 1972). In this view, each of a large number of ordinary workers carries out a task that by itself appears mundane or unremarkable. However, the total result of all such efforts supports the elite (e.g., the queen and drones), who carry the colony into the future, in the insect world through reproduction and in the scientific realm through new discoveries or, even more fundamental, the development of new paradigms. A **paradigm** is a shared set of theoretical structures, methods, and definitions that supports the essential activity of puzzle solving, the posing and working out of problems under the paradigm. Given a paradigm, lesser researchers are enabled to carry out the more day-to-day, problem-solving phase of science, although they may have been incapable of developing a new paradigm in the first place.

Wide Gap between Research and Policy or Practice

There is too often a disconnect between policy or practice in applied areas and related research in the behavioral sciences. For example, Miller (1999) described the "black hole" of educational research into which vast resources invested in empirical studies disappear with little impact on efforts to reform schools. Specifically, the formation of education policy is infrequently informed by the results of education research. Even when numerous empirical studies in some area exist, the results are often contradictory or based on research methods that are so weak that no clear conclusion can be drawn. Consequently, policymakers do not reflexively ask, What does the research say?, before making decisions that affect how schools are organized or funded.

There are also situations in which education research follows education policy instead of the other way around. One example concerns the concept of a learning disability. In the United States, a learning disability is defined in federal law based on an IQ–achievement discrepancy model, in which children are identified as learning disabled when their IQ scores are in the normal range but their scores on scholastic achievement tests are much lower. Children so identified are entitled to remedial services under federal law. However, children with poor achievement skills who have below-average IQ scores may not qualify for remedial assistance. This is because such children may be considered as "slow learners" whose low achievement is consistent with low overall ability. For the same reason—low overall ability—it is also assumed that "slow learners" are less likely to benefit from intervention than children classified as learning disabled. Unfortunately, there is little evidence that IQ scores measure one thing (ability, potential; i.e., fluid intelligence) and achievement scores another (school-related or crystallized intelligence). And there is virtually no evidence that "slow learners" are less likely to benefit from special education than the learning disabled in the long run. The IQ–achievement discrepancy model just described is under review, but, predictably, there is little consensus about an alternative definition of a learning disability (Dombrowski, Kamphaus, & Reynolds, 2004).

Dawes (1994) described similar examples in the mental health field where doctoral-level psychologists—all of whom have research backgrounds—engage in practices without empirical support or, worse, continue a practice in the face of negative evidence. One example is the interpretation of children's drawings of human figures as projective tests of personality. In this approach, drawing features are taken as "signs" of

internal personality characteristics. The absence of visible hands in a drawing would be considered a sign of helplessness, for instance, and the presence of visible teeth or fingernails would be seen as indicating aggression.
However, the results of numerous studies have indicated that such signs
are generally uncorrelated with child adjustment or mental health, yet too
many professional psychologists still view drawings as valid measures of
personality. There is a similar problem with the Rorschach inkblot test:
The evidence for its validity is mostly negative, but it is still widely used
(Wood, Nezworski, Lilienfeld, & Garb, 2003). Likewise, the results of a
survey by Woody, Weisz, and McLean (2005) indicated that doctoral clinical psychology programs made relatively little progress in teaching empirically supported treatments in the previous decade.

The situation concerning the practical impact of research in psychology or education is not entirely bleak, however. For example, the "whole-
language" philosophy of reading instruction was widely accepted in educational circles in the middle 1970s in the United States. In this model,
the explicit teaching of phonemic awareness, phonics, and spelling was
deemphasized in favor of "natural" learning of entire words in context.
However, at the time there was ample evidence in the education research
literature that children do not learn to read "naturally" and that many
need systematic instruction in the correspondence between letters and
sounds (Lyon, Shaywitz, Shaywitz, & Chhabra, 2005). Although it took
more than 20 years before limitations of the whole-language approach
were recognized, the education research literature did play a role. Also,
the very fact that the hoary IQ–achievement discrepancy model of learning disabilities is now in question at the policy level in the United States
is encouraging.

Lack of Relevance for Practitioners

Some barriers to basing practice on research findings in applied settings
are considered next. In general, researchers communicate poorly with practitioners. This can happen when researchers report their findings using
language that is pedantic or unnecessarily technical. The use of excessively
complicated statistical techniques and the description of results solely in
terms of their statistical significance are examples of the latter. Unfortunately, one tends to obscure rather than illuminate through the overuse of
academic or technical jargon. There is an expression that goes something
like this: The more you know, the more simply you should speak. Unfortunately, too few of us as researchers follow this prescription.

Behavioral science researchers are sometimes overly enthusiastic about the potential for applying their results as cures for societal ills. Part of the problem is that they may be rather oblivious to the problem of sampling error and the effects of specific settings on the outcomes of interventions (Pedhazur & Schmelkin, 1991). Another is that they may not realize the importance of organizational support needed by practitioners for changing established procedures (Retsas, 2000). In a survey by Beutler, Williams, Wakefield, and Entwistle (1995), clinical psychology practitioners said that they valued clinical research and considered their practices to be augmented by such research. But many also said that research topics are sometimes too narrow or specific to be of much practical value. Also, the practitioners tended to look more often to the applied or clinical literature for information about research than to more traditional, hard-core journals with stronger scientific bents. It seems that we as researchers have much work to do in order to improve the chances that our findings will have relevance outside academia.

Incorrect Statistical Results

The issue discussed next does not refer to the use of less-than-optimal-but-still-acceptable statistical techniques. Instead, it concerns outright errors in the reporting of results from statistical tests in articles. The results of a study by Rossi (1987) about this question are both surprising and distressing. Rossi assigned students enrolled in two different psychology statistics classes, one at the undergraduate level and the other at the graduate level, to recompute values of statistical tests based on summary statistics reported in journal articles. The students' recalculations were checked by the instructor for accuracy. In about 15% of the recalculations, results originally reported as statistically significant were not when recomputed from article summary statistics. Now, it is possible that some of the disagreements between original and recalculated test statistics were due to errors in the reporting of summary statistics. Another possibility is typographical errors in printed values of test statistics. As noted by Rossi, neither explanation is much of a consolation. This is because such errors are supposed to be caught in the production process by careful review of galley proofs by authors. In any event, these results suggest that the reporting of incorrect statistical results may be much more common than we would like to believe. These results mirror my own experiences: It has happened several times that I have been unable to reproduce the original statistical results based on the summary statistics reported in an article. I check and recheck my calculations whenever this happens. A few times the mistake was mine, but usually not.

The (Really) Ugly

The three problems described next are catastrophic concerning the scientific merit of our research literature. They are also interrelated in that weakness in one area negatively affects quality in other areas. Again, these problems afflict "soft" research areas more than "hard" research areas.

Little Real Contribution to Knowledge

It was said earlier that most manuscripts submitted to journals are rejected and that most published articles are never cited. Even among the cited articles, most are generally uninformative. That is, after reading even a cited work, one is likely to feel that little new was just learned. Lykken (1991) and others have estimated that about 90% of all published articles in the psychology research literature could be classified as either "utterly inconsequential" or "run of the mill" in terms of actual contribution to

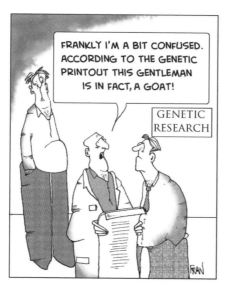

Even natural scientists have embarrassing moments. Copyright 2008 by Fran Orford. Reprinted with permission of CartoonStock Ltd.

knowledge. Such works may be characterized by the study of the obvious (e.g., whether poverty is a risk factor) or the touting of results that would be expected even by laypersons. These studies help academicians by boosting their publication counts, but otherwise there is little intrinsic scientific value. Only about 10% (or less) of all published articles may be considered "worthwhile" by those who read and cite them in other works. These works reward the effort of reading by illuminating truly new perspectives or findings. Such works are a source of intellectual joy, but they are an exception. The same low proportion of worthwhile articles probably holds in other behavioral science areas besides psychology. To be fair, perhaps only about 10% of articles published in the natural sciences may be viewed by readers in those fields as genuinely enlightening, too, so this problem is not unique to the behavioral sciences. Not so with the two problems described next, however.

Lack of Cumulative Knowledge

A hallmark of a true science is that knowledge is cumulative. This means that empirical and theoretical structures build on one another in a way that permits results of current studies to extend earlier work. Hedges (1987) referred to this characteristic as **theoretical cumulativeness**; a more colloquial expression is "standing on the shoulders of giants." Unfortunately, the research literature in the behavioral sciences is too often just the opposite. This means that we tend to study something for a relatively short period of time, discover that the results are inconsistent, attempt to resolve these inconsistencies by conducting additional studies that fail to yield any more conclusive answers, and then just lose interest in the problem before going on to study something new. In other words, what is "hot" in our research literature today is quickly forgotten and soon replaced by another fad topic with an equally short shelf-life that eventually suffers the same fate. This cycle is consistent with Meehl's (1978) observation that theories in "soft" areas of psychology tend to be neither refuted nor corroborated but instead just fade away as we lose interest. Lykken (1991) used the following analogy about psychology research: Instead of building cumulative knowledge, we build mostly sand castles with little durability. The failure to develop cumulative knowledge in the behavioral sciences is not specific to just psychology, though; it is also a shortcoming in other "soft" areas of the behavioral sciences.

A related problem is that we rarely seem to come to any particular conclusion across our empirical studies except that "more research is needed" about the topic. Indeed, one sees this phrase at the conclusion of so many behavioral science journal articles that it is almost a self-parody. The quote from Kmetz (2002) presented next poignantly expresses a similar idea—note that the term "s³m" below refers to the "soft social science model":

> After publishing nearly 50 year's worth of work in s³m, the three terms most commonly seen in the literature are "tentative," "preliminary," and "suggest." As a default, "more research is needed." After all these years and studies, we see nothing of "closure," "preponderance of evidence," "replicable," or "definitive." (p. 62)

The lack of cumulative knowledge also means that it is difficult to point to clear examples of progress in many areas of behavioral science research. Lykken (1991) offered a variation on this analogy: Suppose that a time machine is capable of transporting a person back in time 50 or so years in the past. Two university professors are selected as passengers for time travel, an engineering professor and a psychology professor. Both are asked to give a 20-minute colloquium about *real* advances over the last 50 years to his or her colleagues in the past. Without a doubt the engineering professor would amaze his audience with tales of our modern technical prowess in any number of areas. Indeed, it would be hard to fit everything into only 20 minutes. Depending on the research area of the psychology professor, though, it might actually be difficult to think of what to say. For example, how much *real* progress has been made over the last 5 decades in, say, our understanding of the nature of intelligence? For the example just mentioned, not much; perhaps there is more for other areas of psychology research, but the number of true scientific breakthroughs in psychology over the last few decades is very modest.

Paucity of Replication

Replication is a gold standard in science. It is also the ultimate way to deal with the problem of sampling error and that of spurious claims. I speculated elsewhere that a survey would find just as many behavioral scientists as their natural science colleagues who would endorse replication as a critical activity (Kline, 2004). However, it clear that replication is paid scant attention in the behavioral science research literature. This is because only small proportions—in some cases < 1%—of all published studies in the behavioral sciences are specifically described as replications. So our actions rather than our words make it clear that replication is grossly undervalued in the behavioral sciences. This is a devastating flaw of our research literature.

Taken together, the general absence of cumulativeness and replication in our research literature mean that it is often unnecessary to read journal articles until one is ready to write up one's own work for publication and needs citations for the introduction and discussion (Lykken, 1991). This is a stinging criticism, and one that contradicts what we tell students all the time: Stay current, read the research literature. It does ring true, though, especially when fads dominate the attention of researchers in some area (i.e., there is little cumulative knowledge). However, I am *not* recommending here that you pay no attention to the research literature in your area except when you are writing up your results. To do so would mean that you will miss that occasional and exceptional work from the upper 10% of the literature that is truly worthwhile. In this sense, reading our research literature is analogous to prospecting for gold: One must sift through a lot of uninteresting rubble before finding that rare and precious nugget that rewards the search.

Why?

Considered next are three possible reasons for the overall poor state of behavioral science research.

Soft Science Is Hard

As mentioned, problems outlined in previous sections are more severe in "soft" areas of behavioral science research than in "hard" areas. However, it is arguably more difficult to conduct "soft" research than "hard" research. A big reason is that true experimental designs are simply impossible to use in many types of studies with human research participants. For instance, although it is theoretically possible to experimentally study the effects of lead exposure on children's learning ability—all that would be required is the random assignment of children to various controlled levels of exposure, including none—such a study is obviously forbidden on ethical grounds. Also, it is impossible to study some characteristics of people in laboratories instead of natural settings. One example concerns the evaluation of whether community characteristics, such as levels of income or crime, predict reading achievement among elementary school children. There are types of quasi-experimental designs for situations in which random assignment is not feasible that permit causal inference on a level comparable with that in experimental designs (Chapter 4), but they are more difficult to apply than experimental designs.

Some additional reasons why the "soft" sciences may be more difficult than the "hard" sciences are listed next (Berliner, 2002; Lykken, 1991; Pedhazur & Schmelkin, 1991):

1. Human behavior may be much more subject to **idiographic factors** than to **nomothetic factors** than physical phenomena. The latter refers to general laws or principles that apply to every case and work the same way over time. In contrast, idiographic factors are specific to individual cases. They concern discrete or unique facts or events that vary across both cases and time. If human behavior is more controlled by idiographic factors (e.g., experiences and environments) than by nomothetic factors (e.g., genetics and common neural organization), then there is less potential for prediction. As noted by Lykken (1991), a natural scientist would not be upset if he or she could not exactly predict where each and every leaf from a tree will hit the ground in autumn. Instead, understanding the general life cycle of the tree may be sufficient.

2. Context effects tend to be relatively strong for many aspects of human behavior. That is, how a behavior is expressed often depends on the particular familial or social context. This is another way to describe interaction effects, which concern conditional or joint associations between two or more variables with other variables. For example, the effectiveness of a particular kind of school reform may depend on local conditions in the surrounding community. Context effects may also be era-dependent. For example, social conditions concerning the status of women have changed dramatically over the last few decades, and certain effects of the differential socialization of girls versus boys may be different today than in the past. Finally, strong context effects tend to reduce the chance that a result will replicate across different situations, samples, or times.

3. Our practices concerning measurement in the behavioral sciences are too often poor, especially when we try to assess the degree of a hypothetical construct, such as "verbal reasoning" or "anxiety," present in human research participants. In any area of science, if the subject of interest cannot be measured with precision, then it cannot be understood with any

degree of precision. The topic of measurement is so important that a later chapter is devoted entirely to it (Chapter 7).

4. The "soft" behavioral sciences lack a true paradigm, and a paradigm in science is necessary for theoretical cumulativeness. Note that our use of a common set of statistical techniques across the behavioral sciences does not by itself constitute a paradigm. The use of common tools is only a small part of a paradigm. The rest involves a set of shared assumptions and methods that together identify the main problems of interest (i.e., the puzzles to be solved) and how to go about solving them. In contrast, there is little agreement in the "soft" behavioral sciences about just what the main problems are and exactly how to study them. This disagreement reflects the preparadigmatic (i.e., prescientific) state of much of the behavioral sciences.

Overall, researchers in "soft" sciences work under conditions that researchers in the "hard" sciences may find intolerable. This is why Berliner (2002) suggested that a better distinction than "hard" versus "soft" for the sciences would be one between the "hard-to-do" sciences versus the "easy-to-do" sciences in terms of the available degree of experimental control. Under this distinction, "soft" science would be considered the hardest of all.

Overreliance on Statistical Tests

The problem discussed now is entirely of our own making; therefore, it is a possible area for reform, especially for those who are about to enter the discipline (i.e., you). The use of statistical tests has dominated the way that hypotheses have been tested in the behavioral sciences for the last 40 years or so. Also, results of statistical tests are reported in virtually all empirical studies in the behavioral science literature, and these tests are taught in virtually all statistics courses in psychology, education, and related disciplines. Thus, you may be surprised to learn that this status quo in the behavioral sciences is now very controversial. Specifically, increasing numbers of authors in many different fields now argue that we (1) rely too much on statistical significance tests and (2) typically misinterpret outcomes of statistical tests. It is also argued that our collective misunderstandings of statistical tests are responsible for some of what ails behavioral science research; that is, research progress has been hindered by our dysfunctional preoccupation with statistical tests. You may know that statistical tests are used infrequently in the natural sciences, and yet the natural sciences continue to thrive. Whether this association is causal or not is a matter of critical debate, one that is considered in Chapter 5.

Economy of Publish or Perish

You already know that "publish or perish"—the pressure to publish constantly in order to demonstrate scientific merit—is a reality for new, tenure-track professors, especially in research-oriented universities. Accordingly, junior faculty members are sometimes counseled to break their research down into pieces and publish those pieces in multiple articles, which would boost a researcher's publication count if successful. A related idea is that of the **least publishable unit** (LPU), which refers to the smallest amount of ideas or data that could generate a journal article. This term is used in a derogatory or sarcastic way to describe the pursuit of the greatest quantity of publications at the expense of quality. Now, it is true that publication in prestigious journals will usually benefit a tenure-track professor, but the total quantity of published articles across journals at different levels of prestige is also important.

The emphasis on quantity that is part of the publish-or-perish reality may be in part responsible for the low overall quality of many articles. This same point was made in physics by Gad-el-Hak (2004), who noted that the economy of publish or perish is driving the information explosion in science as much as advances in computer technology; that is, academics need publications (i.e., demand), it is easier than ever to publish articles (i.e., supply), and those newly created journal spaces must be filled. As more and more journals have entered this marketplace, Gad-el-Hak argued, quantity is ever more trumping quality. Perhaps another indication is the proliferation of large numbers of coauthors (e.g., > 10) on journal articles, not all of whom may be deserving in terms of actual contribution.

Sometimes the publish-or-perish economy for tenure-track academicians is rationalized by the following: Active researchers make better teachers. This explanation makes intuitive sense for a few reasons. For example, researchers may be closer to the forefront of new knowledge and thus are in a better position to convey this information. Another is that researchers-as-teachers may be better able to encourage critical thinking instead of the mere passive acceptance of facts. However, there is actually very little evidence that supports the idea that research productivity makes for better teachers (i.e., it is a myth). For example, using state-of-the-art statistical techniques that control for the lack of independence in data about research productivity and teaching effectiveness, Marsh and Hattie (2002) found that the corrected correlation between these two domains among university professors is about zero. That is, professors who publish many articles are not any more effective teachers than professors who do not publish many articles.

Summary

The rapidly growing research literature in the behavioral sciences has been part of the information explosion, but all is not well with our research tradition. For example, most manuscripts submitted to behavioral science journals are never published, most published articles are never cited, and the quality of most published articles is mundane. In general, very little of our research literature is dedicated to replication, and there is a general lack of cumulative knowledge in psychology and related disciplines. As researchers, we tend to communicate poorly with practitioners about our results, often by using excessive jargon or emphasizing unnecessarily complicated statistics that obscure rather than enlighten. The result is that behavioral science research too often plays a small or nonexistent role in public discourse about social policy alternatives. So we have relatively little to show for the rapid, recent growth in our research literature. One causal factor may be the publish-or-perish mentality, which emphasizes quantity over quality. Another factor specific to the behavioral sciences is our collective overreliance on tests of statistical significance as basically the only way to test hypotheses. There are many potential benefits for research-based education, but perhaps we in the behavioral sciences need to "grow up" in some important ways in order to realize them. Perhaps today's students, with proper guidance and awareness of these problems, will become tomorrow's reformers in the behavioral sciences. Let us continue this process with an integrated review of design, measurement, and analysis in the next part of this book.

RECOMMENDED READINGS

The Lykken (1991) and Miller (1999) articles are hard-hitting critiques of, respectively, psychology research and education research. Although directed at different disciplines, they describe many of the same shortcomings. These same problems plague the research literatures in other areas of the behavioral sciences, too; that is, they are not unique to psychology or education.

Lykken, D. T. (1991). What's wrong with psychology, anyway? In D. Cicchetti & W. Grove (Eds.), *Thinking clearly about psychology* (Vol. 1, pp. 3–39). Minneapolis: University of Minnesota Press.

Miller, D. W. (1999, August 6). The black hole of education research: Why do academic studies play such a minimal role in efforts to improve the schools? *Chronicle of Higher Education, 45*(48), A17–A18.

PART II

CONCEPTS

CHAPTER 3

The Research Trinity

Science is more than a body of knowledge; it is a
way of thinking.

—CARL SAGAN (1996, p. 25)

This chapter is intended to help you to better understand the connections
among the three fundamentals—the trinity—of research: design, measurement, and analysis. This discussion emphasizes the integration of these
elements, specifically, (1) how they combine and complement one another to form the logical framework of empirical studies; and (2) how each
is concerned with a particular type of validity regarding the accuracy of
inferences. An integrative perspective contrasts with a fragmentary one
where each element is taught in a separate course, such as statistics in one
course and research methodology in another. This is standard practice
in many academic programs, but a piecemeal approach may not foster a
sense of how each of design, measurement, and analysis gives context and
meaning to the others.

Trinity Overview

This adage attributed to the physician and professor Martin Henry Fischer
(1879–1962) is an apt starting point: Knowledge is a process of piling up
facts; wisdom lies in their simplification. You already know lots of facts

39

about research methodology and statistics—maybe even piles of facts—but perhaps less so about measurement. Let us now arrange those facts in a more cohesive way that I hope ends up closer to the ideal of knowledge. We will do so by first reviewing familiar but important concepts about design. Later presentations about measurement and analysis may cover ideas less familiar to you, but this is part of building a broader understanding about research.

Presented in Figure 3.1 is a schematic that represents the essential roles of design, measurement, and analysis and the main type of validity associated with each. These types of validity refer to the *approximate truth* of inferences about causal relations, or **internal validity**; whether such inferences hold across variations in cases, treatments, settings, or measures, which is referred to as **external validity**; the correct measurement of variables that the researcher intends to study, or **construct validity**; and the appropriate use of statistical methods in the analysis to estimate relations between variables of interest, or **conclusion validity**, also called **statistical conclusion validity**. The phrase "approximate truth" was emphasized

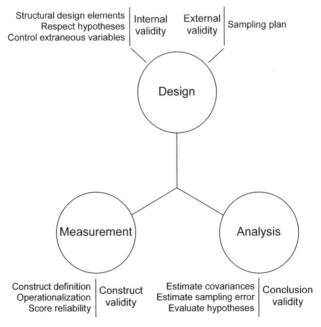

FIGURE 3.1. Essential characteristics and the major type(s) of validity addressed by design, measurement, and analysis.

in the previous sentence because judgments about validity are not absolute. This is because it is virtually impossible in a single study to falsify all alternative explanations of the results. This reality also highlights the importance of replication. Note that external validity is mainly a function of sampling and, specifically, whether sampling is representative. Some studies in the behavioral sciences include specific sampling plans as part of the design in order to maximize external validity, but such studies may be a minority. Accordingly, external validity and sampling are considered later.

Design

Design provides the conceptual framework that holds together the five structural elements of an empirical study (Trochim & Donnelly, 2007), including:

1. Samples (groups)

2. Conditions (e.g., treatment or control)

3. Method of assignment to groups or conditions (i.e., random or otherwise)

4. Observations (i.e., the data)

5. Time, or the schedule for measurement or when treatment begins or ends

The third element deals with case assignment. If cases are randomly assigned to either treatment or control conditions—a process known as **randomization**[1]—then the design is an **experimental design**. Studies based on experimental designs are referred to in the behavioral sciences as **randomized experiments** and in medicine as **randomized control trials** or **randomized clinical trials**. If either (1) cases are divided into groups that do or do not receive treatment using any other method (i.e., nonrandom assignment), or (2) there is no control group but there is a treatment group, then the design is a **quasi-experimental design**. In both experiments and quasi-experiments, a presumed cause (treatment; i.e., the

---

[1]Randomization is not the same thing as random sampling, which concerns how cases are selected for inclusion in the sample.

independent variable) is implemented before its presumed effects on the dependent (outcome) variable(s) are measured. Accordingly, both designs just mentioned are referred to as **cause-probing designs** where inferences about cause–effect relations (i.e., internal validity) are of paramount interest. However, the absence of randomization in quasi-experimental designs makes it more difficult to reject alternative explanations of the results compared with experimental designs.

Presumed causes and effects may be identified and measured in **nonexperimental designs**—also referred to as **passive observational designs** or **correlational designs**[2]—but the design elements of random assignment, control groups, and the measurement of presumed causes before presumed effects are usually absent in these designs (Shadish, Cook, & Campbell, 2001). Consequently, it is difficult or even well-nigh impossible to make plausible causal inferences in nonexperimental designs. Accordingly, the term "predictor" is often used in these designs instead of "independent variable." This distinction highlights the fact that presumed causes are not directly manipulated in such designs. For instance, studies of gender differences are inherently nonexperimental because researchers cannot somehow "assign" research participants to be either a woman or a man. Likewise, the term "criterion" is often used in nonexperimental designs to refer to presumed effects instead of "dependent variable."

The categories of experimental, quasi-experimental, and nonexperimental designs are not mutually exclusive. This is because one can design a study with elements from at least two of these three categories. Suppose that men and women are randomly assigned to either treatment or control conditions. Gender is treated as a factor in the analysis along with the treatment–control distinction. The former is a nonexperimental variable, but the latter is an experimental one. Also, the goal in nonexperimental designs is not always to evaluate hypotheses about causality. Sometimes the aim is limited to the study of associations between variables of interest with no distinction between presumed causes and effects. For example, a researcher may wish to estimate the correlation between the traits of "extraversion" and "impulsivity" without assuming that one causes the other.

The combination of the five structural elements of design specified by the researcher sets the basic conditions for evaluating the hypotheses. This combination is typically far from ideal. That is, few (if any) real-world

---

[2]Pedhazur and Schmelkin (1991) argued that "correlational design" is a misnomer because "correlational" refers to an analytical technique, not a design, and correlations can be calculated in experimental designs, too.

researchers can actually measure all relevant variables in large, representative samples tested under all pertinent conditions. Instead, researchers must typically work with designs given constraints on resources (i.e., time and money). Accordingly, the real task is to specify the best possible design, given such compromises *and* respecting the hypotheses (Figure 3.1). Trochim and Land (1982) noted that a best possible design is:

1. Theory-grounded because theoretical expectations are directly represented in the design.

2. Situational in that the design reflects the specific setting of the investigation.

3. Feasible in that the sequence and timing of events, such as measurement, is carefully planned.

4. Redundant because the design allows for flexibility to deal with unanticipated problems without invalidating the entire study (e.g., loss of one outcome measure is tolerable).

5. Efficient in that the overall design is as simple as possible, given the goals of the study.

Research hypotheses can often be expressed as questions or statements (predictions) about the existence, direction, and degree (i.e., effect size) of the relation—or covariance—between two variables. For example, in a study of the effectiveness of a new reading program for grade 1 students, the research question could be phrased as follows: How much of a difference (if any) does the new program make in terms of reading skill compared with standard instruction? In this case, the question concerns the covariance between the variables of participation in the new program (yes or no) and outcome (reading skill). Hypotheses can also concern covariances among three or more variables, too. For example, one could evaluate whether reading skill covaries with participation in the new reading program and gender.

Design should also provide the context to precisely study and subsequently estimate covariances by controlling **extraneous variables** (Figure 3.1), or uncontrolled variables other than the independent variable that may affect the dependent variable. There are two kinds: One is **nuisance (noise) variables** that introduce irrelevant or error variance that reduces measurement precision. For example, testing grade 1 students in chilly, noisy rooms may not yield precise reading skill scores. The administration of a good measure, but by poorly trained examiners, could also yield imprecise scores. Nuisance variables are controlled through a measurement plan that specifies proper testing environments, tests, and examiner qualifications. **Confounding variables**—also called **lurking variables** or **confounders**, is the other kind. Two variables are confounded if their effects on the dependent variable cannot be distinguished from each other. Suppose that parents are excited by the enrollment of their children in a new reading program. Unbeknown to the researcher, they respond by spending even more time reading books at home. These same children read appreciably better at program's end, but we do not know whether this result was due to the program or extra at-home reading. This is because the researcher did not think in advance to measure at-home reading.

Design must also generally guarantee the **independence of observations**, which means that the score of one case does not influence the score of another. For instance, if one student copies the work of another during a group-administered reading test, their scores are not independent. It is assumed in many standard statistical techniques, such as the analysis of variance (ANOVA), that the scores are independent. *This assumption is critical because the results of the analysis could be inaccurate if the scores are not independent.* This is especially true concerning the results of tests of statistical significance. Also, there is no such thing as a magical statistical fix or adjustment for lack of independence. *Therefore, the requirement for independence is generally met through design and measurement, not analysis.*

In cause-probing studies of treatment effects, the question whether observed posttreatment differences between treated and untreated cases are the result of treatment versus extraneous variables is a matter of internal validity. Shadish et al. (2001) used the term **local molar causal validity** when referring to internal validity. This alternative term emphasizes that (1) any causal conclusions may be limited to the particular samples, treatments, outcomes, and settings in a particular investigation (local); and (2) treatment programs are often complex packages of different elements, all of which are simultaneously tested in the study (molar). The term "molar" also emphasizes the fact that most experiments are better at permitting the attribution of variation in outcomes to deliberately varying a treatment, or **causal description**, than at clarifying the specific, underlying mechanisms through which a causal effect operates, or **causal explanation**. For example, most of us know that flicking a light switch is a cause of illuminating a room (description), but few really understand the underlying electrical and mechanical causal pathways between the two events (explanation) (Shadish et al., 2001).

Three general conditions must be met before one can reasonably infer a cause–effect relation (e.g., Cook & Campbell, 1979; James, Mulaik, & Brett, 1982; Pearl, 2000, describe these requirements from a more mathematical perspective):

1. **Temporal precedence:** The presumed cause must occur before the presumed effect.

2. **Association:** There is observed covariation, that is, variation in the presumed cause must be related to that in the presumed effect.

3. **Isolation:** There are no other plausible alternative explanations (i.e., extraneous variables) of the covariation between the presumed cause and the presumed effect.

Temporal precedence is established in experimental or quasi-experimental designs when treatment clearly begins (and perhaps ends, too) before outcome is measured. However, if all variables are simultaneously

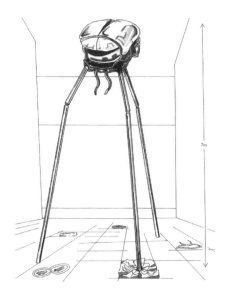

The Martian war machines in the H. G. Wells novel *The War of the Worlds* also stood on three legs, a trinity of sorts. This sketch by Michael Condron is of his sculpture "Martian Walking Engine" (1998), which was commissioned by the Woking Council (England) to mark the centenary of Wells's novel. Reproduced with permission of the artist (personal communication, June 6, 2007).

measured—as is generally true in nonexperimental designs—then temporal precedence may be ambiguous; that is, which variable is the cause and which is the effect? The condition about the absence of plausible alternative explanations (isolation) is typically the most challenging. This is so because it is virtually impossible to control all plausible extraneous variables in a particular study. A plausible alternative explanation is also a threat to internal validity. Common threats to internal validity and how to manage them through design—and through measurement and analysis, too—are considered later.

Measurement

The role of measurement in empirical studies is critical, no less so than that of design and analysis. It serves three essential purposes (see Figure 3.1), including (1) the identification and definition of variables of interest. In human studies, these variables often correspond to hypothetical constructs that are not directly observable. Suppose that a researcher intends to measure quality of life among patients with schizophrenia. This requires a definition of just what is meant by life quality. The next step requires (2) an operational definition, which specifies a set of methods or operations that permit the quantification of the construct. This in turn generates (3) scores (i.e., the data), which are the input for the analysis. It is critical that these scores are reliable, which means that they are relatively free from random error; otherwise, the analysis may not yield useful information. As noted by Pedhazur and Schmelkin (1991):

> Unfortunately, many readers and researchers fail to recognize that no matter how profound the theoretical formulations, how sophisticated the design, and how elegant the analytic techniques, they cannot compensate for poor measures. (p. 3)

Construct validity is the main focus of measurement (Figure 3.1). Briefly, construct validity concerns whether the scores reflect the variables of interest, or what the researcher intended to measure. A requirement for construct validity is score reliability. Unreliable scores are basically random numbers, and random numbers cannot measure anything in particular. Chapter 7 deals with measurement in more detail, including how to select good measures for use in your study. Other potential threats to construct validity are considered later in this chapter.

Analysis

There are three main goals in the analysis (Figure 3.1). These include (1) estimating covariances between variables of interest, controlling for the influence of other relevant, measured variables; (2) estimating the degree of sampling error associated with this covariance; and (3) evaluating (test) the hypotheses in light of the results. Each of these goals is discussed next.

In experimental or quasi-experimental designs, the covariance to be estimated is between the independent variable of treatment and the dependent variable, controlling for the effects of other independent variables or covariates in the design, if any. (A covariate is defined momentarily.) This covariance is a **point estimate** of a population parameter with a single numerical value. It is most informative if this covariance is scaled so that its value clearly indicates the strength of the association, or effect size, between the independent and dependent variables. That is, if treatment had some effect relative to control, just how large is it? The estimation of effect size is part of statistics reform, and Chapter 6 deals with this topic in detail.

Estimation of the degree of sampling error associated with the covariance refers to **interval estimation**, and it involves the construction of a confidence interval about a point estimate. A **confidence interval** can be seen as a range of values that *may* include that of the population covariance within a specified level of uncertainty. It also expresses a range of plausible values for the covariance that *may* be observed in hypothetical replication samples with the same number of cases drawn from the same population. In graphical displays, confidence intervals are often represented as **error bars** represented as lines extending above and below (or to the left and right, depending on graph orientation) around a single point. Sagan (1996) called error bars "a quiet but insistent reminder that no knowledge is complete or perfect" (pp. 27–28), a fitting description. Reporting point estimates with confidence intervals is also part of statistics reform.

The evaluation of the hypotheses in light of the results is conducted with the best research computer in the world: your brain. That is, the researcher must consider the degree of support for the hypotheses, explain any unexpected findings, relate the results to those of previous studies, and reflect on implications of the results for future work in the area. These are all matters of human judgment, in this case based on the researcher's substantive expertise about the research problem. A statistician could help select appropriate statistical tools, but not with the rest without relevant domain knowledge. As aptly put by Huberty and Morris (1988), "As in all statistical inference, subjective judgment cannot be avoided. Neither can reasonableness!" (p. 573).

You may be surprised to see that "conduct statistical tests" is *not* listed among the three primary goals of the analysis. This is because it is quite possible to evaluate hypotheses *without conducting statistical tests at all!* This is done in the natural sciences all the time, and recent events point to a diminishing role for statistical tests in the behavioral sciences. The likelihood that our collective overreliance on statistical tests explains in part the limited impact of behavioral sciences research was discussed in the previous chapter. In some sources, conclusion validity is defined as whether inferences about the null hypothesis based on results of statistical tests are correct. However, this view is too narrow, for the reasons just given.

Conclusion validity is associated mainly with the analysis (Figure 3.1). In a broad sense, it concerns whether inferences about estimated covariances are correct. Specifically, this means (1) whether the correct method of analysis was used, and (2) whether the value of the estimated (sample) covariance approximates that of the corresponding population value. Obviously, the incorrect use of statistics or techniques under conditions where the results are likely to be inaccurate could adversely affect the accuracy of inferences about covariances. Some authors argue that conclusion validity also includes whether a treatment program has been properly implemented (Shadish et al., 2001). The rationale is as follows: If an intervention or program has been poorly carried out (e.g., due to lack of protocol standardization), then its observed covariance with outcome may be inaccurate. In this view, conclusion validity does not fall exclusively within the realm of statistical analysis; instead, it is also part of the correct implementation of the design, here the independent variable.

A few words are needed about the choice of statistical techniques: There is no one-to-one correspondence between a design and a statistical technique. The selection of a technique depends in part on the dependent variable. For example, categorical outcomes—especially dichotomous ones, such as relapsed–not relapsed—may require specialized statistical methods. Some of these techniques are relatively complicated and ordinarily are taught at the graduate level (i.e., they are not good choices for undergraduate-level studies without proper supervision). However, some straightforward effect size statistics for categorical outcomes are described in Chapter 6. See Agresti (2007) for more information about statistical options for categorical data analysis.

Many outcome variables in behavioral science studies are continuous and for which means are appropriate measures of central tendency. You are probably familiar with standard statistical methods for analyzing means, including ANOVA. The family of ANOVA methods is flexible and can be used in designs with continuous outcomes and any combination of these design elements: multiple groups (i.e., a between-subject design), multiple independent variables (e.g., a factorial design), matching or repeated measures (i.e., a within-subject design), and covariates. It is no wonder that ANOVA is one of the most widely used statistical methods in the behavioral sciences, especially in student research projects. There are five fundamental things you need to know about ANOVA. First, if someone uses ANOVA mainly to conduct *F*-tests of mean differences, then that usage is much too narrow. This is because there is even more valuable information in the rest of the ANOVA source table besides the column in which *F*-values and asterisks (for indicating levels of statistical significance) are listed. This other information includes the values of the sums of squares and mean squares for various effects or error terms, which can be easily recombined in the calculation of effect sizes.

Second, a drawback of ANOVA is that it is awkward to include a continuous variable, such as age in years or weight in pounds, as a factor (independent variable) in the analysis. One way to do so is to convert a continuous variable into a dichotomous one by splitting the cases into two groups, one with scores below a cutting point and the other with scores above the cutting point. A common cutting point is the sample median. For example, in a **median split**, one group has scores below the 50th percentile on the original variable, and the other group has scores above the 50th percentile. After the median split, the groups (below vs. above median) are represented as two levels of a single factor in an ANOVA. Alternatively, low versus high groups could be formed relative to different cutting points, such as the sample average in a **mean split** or any other point in the distribution (e.g., 1 standard deviation above the mean). *However, dichotomization of a continuous predictor is generally a bad idea.* One reason is that most of the numerical information about individual differences in the original distribution is discarded when a continuous variable is dichotomized. Other drawbacks described by MacCallum, Zhang, Preacher, and Rucker (2002) for the case of a single independent variable are outlined next:

1. Assuming normal distributions, dichotomization reduces population correlations, and the degree of this reduction is greater as the cutting point moves further away from the mean.

2. Sample correlations based on the dichotomized variable are generally lower in absolute value compared with the corresponding correlations based on the original variables.

3. When the population correlation is low or the sample size is small, dichotomization can actually *increase* the sample correlation. However, this result is probably due to sampling error and thus is not generally evidence that dichotomization was appropriate.

MacCallum et al. (2002) noted that dichotomization of two continuous independent variables so that the data can be analyzed in a 2 × 2 factorial ANOVA can result in spurious main or interaction effects (i.e., they are statistically significant but artifactual results). See Thompson (2006, pp. 386–390) for more information about negative effects due to categorizing continuous predictor variables.

Third, the problem just mentioned about representing continuous variables as factors in the analysis goes away once you realize that all forms of ANOVA are nothing more than a restricted case of multiple regression (MR) (J. Cohen, 1968), which itself is just an extension of bivariate regression that analyzes one or more predictors (independent variables) of a continuous criterion (dependent variable). Any predictor in MR can be continuous or categorical, and both types of predictors can be analyzed together. Thus, there is no need to categorize a continuous predictor in MR. It is also possible in MR to estimate interaction effects between continuous or categorical factors; ANOVA is limited to interactions between categorical factors only. Both ANOVA and MR are based on the same underlying mathematical model—the **general linear model**—but MR is much more flexible. Another advantage is that computer output for regression analyses includes correlations or squared correlations (proportions of explained variance), which are standardized effect sizes. There are whole books that deal with the relation between ANOVA and MR. One of these is Cohen, Cohen, West, and Aiken (2003), which many consider to be a kind of "bible" about MR (i.e., it is an essential reference work). A related book is by Keppel and Zedeck (1989), which explains how to carry out many standard types of analyses for comparing means from both an ANOVA perspective and an MR perspective.

Fourth, the technique of ANOVA (and MR, too) permits the distinction between random effects and fixed effects. The levels of a **random-effects factor** are randomly selected by the researcher. Suppose that participants are required to learn a list of words. If only a single word list is used, it is possible that the results are specific to that word list. Using several word lists matched on characteristics such as relative word frequency and randomly selecting a particular list for the sake of generality would enhance external validity. In contrast, levels of a **fixed-effects factor** are intentionally selected by the researcher, such as when four different dosages of a drug that form an interval scale (e.g., 0 [control], 5, 10, and 15 mg $\times$ kg^{-1}) are chosen for study. The specification of random factors in the behavioral sciences is relatively rare, but it can be directly represented in ANOVA and MR. Implications of the specification of factors as fixed versus random for external validity are considered later.

Fifth, the statistical assumptions of ANOVA (and MR, too) are critical. In between-subject designs, these include the requirement for independence of the observations, normal population distributions, and equal population variances, or **homogeneity of variance**. The independence assumption was discussed earlier. You may have heard in a previous statistics course that the F-test in ANOVA is robust against violations of the normality and homogeneity of variance assumptions. However, this is generally true only in large and representative samples with equal group sizes. Otherwise, even slight departures from normality can greatly reduce statistical power (Wilcox, 1998). There can be serious **positive bias** when the ratio of the largest over the smallest within-group variance is greater than 9 or so, especially when the group sizes are unequal or when heterogeneity is associated with one outlier group than when it is spread across all groups (Keppel & Wickens, 2004). Positive bias means that the null hypothesis is rejected more often than it should be because the probabilities associated with the F-test are too low. There are special statistical tests for detecting heterogeneity of variance, but they have restrictive assumptions, such as normality, and thus are not generally recommended (Thompson, 2006; Wilkinson & Task Force on Statistical Inference, 1999). Additional statistical assumptions for within-subject designs are explained in the next chapter, and those for covariate analyses are outlined next. Overall, the statistical assumptions of ANOVA are much more demanding than many of us realize. They also cannot be ignored.

A related technique is the analysis of covariance (ANCOVA), which is just an ANOVA conducted with covariates. A **covariate** is a variable that predicts outcome but is ideally unrelated to the independent variable. In ANCOVA, the variance explained by a continuous covariate is statistically removed, which reduces error variance. Suppose that a test of prereading skill (e.g., phonemic awareness) is administered to grade 1 students before they either enter a new reading program or receive standard reading instruction. It is likely that scores on the pretest will covary with those on the outcome measure, a reading skill test. This covariance is statistically removed from the reading skill test in ANCOVA. This adjustment may substantially reduce unexplained variance in the reading skill test, which in turn increases precision in the estimation of treatment effects.

In experimental designs where the treatment and control groups have similar means on the covariate, the only appreciable statistical correction in ANCOVA is the reduction of error variance. Otherwise, group means on the dependent variable are also adjusted, given the observed group differences on the covariate and the statistical association between the covariate and outcome variable. These adjusted means are also referred to as **predicted means**. Relative to the observed (original, unadjusted) means, the predicted means could indicate a smaller or larger group mean difference. It is even possible that the direction of group mean differences is not the same across the observed and predicted means. Suppose that the treatment group in a study about a new grade 1 reading instructional program has a higher mean on a reading pretest than does the control group. That is, the treatment group starts off with an advantage even before the new reading program begins. With no adjustment, this group would be expected to have a higher mean on the outcome measure of reading skill even if the treatment effects were nil. In ANCOVA, group means on the reading skill test would be corrected for the initial difference on the pretest, perhaps by reducing the magnitude of the group difference on the predicted means compared with that indicated by the observed means. This is exactly the rationale in the sport of golf of a handicap, which is the numerical measure of an amateur's skill that is used to calculate a corrected score based on the observed number of strokes. This corrected score allows players of different abilities to compete against each other on somewhat equal terms.

Presented in Figure 3.2 is a graphical example of the relation between observed and predicted means in ANCOVA. An experimental design is assumed. Represented in the figure is a scatterplot for the association between the covariate (Z) and dependent variable (Y) for each of two groups. Across both groups, this association is linear and the slopes of the within-group regression lines are identical. The grand mean on the covariate for all cases in both groups combined is M_Z. Relative to Group 2, Group 1 has a higher observed mean on both the covariate ($M_{Z1} > M_{Z2}$) and the dependent variable ($M_{Y1} > M_{Y2}$). In ANCOVA, the predicted means are obtained from the intersection of the within-group regression lines and the vertical line from $Z = M_Z$ (see Figure 3.2). That is, the predicted means

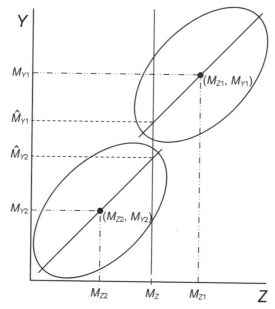

FIGURE 3.2. Observed and predicted means on the dependent variable (Y) in ANCOVA when two groups differ on the covariate (Z).

are the literal statistical answer to the question, if the groups had started with the same scores on the covariate (i.e., $M_{Z1} = M_{Z2} = M_Z$), by how much are they predicted to differ on the dependent variable? Note in Figure 3.2 that the predicted mean for Group 1 is lower than the corresponding observed mean, or $\hat{M}_{Y1} < M_{Y1}$. However, the opposite is true for Group 2, or $\hat{M}_{Y2} > M_{Y2}$. In ANCOVA, the predicted group mean difference equals $\hat{M}_{Y1} - \hat{M}_{Y2}$, which you can see in Figure 3.2 is smaller than the observed mean difference, or $M_{Y1} - M_{Y2}$. In contrast, the observed mean difference $M_{Y1} - M_{Y2}$ is the ANOVA estimate of the group mean difference, but this estimate ignores the covariate.

Because a covariate analysis is a form of statistical control, it can be incorporated into many different types of designs. *However, ANCOVA works best in experimental designs where groups were formed by random assignment, and it is critical to meet its statistical requirements (assumptions).* One requirement is that the scores on the covariate are highly reliable. Another is that the relation between the covariate and the outcome variable is linear for all groups. A third is for **homogeneity of regression**, which means that the slope of the within-group regression lines for the association between the dependent variable and the covariate is the same across all groups (e.g., see Figure 3.2). If these key assumptions are violated, then values of adjusted error variances, predicted means, or statistical tests (i.e., F-ratios) in ANCOVA can be quite inaccurate. For example, the adjusted means could indicate no effect of treatment when there really is one, or they could spuriously indicate a treatment effect when it is actually nil, given violated assumptions.

There are additional complications when ANCOVA is applied in designs where cases are not randomly assigned to groups. This includes quasi-experimental designs where cases are assigned to treatment or control groups through any other method than randomization. In such designs, it often happens that the treatment and control groups differ on relevant variables *before* the treatment is administered. Any subsequent treatment effect is thus confounded with preexisting group differences. In these situations, it might seem that ANCOVA could be applied as a way to correct for initial group differences on covariates when estimating a treatment effect on the outcome variable. This type of analysis is actually fraught with many potential problems that are elaborated in the next chapter. However, I can say now that these problems are often so severe that little confidence may be warranted whenever ANCOVA is used to "correct for" initial group differences in designs without randomization. The same basic point was made by Keppel and Zedeck (1989):

> The method [ANCOVA] also depends on the assumption that individuals have been randomly assigned to the conditions. If this assumption is not met, any adjustment in treatment means cannot be defended or justified statistically. Therefore, most quasi experiments cannot be properly brought into statistical alignment by ANCOVA. (p. 481)

Some alternatives that *may* avoid some of the limitations of ANCOVA in quasi-experimental designs are described in the next chapter. Considered next are various threats to internal validity, construct validity, conclusion validity, and external validity and how to deal with them.

Internal Validity

The critical issue about internal validity is the requirement that there should be no other plausible explanation of the results other than the presumed causes measured in your study. This requirement is addressed through the control of extraneous variables, and there are six basic ways to do so. These strategies involve design, analysis, measurement, and your knowledge of the research area. These methods are listed next and described afterward:

1. Direct manipulation.

2. Random assignment (randomization).

3. Elimination or inclusion of extraneous variables.

4. Statistical control (covariate analysis).

5. Through rational argument.

6. Analyze reliable scores.

In experimental designs, one or more independent variables are directly manipulated, and their effects on outcome or dependent variables are then measured. In the natural sciences, researchers who work in laboratories may be able to precisely manipulate physical variables, such as the level of gamma radiation, and measure their effects with equal precision on other variables, such as the proportion of healthy white blood cells.

In the behavioral sciences, direct manipulation is usually accomplished in experimental designs through the random assignment of cases to groups or levels of independent variables that represent conditions, such as treatment versus control. Because randomization is a chance-based method, it tends to minimize differences between groups by equally distributing cases with particular characteristics across the groups. Some of these characteristics may reflect individual difference variables that are confounded with the effects of treatment. For example, if children assigned to a new reading program are already better readers than those given standard instruction, program effects are confounded with initial differences. Randomization tends to equate groups on all variables before treatment, whether these variables are directly measured or not (Shadish et al., 2001). In the example just mentioned, randomization would tend to evenly distribute initial reading skill and all other individual difference variables across the two conditions. This property of randomization plays a crucial role in minimizing threats to internal validity in experimental designs.

It is critical to understand that randomization equates groups *in the long run* (i.e., on expectations), and it works best when the overall sample size (*N*) is large. However, there is no guarantee that groups formed through randomization in a *particular study* will be exactly equal on all measured or unmeasured variables, especially when *N* is not large. That is, randomization equates groups *on average* across independent replications of the study. Sometimes it happens that groups formed through randomization in a particular study are clearly not equal on some characteristic before the treatment is administered. The expression **failure of randomization** is used to describe this situation, but it is a misnomer because it assumes that randomization should guarantee equal groups every time it is used. However, when (not if) unequal groups are formed by randomization, it is the result of chance. Any chance difference can be accounted for by (1) administering pretests to all cases before treatment and (2) using statistical control to adjust for differences indicated on the pretests (e.g., ANCOVA).

The **elimination of an extraneous variable** basically involves converting it to a constant. For example, testing animals under constant temperature and lighting conditions isolates these variables from having influence on the outcome variable. **Inclusion of an extraneous variable** involves the direct measurement of such a variable and its addition as a distinct factor (independent variable) in the design. For example, the amount of time that parents read books to their children at home could be measured in a study where outcomes of a new reading program are also directly measured. In this way, it should be possible in the analysis to separate out the effects of home and program variables on children's reading skill. The principle of inclusion is also part of the rationale for blocking designs, which are hybrids of experimental designs and quasi-experimental designs. Blocking designs are described in the next chapter.

The rationale of **statistical control** is exactly that of a covariate analysis, which was described earlier. In this context, an extraneous variable is directly measured, but it is not explicitly represented as a factor in the design. Instead, the influence of this variable on the outcome variable is removed in the statistical analysis, such as ANCOVA. Some methodologists advocate the use of statistical correction *after* other design controls—especially inclusion—have been used (e.g., Shadish et al., 2001). This is a sensible view, especially in designs where randomization is not used to form treatment and control groups.

Sometimes researchers can offer rational arguments about why the effects of a potential extraneous variable may not be substantial. These arguments can be made either a priori (before the study is conducted) or a posteriori (afterward). As noted by Trochim and Land (1982), (1) a priori arguments tend to be more convincing than a posteriori arguments, and (2) argument by itself is weaker than design controls and statistical correction in dealing with extraneous variables. For instance, the researcher can present a stronger case that an increase in at-home reading in the treatment group does not explain the apparent benefits of a new grade 1 reading instruction program by actually measuring this variable in all groups than by simply offering arguments that this explanation is implausible. The final way to reduce irrelevant variance is to use outcome measures that generate reliable scores, which is a measurement issue.

In nonexperimental studies where causal hypotheses are evaluated, threats to internal validity are dealt with mainly through the direct measurement of alternative explanations and the use of statistical control in the analysis. However, this process relies heavily on the researcher to specify these alternative explanations in the first place and then to measure them with precision. Both of these steps require strong knowledge about which alternative explanations are plausible. If the researcher cannot give a good account of both specification and measurement, then causal inferences in nonexperimental designs are probably unwarranted. This is why some methodologists are skeptical about the strength of causal inferences in nonexperimental designs (e.g., Pedhazur & Schmelkin, 1991). An example follows.

Lynam, Moffitt, and Stouthamer-Loeber (1993) hypothesized that poor verbal ability is a cause of delinquency, but both variables were measured simultaneously in their sample, which raises some questions: Why this particular direction of causation? Is it not also plausible that certain behaviors associated with delinquency, such as drug use, head injuries due to fighting, or dropping out of school, could impair verbal ability? And, what about other causes of delinquency besides verbal ability? The arguments offered by Lynam et al. for their hypothesis included the following: Their participants were relatively young (about 12 years old), which may rule out delinquent careers long enough to affect verbal ability; the authors also cited results of prospective research which indicated that low verbal ability precedes antisocial acts. Lynam et al. also measured other presumed causes of delinquency, including social class, motivation, and scholastic achievement, and controlled for these variables in the analysis. Although the particular arguments given by Lynam et al. that poor verbal ability is a cause of delinquency are not above criticism, they at least exemplify the types of arguments that researchers should provide when estimating presumed causal associations in nonexperimental designs. Unfortunately, too few authors of nonexperimental studies give such detailed explanations of their specifications of directional causal effects among variables simultaneously measured.

Summarized in Table 3.1 are major threats to internal validity, listed both for studies in general and in particular for studies with multiple groups (e.g., treatment vs. control). Perhaps the most basic threat is **ambiguous temporal precedence**, or the lack of understanding about which of two variables, a presumed cause and a presumed effect, occurred first. Another general threat is that of **history**, which refers to events that occur at the same time as treatment and that could cause the observed effects. Suppose that the local community launches a public campaign to encourage the development of early reading skills during a study about a new grade

TABLE 3.1. Descriptions of Major Threats to Internal Validity

Threat	Description
General	
Ambiguous temporal precedence	Lack of understanding about which of two variables occurred first (i.e., which is cause and which is effect?)
History	Specific events that take place concurrently with treatment
Maturation	Naturally occurring changes are confounded with treatment
Testing	Exposure to a test affects later scores on outcome variable
Instrumentation	The nature of measurement changes over time or conditions
Attrition	Loss of cases over conditions, groups, or time
Regression	When cases selected for extreme scores obtain less extreme scores on the outcome variable
Multiple-group studies	
Selection	Groups differ before treatment is given
Treatment diffusion or imitation	Control cases learn about treatment or try to imitate experiences of treated cases
Compensatory rivalry	Control cases learn about treatment and become competitive with treated cases
Compensatory equalization of treatment	Cases in one condition demand to be assigned to the other condition or be compensated
Resentful demoralization	Control cases learn about treatment and become resentful or withdraw from study
Novelty and disruption effects	Cases respond extraordinarily well to a novel treatment or very poorly to one that interrupts their routines

1 reading instructional program. In this case, the effects of treatment may be confounded with those of the community program. The threat of **maturation** concerns the possibility that natural changes that would occur even without treatment, such as growing older or more experienced, account for changes on outcome variables. For example, grade 1 students mature a great deal during the school year, and with simple maturation may come better reading skills. The threat of **testing** concerns designs where cases are tested more than once (e.g., pretest–posttest designs). Testing effects occur when taking a test on one occasion influences scores when either the same test or a similar one is taken again. These effects may be due to practice or reactivity, which can occur when exposure to test items alters subsequent behavior. For instance, the act of weighing adults at the start of a weight-loss program may be sufficient to motivate changes in eating or exercise habits.

The threat of **instrumentation** concerns the problem when the use, scoring, or interpretation of scores from a test change over time (Table 3.1). An example is the problem of **rater drift**, which refers to the tendency for raters to unintentionally redefine criteria or standards across a series of observations. These instrumentation changes could be confounded with effects of treatment. **Attrition** refers to the loss of cases from the study and subsequently their scores on the outcome measure. If the attrition rate is high or the data loss pattern is systematic instead of random, then the results may not accurately reflect the true effect of treatment. In longitudinal studies, attrition may also affect external validity because the results based on cases with no missing observations may not generalize to all those who began the study. The threat of **regression** concerns the phenomenon of statistical regression to the mean, which refers to the tendency for cases with extreme scores to obtain less extreme scores when retested on the same or similar measures. Regression artifacts are a concern whenever cases are selected because they had scores lower or higher than average and in studies where cases with extreme scores are matched across different conditions.

Summarized in the bottom part of Table 3.1 are major internal validity threats in multiple-group studies. Perhaps the most basic threat is that of **selection**, which happens when treatment and control groups differ systematically before the treatment is administered. For example, if control cases have a more serious form of an illness than treated cases, the treated cases may look better at the end of the study even if treatment had no positive effects. Selection bias also combines with all of the other types of general internal validity threats listed in the top part of Table 3.1 except for ambiguous temporal precedence. These combinations are actually interaction or differential effects where the threat is more serious or in a different direction in one group than in another. For instance, a **selection-maturation** threat results from differential rates of normal growth across the treatment and control groups that could mimic a treatment effect. A **selection-attrition** threat is due to differential data loss, which happens when the rate of missing data is higher in one group than in another. This can result in different kinds of cases remaining to be measured across the conditions. A **selection-regression** threat happens when there are different rates of regression to the mean across the groups. Suppose that treated cases are selected because they have the highest scores on a pretest of the number of illness symptoms (i.e., they are the sickest), but not control cases. Because of regression to the mean, we expect the treated cases to obtain less extreme scores when tested again, even apart from any beneficial effects of treatment. Selection bias combines with the remaining general external validity threats listed in Table 3.1 in similar ways.

The rest of the internal validity threats in multiple-group studies listed in the bottom part of Table 3.1 are described by some authors as **social interaction threats** (Trochim & Donnelly, 2007). These refer to various kinds of social phenomena that can happen when people in treatment versus control conditions are aware of each other's existence or have direct contact with each other. Note that some authors consider social interaction effects as threats to construct validity, not internal validity (e.g., Shadish et al., 2001). More important than their classification, however, is that the researcher should try to minimize social interaction threats. One type is **treatment diffusion**, which occurs when people in the control conditions receive some or all of the treatment in the other condition. A related threat is **treatment imitation**, which happens when people in control conditions set up their own experiences to approximate those in the treatment condition. One example is when control cases learn certain key information from treated cases (diffusion), such as dietary contributions to an illness, and then act on that information in a way that mimics treatment (imitation), such as by following a healthier diet. **Compensatory rivalry** can have similar consequences, and it happens when control cases feel they must compete with treated cases, perhaps by working harder or taking better care of themselves. Control cases may also demand of researchers or administrators for **compensatory equalization of treatment**. This could involve "switching" a case from the control condition to the treatment condition or offering some type of other compensation for not receiving the treatment. Awareness of the treatment condition can also lead to **resentful demoralization**, which happens when control cases become so bitter about not receiving treatment that they stop trying or drop out of the study. **Novelty and disruption effects** can also affect scores on outcome measures in ways that have nothing to do with treatment. Specifically, people tend to respond with enthusiasm to interventions that are perceived as novel or stimulating but not so well to interventions that disrupt their daily routines, especially if the intervention interferes with current effective practices. A specific instance of the novelty effect is the **Hawthorne effect**, which refers to the tendency of some people to work harder or perform better when they are participants in an experiment. That is, perhaps the special attention that comes with participating in a study is enough to effect behavior changes in ways that mimic a treatment effect.

Randomization is the clearest way to eliminate selection bias in its various forms. However, it is not always possible to use randomization, especially in field studies. For example, sometimes treatment and control groups are already formed (i.e., they are intact) at the start of the study. Suppose that a new reading program will be implemented on a trial basis in just one school. This decision is a matter of policy and is not at the researcher's discretion. At the end of the program, reading test scores will be compared with those of students who attended a different school and received standard reading instruction. This design is quasi-experimental due to the absence of randomization to form the groups. It is possible that the two intact groups in this example (new program vs. standard instruction) could differ on many variables, such as level of prereading skills, family income, or school quality, that are confounded with effects of reading instruction. This is why it is more difficult to attribute differences between treated and untreated cases to treatment in quasi-experimental designs.

To reduce threats due to history and maturation, treatment and control groups should be selected from the same general geographic area. Both groups should be roughly the same age so that their maturational status is comparable, and they should share the same measurement schedule. These commonalities help to control for local events which may differentially affect the groups (Shadish et al., 2001). Testing effects are of concern only when pretests are administered, especially when the interval between the pretest and posttest is short. The degree of testing effects can be explicitly estimated in designs where some treatment and control cases are administered a pretest but others are not. This type of design is referred as a Solomon Four-Group Design and is described in the next chapter. An instrumentation threat is relevant when cases are tested over time on the same variable, such as in repeated-measures designs. To minimize this threat, the same measure should be given at each occasion under constant conditions, and raters (if any) should be retrained periodically to maintain accurate scoring.

Regression artifacts are plausible whenever cases are selected due to extreme scores. The use of reliable scores to classify cases helps to minimize regression to the mean. It may also help to measure status on a selection variable more than once and then average the scores together before classifying cases. This reduces error in selection, in part because effects of individual outlier scores tend to cancel out when scores are summed. D. T. Campbell and Kenny (1999) described various other ways to handle regression artifacts. Prevention is the best way to deal with attrition (missing data) through the specification of a measurement process in which questionnaires have clear instructions and there are built-in checks for incomplete protocols. However, missing data still occur, despite our best efforts. Social interaction threats may be minimized by isolating treatment and control groups so that they are unaware of each other and by encouraging administrators to not compensate control cases (Trochim & Donnelly, 2007).

Construct Validity

Summarized in Table 3.2 are major threats to construct validity, or the correct assessment of variables that the researcher wishes to measure. One was mentioned earlier: score unreliability. The threats of **poor construct definition** and **construct confounding** involve problems with, respectively, how constructs are defined or operationalized. Incorrect definition could include mislabeling a construct, such as when low IQ scores among minority children who do not speak English as a first language are attributed to low intelligence instead of to limited language familiarity. Another problem is to define the construct at the wrong level of analysis, such as when a researcher believes that a measure of work satisfaction also reflects general life satisfaction (too narrow) or vice versa (too broad). **Monomethod bias** can occur when different outcome measures are all based on the same measurement method, such as self-report, or the same informant, such as parents in studies of children. There may be effects due to that particular method or informant known as **common method variance** that can mask the assessment of underlying traits. Accordingly, it is best to use different

TABLE 3.2. Descriptions of Major Threats to Construct Validity

Threat	Description
Unreliable scores	Scores are nor precise or consistent
Poor construct definition	Construct may be mislabeled or defined at the wrong level (e.g., too general or too specific)
Construct confounding	Definition or study operational definitions confounded with other constructs
Monomethod bias	Measurement of different outcome variables all rely on the same method (e.g., self-report) or informant (e.g., parents)
Mono-operation bias	Refers to the use of a single operationalization of the independent or dependent variables
Evaluation apprehension	Anxiety about measurement and evaluation adversely affects performance
Reactive self-report changes	Motivation to be in a treatment condition affects responses, and this motivation can change over time
Researcher expectancies	The researcher conveys (consciously or otherwise) expectations about desirable responses

measurement methods or informants across a set of outcome measures. In studies with single operationalizations of each construct, there is the possibility of **mono-operation bias**. The use of a single outcome measure when effects of treatment are expected across multiple domains is one example. Another is when a single version of a treatment is studied. A particular version may include just one exemplar of a manipulation, such as when just one dosage of a drug is studied.

The threat of **evaluation apprehension**, or the possibility that nervousness about being tested may adversely affect scores, can be managed by good "test-side manner" on the part of examiners (Table 3.2). The threat of **reactive self-report changes,** or **reactivity**, refers to a type of demand characteristic where participants' motivation to be in treatment or their guesses about the nature of the study affects their responses in ways that mimic treatment effects. Such effects may be reduced by measuring outcome outside the experimental setting, avoiding the use of pretests that give hints about expected outcome, using unobtrusive measures (Webb, Campbell, Schwartz, & Sechrest, 1966), or applying masking (blinding) procedures that try to prevent participants from learning research hypotheses. Use of masking to prevent examiners or raters from knowing the hypotheses may reduce the threat of **researcher expec-**

tancies, where expectations about desirable responses are conveyed to participants, perhaps unintentionally so. This is why double-blind procedures are routinely used in randomized clinical trials for medications: They control for expectancy effects on the part of both participants and researchers.

Conclusion Validity

Described in Table 3.3 are major threats to conclusion validity, or the correct estimation of covariances. The first four threats listed in the table concern uncontrolled sources of error variance, which reduces the power of statistical tests and attenuates effect sizes. One is score unreliability, which is also a threat to construct validity (see Table 3.2). Thus, the analysis of unreliable scores has many deleterious consequences. Another source of imprecision is **unreliability of treatment implementation**, which was already discussed. The threat of **random irrelevancies in study setting** refers to the effects of uncontrolled nuisance variables in the experimental setting

TABLE 3.3. Descriptions of Major Threats to Conclusion Validity

Threat	Description
Unreliable scores	Scores are not precise or consistent
Unreliability of treatment implementation	Treatment delivery does not follow prescribed procedures
Random irrelevancies in study setting	Obscure, irrelevant events in setting, such as noise, that distract cases or researchers, adding to error
Random within-group heterogeneity	High variability on the outcome measure increases error variance
Range restriction	Reduced range of scores on a variable restricts its correlation with another variable
Inaccurate effect size estimation	Systematic overestimation or underestimation of effect size
Overreliance on statistical tests	Failure to consider other aspects of the results, such as effect size or substantive significance
Violated assumptions of statistical tests	Results of statistical tests (i.e., p values) inaccurate due to violation of distributional or other assumptions
Low power	Low probability of correctly rejecting the null hypothesis when it is false
Fishing and inflation of Type I error rate	Failure to correct for experimentwise rate of Type I when multiple statistical tests are conducted

that could obscure the correct estimation of covariances. The threat of **random within-group heterogeneity** can arise when treatment or control groups are heterogeneous. Some of these individual differences could be related to outcome. Suppose that a treatment is more effective for women than for men. If gender is represented as a factor in the design, then error variance is reduced; otherwise, there is greater error. Another strategy is to match groups on relevant characteristics or treat those variables as covariates in ANCOVA or related types of analyses. However, other types of individual differences may be simply irrelevant to outcome, and this random variability also contributes to the error term.

Assuming a true linear relation between variables X and Y, the absolute value of the Pearson correlation r_{XY} can be reduced through **range restriction** (Table 3.3). This can happen when either sampling (case selection) or attrition (missing data) results in reduced inherent variability on X or Y relative to the population. For example, there is generally a positive linear relation between weight loss and systolic blood pressure reduction among adults. However, the observed correlation between these two variables in a sample of obese adults only may be close to zero due to range restriction in weight. The same outcome would be expected if only hypertensive adults are selected for the sample due to range restriction in systolic blood pressure. Low score reliability on either X or Y also tends to lower absolute values of sample correlations. See Thompson (2006, pp. 114–116) and Huck (1992) for more information about range restriction. Both range restriction and low score reliability can also cause **inaccurate effect size estimation**. In general, effect size is underestimated, given range restriction or low score reliability. Overestimation of effect size is also possible, too, but it may happen less often than underestimation when the sample size is not small. The problem of **overreliance on statistical tests** has already been noted. A related concern is **violated assumptions of statistical tests**. The critical assumption of score independence was mentioned earlier. Many statistical tests also assume normal distributions. If distributional assumptions are violated, then the results of statistical tests (i.e., probabilities, or p values) may be incorrect.

Low statistical power also adversely affects conclusion validity (Table 3.3). In studies of treatment effects, **power** is the probability of finding a statistically significant difference between the treatment and control conditions when there is a real population treatment effect. Power varies directly with the magnitude of the real effect and sample size. Other factors that affect power include the level of statistical significance (e.g., .05 vs. .01), the directionality of the test of the alternative hypothesis (i.e., one- or two-tailed test), whether the design is between-subject or within-subject, the particular test statistic used, and the reliability of the scores. The following combination leads to the greatest power: a large population effect size, a large sample, the .05 level of statistical significance, a one-tailed test, a within-subject design, a parametric test statistic (e.g., t) rather than a nonparametric statistic (e.g., Mann–Whitney U), and highly reliable scores. We will see in Chapter 5 that power is generally low in the behavioral sciences, but many times there may be little that researchers can do to substantially increase power. This is another problem when we rely too much on statistical tests.

The last threat to conclusion validity listed in Table 3.3 concerns the problem of **fishing**, which refers to analyzing the data under slightly different conditions, assumptions, or subsets of variables. One negative consequence of fishing is the inflation of Type I error rate across a whole set of statistical tests. Recall that a (1) Type I error happens when a result is statistically significant but there is no real effect in the population; and (2) the researcher sets the risk for Type I error through the specification of the value of alpha (α), which is usually either .05 or .01. You should know that α sets the risk for a Type I error for a single statistical test. When multiple tests are conducted, there is also **experimentwise (familywise) rate of Type I error**, designated below as α_{EW}. It is the probability of making at least one Type I error across a set of statistical tests. If each individual test is conducted at the same level of α, then

$$\alpha_{EW} = 1 - (1 - \alpha)^c \qquad (3.1)$$

where c is the number of tests. Suppose that 20 statistical tests are each conducted at $\alpha = .05$ in the same dataset. The experimentwise Type I error rate is

$$\alpha_{EW} = 1 - (1 - .05)^{20} = .64$$

That is, the probability of making one or more Type I errors across the whole set of 20 tests is .64. However, Equation 3.1 cannot tell us exactly how many Type I errors may have been committed (it could be 1, or 2, or 3 ...) or on which statistical tests they occurred. Note that Equation 3.1 assumes that the tests are independent, that is, what is observed in one test is unrelated to what is observed in another. Otherwise, Equation 3.1 may underestimate the rate of experimentwise Type I error.

External Validity and Sampling

Recall that external validity concerns inferences about whether the results of a study—or about causal relations in the case of experimental or quasi-experimental designs—will hold over variations in persons, treatments, settings, and outcomes (measures). One facet of external validity is **population validity**, which concerns variation over people and, specifically, whether one can generalize from sample results to a defined population. Another is **ecological validity**, which concerns whether the combination of treatments, settings, or outcomes in a particular study approximate those of the real-life situation under investigation. Both facets of external validity just mentioned fall under the **principle of proximal similarity**, which refers to the evaluation of generalizability of results across samples, settings, situations, treatments, or measures that are more or less similar to those included in the original study (Shadish et al., 2001).

Suppose that a new treatment is evaluated and the results look promising. It is natural to wonder: Would the treatment be just as effective in other samples drawn from the same population but tested in other settings or with reasonable variations in the treatment or outcome measures? With sufficient replication of the original study, we will eventually have the answers, but replication takes time. Is there any way to "build in" to the original study some kind of reassurance (but not a guarantee) that the results may generalize?

Yes, and it is achieved through representative sampling of persons, treatments, settings, or outcomes. One way to obtain representative samples is through **probability sampling** where observations are selected from a population by a chance-based method. There are a few different types of probability sampling. In **simple random sampling**, for instance, all observations in the population have an equal probability of appearing in the sample. In **stratified sampling**, the population is divided into homogeneous, mutually exclusive groups (strata), such as neighborhoods, and then observations are randomly selected from within each stratum. In **cluster sampling**, the population is also divided into groups (clusters), but then only some clusters are randomly selected to represent the population. All observations within each selected cluster are included in the sample, but no observations from the unselected clusters are included.

The use of random sampling supports inferences about external validity, just as randomization does for inferences about internal validity. The use of random sampling and randomization together in the same study—

the so-called **statistician's two step**—guarantees that the average causal effect observed in the study is the same as that in any other random sample with the same number of cases drawn from the same population (Shadish et al., 2001). However, this two-step ideal is almost *never* achieved in behavioral science studies. This is because random sampling requires a list of all observations in the population, but such lists rarely exist. Also, the idea of probability sampling does not even apply in animal research, where samples are virtually never randomly selected from known populations.

It is **nonprobability sampling**, which does not involve random selection, that is the rule in the behavioral sciences. There are two general types, accidental and purposive. In **accidental sampling**, cases are selected because they happen to be available. These types of samples are called **ad hoc samples**, **convenience samples**, or **locally available samples**. A group of patients in a particular clinic who volunteer as research participants is an example of an ad hoc sample. When researchers study a convenience sample, the design really has no sampling plan whatsoever. A big problem with convenience samples is that they may not be representative. For instance, it is known that volunteers differ systematically from nonvolunteers, and patients seen in one clinic may differ from those treated in others. Perhaps the best way to mitigate bias in convenience samples is to measure a posteriori a variety of sample characteristics and report them along with the rest of the results. This allows readers of the work to compare its sample with those of other studies in the same area. Another option is to compare the sample demographic profile with that of the population (if such a profile exists) in order to show that a convenience sample is not grossly unrepresentative.

In **purposive sampling**, the researcher intentionally selects cases from defined groups or dimensions. If so, then sampling is part of the study design, and groups or dimensions according to which cases are selected are typically linked to the research hypotheses. For example, a researcher who wishes to evaluate whether the effectiveness of a new medication differs by gender would intentionally select both men and women patients with some illness. After collecting the data, gender would then be represented as a factor in the analysis along with the distinction of treatment (medication) versus control (e.g., placebo). Used in this way, purposive sampling may facilitate generalization of the results to both men and women.

Purposive sampling of cases is used much more often in the behavioral sciences than probability sampling. As noted by Shadish et al. (2001), it is not backed by a statistical logic that justifies formal generalizations as is probability sampling. Some authors, such as Pedhazur and Schmelkin

(1991), are skeptical about statistics from nonprobability samples having anything to do with statistics from probability samples, but, as mentioned, study of the latter is typically not an option. The random selection of treatments, settings, or measures is even rarer still. There is almost never a list of all possible treatments, nor do researchers typically select measures or settings at random (Shadish et al., 2001). The possibility to represent factors in ANOVA or MR as random instead of fixed accommodates the relatively rare occasions when levels of a factor are randomly selected. This specification also has implications for external validity. For fixed factors, the results may not generalize to other levels not included in the original study. If the levels of a fixed-effects drug factor are dosages of 0, 5, 10, and 15 mg $\times$ kg^{-1}, then the results may not generalize to higher dosages or even to intermediate dosages within this range but not directly tested, such as 12.5 mg $\times$ kg^{-1}. In contrast, selecting dosages at random may give a representative sample from all possible levels; if so, then the results may generalize to the whole population of dosages. See Shadish et al. (2001, Chs. 11–13) for discussion of a theory of generalized causal inference that allows for nonprobability samples.

Threats to external validity concern any characteristic of a sample, treatment, setting, or measure that leads the results to be specific to a particular study (i.e., they do not generalize). Major types of such threats are listed in Table 3.4. Many of these threats can be viewed as conditional or interaction effects where the results depend on the levels of some characteristic. For example, results found in samples of men may not hold over samples of women, and vice versa. If so, then a **treatment × unit interaction** is indicated. A related threat is a **treatment × setting interaction**, which is apparent when a treatment is more effective in one setting than in another, such as private practice versus outpatient clinics. If a treatment has different effects on different outcome variables, then a **treatment × outcome interaction** is indicated. The term **treatment × treatment interaction** in Table 3.4 refers to situations in which effects of some treatment either (1) do not hold over variations in that treatment or (2) depend on exposure to previous treatments (including none). A related threat is that of **multiple treatment interference**, which concerns whether we can generalize the effects of a single independent variable when cases are exposed to several independent variables, perhaps simultaneously as in factorial designs. Note that some authors classify unreliability of treatment implementation, experimenter expectancies, testing effects, and novelty effects as threats to external validity (Martella, Nelson, & Marchand-Martella, 1999). But, again, more important than the classification of these threats is that

TABLE 3.4. Descriptions of Major Threats to External Validity

Threat	Description
Treatment × unit interaction	An effect holds only for certain types of units, including characteristics of cases
Treatment × setting interaction	An effect holds only in certain settings
Treatment × outcome interaction	An effect holds for some types of outcome variables but not others
Treatment × treatment interaction	An effect does not hold over variations in treatment or depends on exposure to previous treatments
Multiple treatment interference	Whether we can generalize the effects of a single independent variable when participants are exposed to multiple independent variables

you take preventive action to deal with them. The best way to address threats to external validity is to conduct replication studies across variations in samples, treatments, settings, or outcomes. That is, replication is the ultimate arbiter of external validity.

Summary

A successful scientific study is the result of a series of well-planned decisions. The starting point in this process is your research question, or hypotheses. Without a clear and meaningful question, all that follows may be for naught, so first think long and hard about the rationale of your hypotheses before considering specifics of design, measurement, or analysis. The design sets the logical framework of the study, and in cause-probing studies it sets basic conditions for internal validity, too. In planning the number of groups or conditions, sample size, the schedule for interventions or measurements, and other design details, you must balance what is ideal against what is possible, given limitations on resources but still respecting the hypotheses. How your cases are selected, or sampling, plays a crucial role in external validity. This is especially true if it is uncertain whether your sample is representative. Because most samples studied in the behavioral sciences are nonprobability samples, concern about generalizability is usually warranted. Consequently, always describe in detail the characteristics of your sample, and be cautious about the potential generalizability of your findings without evidence from replication studies. Measurement requires special attention because the analysis of scores that are unreliable or lack construct validity—they do not measure what you intended to measure—is not likely to yield meaningful results. In the analysis, the main goal is not to conduct statistical tests of your hypotheses. Instead, you should aim to estimate accurate covariances between variables of interest, express these estimates in a way that conveys both effect size and the degree of sampling error, and then interpret these results in light of your hypotheses. The next chapter considers options for design and analysis in more detail.

RECOMMENDED READINGS

Trochim and Donnelly (2007) is an introductory-level research methods book that offers a comprehensive, well-balanced treatment of the major topics discussed in this chapter. van den Akker, Gravemeijer, McKenney, and Nieveen (2006) is oriented toward education students, and it considers methods in different areas of education research. A more advanced treatment of research methods is available in Shadish et al. (2001). It is suitable for graduate students, but advanced undergraduate students with strong methods and statistics backgrounds could also benefit from reading this work. The coverage of quasi-experimental designs in this book is especially strong.

Shadish, W. R., Cook, T. D., & Campbell, D. T. (2001). *Experimental and quasi-experimental designs for generalized causal inference*. New York: Houghton Mifflin.

Trochim, W., & Donnelly, J. P. (2007). *The research methods knowledge base* (3rd ed.). Mason, OH: Atomic Dog.

van den Akker, J., Gravemeijer, K., McKenney, S., & Nieveen, N. (Eds.). (2006). *Educational design research*. New York: Routledge.

EXERCISES

1. Comment: Internal validity, construct validity, conclusion validity, and external validity are the exclusive concerns of, respectively, design, measurement, analysis, and sampling.

2. Comment: Maximizing internal validity in experimental or quasi-experimental designs may reduce external validity.

3. What is the relation between construct validity and external validity? Between conclusion validity and internal validity?

4. Comment: A researcher collects a sample of patients from a local clinic. Half the patients are men, half are women. The resulting sample is a probability sample.

5. Comment: A researcher randomly selects 100 students in a large, introductory-level class of 400 students. The selected students are invited to participate in a research project. The resulting sample will be a random sample.

6. Comment: A sample of 1,000 adults is randomly selected from a community in which 100,000 adults reside. Because the sample is representative, external validity is guaranteed.

7. Describe negative consequences of low score reliability on the dependent variable.

8. In a multiple-group study, explain these internal validity threats: selection-testing, selection-history, and selection-instrumentation.

9. Draw a scatterplot like the one in Figure 3.2 for two groups in an experimental design where the predicted mean difference in ANOVA is *greater* than the observed mean difference on the dependent variable.

10. You collected data in a sample of convenience, and there is no population demographic profile. How do you deal with threats to external validity when reporting the results?

11. Comment: In a study of treatment outcomes, a researcher conducts 50 tests of statistical significance, each at $\alpha = .001$, across multiple dependent variables that are correlated. The researcher claims that the rate of experiment-wise Type I error is $< .05$.

12. Presented next is a small dataset for two independent samples where group membership is coded as $X = 0$ for the treatment group and $X = 1$ for the control group:

$$X = 0: 8, 12, 11, 10, 14$$
$$X = 1: 9, 12, 13, 15, 16$$

Use a computer program to conduct a one-way ANOVA. Using the same data, now conduct a regression analysis where group membership is the predictor and scores on the dependent variable is the criterion. Compare results across the two analyses.

CHAPTER 4

Design and Analysis

Everyone who designs devises courses of action
aimed at changing existing situations into
preferred ones.

—HERBERT A. SIMON (1988, p. 67)

Before selecting a design, think carefully about the research question on
which your study will be based. Think also about the goals (methods) of
the study, and how achieving those goals will address the question. Then
explain your hypotheses and methods to others—your supervisor, obviously, and classmates—until it makes sense to them, too. Only then will you be
ready to consider design details. This chapter is intended to help you do
just that. Considered here are major types of research designs used in the
behavioral sciences. Special attention is paid to experimental designs and
quasi-experimental designs for evaluating the effects of an intervention
or treatment. Strengths and weaknesses of each kind of design are considered, as are options for statistical analyses. Examples of recent empirical
studies based on various designs are also described. Even if none of the
designs considered here corresponds exactly to the one planned for your
research project, you may gain a new perspective or, even better, learn
some ways to improve your design or analysis.

Chapter Overview

It is impossible to review in a single chapter all the types of designs used by behavioral scientists. Instead, core designs with wide application that are also more realistic for student research projects are emphasized. This includes designs for **comparative studies**, in which at least two different groups or conditions are compared on an outcome (dependent) variable. In contrast, longitudinal designs are covered in less detail because they are usually impractical for students. Also stressed here are designs for **quantitative research**, in which there is an emphasis on the (1) classification and counting of behavior; (2) analysis of numerical scores with formal statistical methods; and (3) role of the researcher as an impassive, objective observer. In **qualitative research**, the researcher is often the main data-gathering instrument through immersion in the subject matter, such as in participant observation. There is also greater concern in qualitative research with understanding the subjective perceptions of participants in a social process. However, the distinction between quantitative and qualitative research is not absolute. For instance, participants in a qualitative study can complete objective questionnaires. See Barbour (2007) for an introduction to qualitative research and Creswell (2003) for examples of how to combine elements of both quantitative and qualitative research in the same study. Finally, standard statistical techniques that are more accessible to students are emphasized. These include the ANOVA and MR. Works that describe the application of more advanced techniques are cited, but use of these methods in your project would require help from your supervisor. Otherwise, it is better to use a simpler (i.e., standard) technique.

From Question to Design

There are three basic steps involved in connecting your research question with a possible (candidate) design. First, consider your question, of which there are three basic types (Trochim & Donnelly, 2007):

1. *Descriptive*: This most rudimentary type of question involves the simple description of a sample of cases (people or animals) on a set of variables of interest. Examples of descriptive questions include the following: What proportion in a voting population endorses a particular candidate? What is the survival rate among juvenile animals of a particular species?

However, it is relatively rare when research questions are solely descriptive.

2. *Relational*: This more common kind of question concerns the covariance between variables of interest. In very exploratory research, the most basic question is whether a relation exists at all. However, it is rare that researchers have absolutely no idea in advance about whether two variables are related. Instead, a relational question is more typically one about the direction and degree of covariance. Examples of relational questions include the following: Is support for a particular candidate related to gender and, if so, by how much? Does the survival rate among juvenile animals vary with local levels of pollution and, if so, by how much?

3. *Causal*: A causal question concerns how one or more independent variables affects one or more dependent (outcome) variables. Examples of causal questions include the following: Has a recent advertising campaign had any effect on voter preference? Does reduction in pollution levels increase survival rates among juvenile animals?

These types of questions are cumulative in that a relational question involves description and a causal question involves both description and the estimation of relations (covariances). They also have implications for the design elements of groups or conditions and the schedule for measurement (time). For instance, it is often possible to address a purely descriptive question by measuring variables in a single sample on one occasion. If all relational questions concern pairs of quantitative (continuous) variables, such as weight and blood pressure, then a single sample measured just once may again suffice. However, if some variables are categorical attributes of cases, such as gender, then a multiple-group design may be necessary in order to estimate covariances between these characteristics and other variables, such as blood pressure.

Although causal questions can be evaluated in nonexperimental designs in which variables are simultaneously measured in a single sample, the internal validity of such designs is typically weak (Chapter 3). Instead, it is generally better to evaluate causal questions in designs with either (1) multiple groups, some of which are exposed to an intervention but others are not; or (2) a single sample that is measured across multiple conditions, such as before-and-after treatment. Both variations just mentioned are comparative studies. If assignment to groups or conditions is random, then the design is experimental; if any other method is used and a treatment effect is evaluated, the design is quasi-experimental. If one-to-one matching is used to pair cases across treatment and control groups, then part of the design has a within-subject component; otherwise the design is purely between-subject if each case in every group is tested only once. Testing each case on multiple occasions also implies a design with a within-subject component, in this case a repeated-measures factor. Any causal question concerning change in group status, such as from before to after treatment (i.e., pretest–posttest), generally implies a design with a repeated measure. Levels of a time factor can each correspond to a different condition, such as when incentives change across trials in a learning study. Designs can also have combinations of between- and within-subject factors, which implies the presence of both multiple groups and a time factor. Considered next are basic options for experimental designs.

Experimental Designs

The hallmark of experimental designs is random assignment of cases to conditions (randomization). Because experimental designs generally have at least two conditions, they are inherently comparative. Structural design elements for experimental designs are represented here with a more or less standard notational set where R refers to random assignment, X represents the exposure of a group to a treatment, O refers to an observation or measurement, and each line of symbols corresponds to a separate group. The major types of experimental designs discussed next are represented in Table 4.1 using this notation.

Basic Randomized Experiment

A **basic randomized experiment** or **simple randomized design** has two conditions (treatment, control) and posttest assessment of all cases. Its design elements are represented as follows:

$$R \quad X \quad O$$
$$R \quad \quad O$$

This basic design can be extended by adding treatment or control conditions. The former could correspond to variations on a single treatment, such as different dosages of the same drug, or alternative treatments. There are also different types of control conditions. For example, a **placebo control group** receives all the trappings of treatment except the presumed

TABLE 4.1. Major Types of Experimental Designs

Type	Representation					
Basic	R		X	O		
	R			O		
Factorial	R		X_{A1B1}	O		
	R		X_{A1B2}	O		
	R		X_{A2B1}	O		
	R		X_{A2B2}	O		
Pretest–posttest	R	O_1	X	O_2		
	R	O_1		O_2		
Solomon Four Group	R	O_1	X	O_2		
	R	O_1		O_2		
	R		X	O_2		
	R			O_2		
Switching replications	R	O_1	X	O_2		O_3
	R	O_1		O_2	X	O_3
Crossover	R	O_1	X_A	O_2	X_B	O_3
	R	O_1	X_B	O_2	X_A	O_3
Longitudinal	R	$O \ldots O$	X	O	$O \ldots O$	
	R	$O \ldots O$		O	$O \ldots O$	

Note. R, random assignment; *O*, observation; *X*, treatment.

active ingredient of treatment. In drug studies, a placebo may be an inert pill or a saline injection, which controls for the experience of drug administration but with no specific pharmaceutical agent. In contrast, patients in an **expectancy control group** are told that they will receive a treatment, but they actually get a placebo, which controls specifically for the *belief* in treatment. In a **wait-list control group**, patients are seen for an initial assessment. No treatment is given, but they are promised treatment when they return for a second assessment at a later date, which controls for the *anticipation* of treatment. People in an **attention control group** meet occasionally with research personnel, but no specific treatment is given, which controls for generic social contact with staff. A **no-attention control group** receives no such attention. If there is also no expectation for treatment, then this condition more purely controls for **spontaneous remission**, or the abatement of a disorder without assistance from practitioners. There are other kinds of control groups, and selection among them depends on just for what the researcher wishes to control.

A different extension involves matching, which is a design-based alternative to statistical control (i.e., a covariate analysis). There are two general kinds. In **one-to-one matching**, a separate group corresponds to each condition but where each case is explicitly paired with a case in every other condition on at least one matching variable, such as age, which controls for this variable. Individual cases within each matched set are then randomly assigned to one of the conditions. Equal group sizes is a consequence of one-to-one matching. In the analysis, the design can be treated as a within-subject design instead of a between-subject design, which may increase statistical power. However, there are times when the number of available cases for one group is much smaller than for another group. Suppose that male and female psychology undergraduate students matched by age will be compared on a dependent variable. Because there are many more female than male psychology majors, the use of one-to-one matching would restrict the number of women to be equal to that of men, which would limit the overall sample size. In **group matching**, however, each male student would be matched with all comparable female students on age, which results in unequal group sizes (i.e., there would be more women than men) but increases the overall sample size. Matched-groups designs are subject to regression effects if cases come from extremes of their respective populations. In this case, regression toward *different* means is expected, and this artifact can mimic a treatment effect.

In basic randomized experiments with just two groups or conditions, there is a single **contrast** or **focused comparison**, such as the difference between the treatment and control groups. In designs with three or more conditions, a comparison between any two of them is also a contrast. There is also the **omnibus comparison**, which concerns whether any of the conditions differ. Suppose that there are two treatment groups and one control group. If any of these three groups differ on the dependent variable, there is an omnibus effect. However, this result alone is not often informative. This is because we may be more interested in a series of contrasts, such as whether either treatment group differs from the control group or if the treatment groups differ from each other. Accordingly, it is common practice to either follow an omnibus comparison with contrasts or forego the omnibus comparison and analyze contrasts only.

A standard statistical technique for analyzing data from basic randomized experiments with a continuous dependent variable is one-way ANOVA. Both omnibus comparisons and contrasts can be analyzed using this method. In reporting the results, effect sizes estimated using ANOVA should also be reported (Chapter 6), not just results of *F*-tests of various effects. DeRubeis et al. (2005) randomly assigned a total of 240 depressed adults to one of three conditions, medication (M) (paroxetine), cognitive therapy (CT), and pill–placebo control. Although DeRubeis et al. tested patients at 8 and 16 weeks after treatment, only results at 8 weeks are described here. The basic design is:

$$
\begin{array}{ccc}
R & X_M & O \\
R & X_{CT} & O \\
R & & O
\end{array}
$$

Results of ANOVA contrast analyses on a continuous depression symptoms scale indicated that both treatment groups improved at 8 weeks relative to the pill–placebo group. However, the magnitude of the treatment effect was somewhat larger for medication than for cognitive therapy.

Randomized Factorial Design

In a **randomized factorial design**, cases are randomly assigned to conditions that represent combinations of two or more independent variables, or factors. The basic design has two factors each with two levels that are **crossed**, which means that the levels of each factor are studied in all combinations with the levels of the other factor. Such designs are referred to as 2×2 factorial designs. Suppose that levels of factor A represent instructional set where participants are urged to either compete (A_1) or cooperate (A_2). Levels of factor B represent type of reward, money (B_1) or praise (B_2). A separate group of participants is randomly assigned to each of the four possible combinations of instruction and reward. The structural representation of this **completely between-subject factorial design** follows:

$$
\begin{array}{ccc}
R & X_{A_1B_1} & O \\
R & X_{A_1B_2} & O \\
R & X_{A_2B_1} & O \\
R & X_{A_2B_2} & O
\end{array}
$$

For example, the symbol X_{A1B1} designates the condition in which participants are urged to compete and are rewarded with money. If the same number of cases is assigned to each condition (n), the design is **balanced**; otherwise, it is **unbalanced**. In a balanced 2×2 design, the total sample size is calculated as $N = 4n$. The equation just presented does not apply to an unbalanced 2×2 design due to unequal cell sizes.

A more conventional representation of a balanced 2×2 factorial design is presented in Table 4.2 with observed means shown in their proper places for all cells, rows, columns, or the whole design. For example, the symbol $M_{A_1 B_1}$ in the table represents the **cell mean** for the condition where participants are told to compete before receiving monetary rewards. The mean in each of the two rows or columns is a **marginal mean**, which is just the average of the cell means in that row or column. For example, the symbol M_{A_1} in Table 4.2 represents the average for the compete instruction condition collapsing across the two levels of reward, or $(M_{A_1 B_1} + M_{A_1 B_2})/2$. The symbol for the **grand mean** for the whole design, M_T, is the average of all four cell means in the table. It can also be calculated as the average of the row or column marginal means or as the average across all $4n$ scores.

A **main effect** in a 2×2 factorial ANOVA is estimated by the difference between the marginal means for the same factor. For example, if $M_{A_1} \neq M_{A_2}$ in Table 4.2, then there is a main effect of instructional set (compete vs. cooperate), which is designated here as A. Likewise, there is a main effect of reward (money vs. praise)—designated here as B—if $M_{B_1} \neq M_{B_2}$ in the table. Each main effect is estimated ignoring (collapsing across) the levels of the other factor. The two-way **interaction effect**, designated here as AB, corresponds to the four cell means in Table 4.2. It is a combined or joint effect of both factors beyond their individual main effects. It is also a conditional or **moderator effect** where the impact of one factor on the outcome variable changes across the levels of the other factor, and vice versa. Suppose that the following cell means are observed in a balanced 2×2 design on an outcome variable where a higher score indicates better task performance:

TABLE 4.2. General Representation of a Balanced 2×2 Factorial Design

Instruction	Reward		Row means
	B_1 (Money)	B_2 (Praise)	
A_1 (Compete)	$M_{A_1 B_1}$	$M_{A_1 B_2}$	M_{A_1}
A_2 (Cooperate)	$M_{A_2 B_1}$	$M_{A_2 B_2}$	M_{A_2}
Column means	M_{B_1}	M_{B_2}	M_T

	B_1	B_2
A_1	50.00	25.00
A_2	25.00	50.00

Given these results, we can say that (1) both main effects of instruction (*A*) and reward (*B*) are zero because both sets of row or column marginal means are equal (e.g., $M_{A_1} = M_{A_2} = 37.50$); and (2) there is an interaction effect (*AB*) because the impact of instruction on performance depends on reward, and vice versa. Specifically, instructing participants to compete leads to better performance when there is a monetary reward ($M_{A_1B_1} > M_{A_1B_2}$), but telling them to cooperate is better when the reward is praise ($M_{A_2B_1} < M_{A_2B_2}$).

There are three basic ways to extend a randomized factorial design, including (1) add levels of either factor or add new factors to the design, (2) specify at least one factor as an individual-difference variable, or (3) specify at least one factor as a repeated-measures factor. For example, the main and joint effects of three different types of instruction (compete, cooperate, neutral) and two different types of reward (money, praise) could be estimated in a 3 × 2 factorial design. In a basic three-way factorial design, designated as a 2 × 2 × 2 design, a total of seven basic effects are estimated, including three main effects (*A*, *B*, *C*), three two-way interactions (*AB*, *AC*, *BC*), and one three-way interaction (*ABC*). The latter means that the effects of each factor changes across the levels of the other two factors. It also means that every two-way interaction is different across the levels of the other factor (e.g., the *AB* interaction changes across C_1 and C_2). However, quite large sample sizes may be needed for full factorial designs with three or more factors. For example, there are 16 cells in a 2 × 2 × 2 × 2 factor design, which requires a total of 16*n* cases in a balanced between-subject design.

The second extension concerns a **randomized blocks design**, in which at least one factor is an individual-difference variable, or a **blocking factor**, but the others are manipulated variables. This design is actually a hybrid of an experimental design and a nonexperimental design. Suppose that factor *A* in the 2 × 2 design of Table 4.2 represents gender. Men and women are randomly assigned to receive one of two different drugs, B_1 or B_2. Here, gender is the blocking factor, and a large *AB* effect would indicate that drug effects are different for men versus women. This information about a conditional effect could be invaluable in clinical practice with these drugs. If the individual difference variable is continuous (e.g., weight), however, then it is probably best *not* to categorize it by dividing the cases into two or more groups. (Recall the discussion about potential drawbacks of dichotomizing continuous variables in Chapter 3.) In this case, it may be better to treat a continuous individual-difference variable as a covariate in ANCOVA.

The third variation is to specify at least one factor as a repeated-measures factor. Suppose in the 2×2 design of Table 4.2 that B is a repeated-measures factor where each case in one of two separate groups (A_1 and A_2) is tested twice (B_1 and B_2). In this **mixed within-subject factorial design**—also called a **split-plot design** or just a **mixed design**—one factor is between subject (A), the other within subject (B). If all factors are within subject where a single group is tested across all combinations of at least two factors, then the design is a **factorial repeated-measures design** or a **completely within-subject factorial design**. Compared with between-subject designs, designs with repeated-measures factors may reduce error variance and increase statistical power. These advantages have potential costs, though. One is **order effects**, which happen when the particular order in which cases are exposed to levels of a repeated-measures factor affects their scores. Order effects can be the result of practice, fatigue, sensitization, or carryover. The latter is a special concern in drug studies, and it refers to any effect of treatment which lasts beyond a specific period of treatment or observation. These effects could still be present when the case is administered in a different treatment. In a **counterbalanced within-subject design**, treatments are administered in systematically different sequences, which tends to cancel out order effects. It is also possible to represent order of administration as a factor in the design. This permits the direct statistical estimation of main or interaction effects pertaining to order.

A second potential cost is that the statistical assumptions of ANOVA for within-subject factors with at least three levels are very stringent. These include the standard ANOVA requirements—such as normal population distributions with equal variances—and the additional assumption of **homogeneity of covariance**, also known as **sphericity** or **circularity**. This is the requirement that the variance of the population difference scores between every pair of levels on the within-subject factors are all equal.[1] Another way to express this assumption is that the population covariances between every pair of levels are all equal. The sphericity assumption is

---

[1]The homogeneity of covariance assumption does not apply when there are only two repeated measures. In this case, there is only one set of difference scores.

difficult to meet, so much so that it may be violated most of the time in actual samples. The general consequence of violating this assumption is positive bias in F-tests; that is, the results are statistically significant too often. There is a statistical test, known as **Mauchly's test**, of the sphericity assumption that is based on the chi-square (χ^2) statistic. If the result is statistically significant, then violation of this assumption is indicated. However, Mauchly's test is actually not very useful for deciding if the sphericity assumption is violated. In small samples, it tends to yield too many Type II errors (i.e., it misses true sphericity violations), and in large samples it can be statistically significant even though the degree of violation is slight (e.g., Keselman, Rogan, Mendoza, & Breen, 1980). Another approach involves estimation of the amount of violation of sphericity in the form of a correction factor that reduces the degrees of freedom for the critical value of the F-test of a repeated-measures factor. This correction has the effect of increasing the critical value, which makes it more difficult to reject the null hypothesis (i.e., the F-test is made more conservative). One of these correction factors is the **Geisser–Greenhouse correction**; another is the **Huynh–Feldt correction**. Both are available in the SPSS computer program for general statistical analyses. See Keselman, Algina, and Kowalchuk (2001) for more information about ways to deal with violation of the sphericity assumption.

Sanderson, Wee, and Lacherez (2006) evaluated the learnability and discriminability of melodic alarms for digital medical equipment in a randomized blocks design with repeated measures. Melodic alarms signal various critical events, such as equipment malfunction. Some patients are connected to multiple devices, so it is crucial that caregivers can accurately discriminate between alarms from different devices. A sample of 33 undergraduate students were classified according to whether they had at least 1 year of formal music training or not. Students in each group were then randomly assigned to either mnemonic or nonmnemonic learning conditions. In the former, the melodic alarms for a particular device, such as for drug infusion, were associated with a mnemonic, such as a jazz chord to represent drops falling and "splashing" back up. All participants were exposed to a total of 16 different alarms for eight different devices each at two levels of priority, medium and high priority (crisis). Their ability to discriminate the alarms was tested across eight trials over 2 days. Only about 30% of the participants could identify the alarms with 100% accuracy at the end of training, and accuracy was greater for medium- than for high-priority alarms. As expected, response accuracy of participants with musical backgrounds was greater, but mnemonic training did not increase overall accuracy for either group. These results raise concerns about the learnability and discriminability of melodic alarms. The specification of a mixed factorial design was especially effective here because is allowed for the simultaneous study of the effects of whether the participants had a music background or not, whether they received mnemonic or nonmnemonic training, type of medical device, level of alarm priority, and practice on the ability to remember and discriminate melodic alarms.

Randomized Pretest–Posttest Designs

The absence of a pretest in the experimental designs considered to this point poses a risk if there is a possibility of attrition or loss of cases from the study. The availability of pretest information can help to determine whether participants who left the study differed from those who remained. This risk is reduced in the **randomized pretest–posttest design** where at least one pretest is administered to all cases. The structural representation for a basic pretest–posttest design is

$$
\begin{array}{cccc}
R & O_1 & X & O_2 \\
R & O_1 & & O_2
\end{array}
$$

where O_1 stands for the pretest and O_2 stands for the posttest (outcome measure). Note in this representation that the symbol R appears at the beginning of each line. In actual experiments, however, randomization could occur either before or after administration of the pretest, so the position of the R would accordingly vary. Described next are the three general types of pretests used in experiments:

1. A **proxy pretest** is a variable that should predict the posttest but is not identical to it. Such a pretest can be a demographic variable or, even better, a psychological variable that is conceptually related to outcome. It can also be an archival variable that is collected after the start of the study. An example of a proxy pretest in a study of reading outcomes (posttest) among grade 1 students is a phonological ability test administered at the beginning of the school year. Not only should the two be related, but not all children can read at the beginning of grade 1.

2. A **repeated pretest** is identical to the posttest. This is because all cases are tested twice, before and after treatment, using the same measure. This type of pretest offers a more precise way to index group differences

prior to the start of treatment than proxy pretests. It also helps to identify maturational trends or regression artifacts, but (1) these threats are usually greater in quasi-experimental designs than experimental designs, and (2) it is easier to detect such effects when a pretest is administered at least twice before treatment is given. There are also ways to detect testing or instrumental effects due to repeated administration of the same measure. Both of these points are elaborated later.

3. A **retrospective pretest** is administered at the same time as the posttest, and it requests of participants that they describe their status *before* treatment. For example, at the conclusion of a professional development workshop, participants may be asked to rate what they learned (posttest) and at the same time describe their prior level of knowledge (retrospective pretest). However, such ratings are subject to motivational biases in that participants could indicate that learning took place regardless of whether it did or not. One reason could be to please the instructor; another could be to justify time spent in the workshop. Accordingly, Hill and Betz (2005) argued that retroactive pretests are probably better for evaluating subjective experiences of posttreatment change than for estimating actual treatment effects.

A proxy pretest can be treated as a covariate in an ANCOVA, in which unexplained variance in the posttest will be reduced by a factor related to the predictive power of the pretest. Recall that ANCOVA requires reliable covariate scores and assumes linearity and homogeneity of regression (e.g., Figure 3.2). An alternative is to stratify cases on the pretest and then represent the blocking factor as a distinct factor in the analysis. The resulting design is actually a randomized blocks design, and the data would be analyzed with ANOVA, not ANCOVA. Neither blocking nor ANCOVA is uniformly superior to the other. Briefly, ANCOVA may be preferred when the pretest is a continuous variable, such as age in years, and blocking works best with categorical variables, such as gender. If the statistical assumptions of ANCOVA are not tenable, then blocking may be preferred. From an ANOVA perspective, what is heterogeneity of regression in ANCOVA (i.e., a problem) is just a block × outcome interaction in a randomized blocks design that is estimated along with other effects (i.e., it is not a problem). However, the accuracy of these estimates requires that the researcher has formed the correct number of blocks (e.g., two, three, or more groups?) when categorizing a continuous pretest (Maxwell, Delaney, & Dill, 1984).

There are also two basic analysis options for a repeated pretest. The first is to use ANCOVA where the pretest is treated as a covariate and the data are analyzed as though they came from a between-subject design. The second option is to use ANOVA where the design is treated as a mixed design with a between-subject factor (treatment control) and a within-subject factor (pretest–posttest). That is, the pretest is treated as a level of a time factor and as part of the dependent variable in the analysis of group differences. In this approach, *change* in both groups from before to after treatment is explicitly estimated, and also whether the direction or magnitude of change differs across the groups (i.e., an interaction effect). There is no absolutely clear consensus about which analysis option is best for randomized pretest–posttest designs. Some authors recommend ANCOVA over repeated-measures ANOVA due to expected greater statistical power of the former over the latter (Rausch, Maxwell, & Kelly, 2003). In designs with at least three assessments, such as pretest–posttest–follow-up (PPF) designs, it is possible to combine both analytical methods by specifying the pretest as a covariate and the posttest and follow-up observations as levels of a repeated-measures factor.

The basic pretest–posttest design can be extended by adding pretests, posttests, measurement occasions (e.g., PPF designs), or additional conditions. For example, Justice, Meier, and Walpole (2005) evaluated the effectiveness of a storybook-reading intervention in teaching novel vocabulary words to 57 at-risk kindergarten students. The children were randomly assigned to either intervention or control conditions. Two pretests were administered, one of words specifically elaborated (E) in the intervention and another of words not elaborated (N). The same two measures were administered at posttest. The rationale for the specification of this set of **nonequivalent dependent variables** is that the intervention should affect one (E) but not the other (N). Otherwise, any observed advantage in the treatment group may not be specific to the storybook-reading intervention. The overall design is represented next with the nonequivalent dependent variables enclosed in braces:

$$R \qquad \{O_{1E}, O_{1N}\} \qquad X \qquad \{O_{2E}, O_{2N}\}$$
$$R \qquad \{O_{1E}, O_{1N}\} \qquad\qquad \{O_{2E}, O_{2N}\}$$

In the analysis, the pretests and posttests were treated as levels of repeated-measures factors. The results indicated that children in the reading intervention group learned more of the elaborated words compared with those in the control condition. However, the groups did not differ appreciably in their learning of nonelaborated words. This pattern is consistent with attribution of the overall increase in vocabulary words to the storybook-reading intervention.

Solomon Four-Group Design

Another extension of the pretest–posttest design is the **Solomon Four-Group Design**, which is actually a combination of a pretest–posttest design and a factorial design. The goal is to evaluate testing effects, that is, whether administration of a pretest affects scores on the outcome variable. A basic Solomon Four-Group Design for a randomized experiment is represented as follows:

$$
\begin{array}{cccc}
R & O_1 & X & O_2 \\
R & O_1 & & O_2 \\
R & & X & O_2 \\
R & & & O_2 \\
\end{array}
$$

In this design, there are two treatment groups, of which only one is given the pretest. If these two groups differ appreciably at posttest, then there may be a testing effect for the treated cases. Likewise, there are two control groups, one given the pretest and the other not. A testing effect for the untreated cases is indicated if the two control groups differ appreciably at posttest. Because the basic design is also a 2×2 factorial design, whether the administration of a pretest interacts with the difference between treatment and control can also be estimated. If this interaction effect is relatively large, then there are differential testing effects (e.g., selection-testing bias), which means that effects of giving a pretest are different for treated versus untreated cases.

van Sluijs, van Poppel, Twisk, and van Mechelen (2006) evaluated whether an individually tailored program administered by doctors aimed at increasing physical activity in their patients actually achieved this result. The sample consisted of over 600 adults recruited from general practitioner offices located throughout the Netherlands. Additional outcome variables were also studied by van Sluijs et al., but level of physical activity is the only dependent variable considered here. Using a Solomon Four-Group Design, participants were randomized twice, first to a control or intervention group and then again to a group participating in measurement of physical activity at baseline (pretest), 2 and 6 months (respectively, posttest, and follow-up), or in a group participating in measurement at 6 months only. Because van Sluijs et al. considered measurement of physical activity at pretest as a kind of intervention that might by itself motivate people to become more active, they specified a randomized Solomon Four-Group Design with the following structural representation:

$$
\begin{array}{ccccc}
R & O_1 & X & O_2 & O_3 \\
R & O_1 &   & O_2 & O_3 \\
R &   & X &   & O_3 \\
R &   &   &   & O_3
\end{array}
$$

The results indicated both program and testing effects. Specifically, patients in the physician-directed program were subsequently more active than those in the control condition, and measurement of activity at pretest was associated with increased activity, too. Also, the measurement effect was not modified by randomization to the intervention or control condition; that is, there was no interaction effect. A limitation of this design is that it was possible to estimate testing effects at the 6-month follow-up only. It is plausible that testing effects were even stronger at the 2-month posttest than at the 6-month follow-up evaluation.

Switching-Replications Designs and Crossover Designs

Two other types of randomized designs involve at least two independent implementations of treatment, which permits the direct evaluation of order effects. Both designs also address the potential ethical problem in standard experimental designs that treatment is withheld from control cases. In the basic **switching-replications design**, there are two randomized groups and three measurement occasions. Both groups are administered a pretest. The treatment is then administered to the first group only, and a posttest measure is taken for both groups. Next, the treatment is given to the second group only, and a third measurement is taken for both groups. In this way, the implementation of treatment is replicated, and the two groups switch roles—from treatment to control and vice versa—when the treatment is repeated. At the end of the study, cases in both groups have been treated, but in a different order. Because treatment is given at any one time to just one group, resources are saved compared with treating all cases at once.

The structural representation of a basic switching-replications design is presented next:

$$R \qquad O_1 \qquad X \qquad O_2 \qquad\qquad\qquad O_3$$
$$R \qquad O_1 \qquad\qquad\quad O_2 \qquad X \qquad O_3$$

As in pretest–posttest designs, the pretest O_1 can be identical to O_2 and O_3 for repeated measures across the three times, or the pretest can be a different variable that predicts O_2 and O_3. In the analysis, the pretest O_1 could be specified as a covariate and O_2 and O_3 as two levels of a repeated-measures factor. When O_1–O_3 are identical, an alternative is to specify O_1 as the third level of a repeated-measures factor along with O_2 and O_3. It is also possible in these designs to estimate whether treatment effects in the second group are different from those in the first group. If so, there is an interaction between treatment and order. Such a finding could indicate unreliability of treatment implementation, or the failure to carry out treatment in the same way for both groups. Another possibility is a selection-history threat, or the occurrence of an event between the pretest and posttest that differentially affected the groups. However, this threat may be unlikely in an experimental design where the groups were formed at random.

Stuss et al. (2007) evaluated the effectiveness of a 3-month cognitive rehabilitation program within a sample of 49 healthy adults who were 77–89 years old. The sample was stratified by age, gender, and education before random assignment to a designated treatment order. This design is actually a combination of randomized blocks design and a switching-replications design. Participants in the first condition underwent the cognitive rehabilitation program while participants in the other condition served as the control group. At the end of the program in the first condition, participants in the second condition received the treatment while the first group switched over to the control condition. Measures of cognitive, memory, and psychosocial status were administered to all participants at pretest, after each round of treatment, and finally at a 3-month follow-up (i.e., each participant was tested four different times altogether). There were two advantages of the switching-replications design in this study: (1) both groups of elderly adults were able to participate in the cognitive rehabilitation program, albeit at different times; and (2) it was possible to test whether effects in the first group exposed to treatment were maintained up to 6 months later. Treatment-related gains in cognitive, memory, and psychosocial status were observed for both groups, and these gains generally persisted at follow-up.

In the basic **crossover design**—also known as a **switchback design** or a **reversal design**—all cases receive two different treatments in sequence, so there is no separate control group. Also, each case is randomly assigned to a specific treatment order and is measured three times, at pretest and after each treatment. The notation for this design is written as follows:

$$R \qquad O_1 \qquad X_A \qquad O_2 \qquad X_B \qquad O_3$$
$$R \qquad O_1 \qquad X_B \qquad O_2 \qquad X_A \qquad O_3$$

The crossover design also allows for the direct estimation of order effects. Specifically, the evaluation of possible carryover effects is a special concern in these designs. For example, if scores on O_3 for the first group in the design notation above are affected by both X_A and X_B instead of just by X_B, then there is carryover. One way to prevent carryover is to specify a **washout period** between treatments, during which the effects of the first treatment should dissipate before beginning the second. Options for the statistical analysis of data from crossover designs are basically the same as those for switching-replications designs.

In a randomized crossover design, Kulczycki, Kim, Duerr, Jamieson, and Macaluso (2004) randomly assigned a total of 108 women to use 10 male condoms followed by 10 female condoms or the reverse. This crossover design had the advantages that (1) each woman served as her own control and (2) the design controlled for the possibility that experience with one type of condom may affect subsequent experience with the other type (i.e., a condom type × order interaction). Demographic information was collected at pretest, and measures of user satisfaction were collected after each round of condom use. Just under 90% of the women in both treatment orders disliked using the female condom and generally rated the male condom as easier to apply, use, and enjoy. There were also no apparent order effects. Based on these results, the potential in this sample for acceptance of the female condom for long-term use may be poor.

Randomized Longitudinal Designs

The structural representation for a **randomized longitudinal design** is presented next:

$$R \qquad O...O \qquad X \qquad O \qquad O...O$$
$$R \qquad O...O \qquad \qquad O \qquad O...O$$

A series of observations is collected before treatment for both groups. Another observation may be taken right at the conclusion of treatment, and others are collected later (follow-up). It is critical to try to match the interval between the measurement occasions to the expected temporal properties of the effect of treatment. For example, some treatments show beneficial results only after a certain amount of time (e.g., 12 weeks), and effects of other treatments are temporary and dissipate after a certain time. If observations are collected too soon or too late, then a treatment that actually works may look ineffective.

If the follow-up period after treatment is relatively long (e.g., 5 years), then a longitudinal design can be very expensive in terms of the resources needed to carry it out. The issue of attrition is also a serious challenge. For example, it is not unexpected to lose up to 50% of the participants over the course of a year unless they are carefully screened, such as for motivation, and near-Herculean efforts are made to follow them. For these reasons, longitudinal designs are usually more theoretical than practical even for established researchers, and student participation in such studies is usually limited to the analysis of existing datasets or the collection of scores for a single wave.

Several different kinds of statistical techniques are applied to longitudinal data, especially in studies with at least three measurement occasions. Some advanced (i.e., graduate-level) techniques estimate a **latent growth model**, which captures the initial level and trajectory of behavior change, variation in both initial level and trend, and the covariation between initial level and subsequent change. The latter concerns whether cases that start out at a higher (or lower) level at the initial assessment show a higher (or lower) rate of change across subsequent occasions. Two major techniques used to estimate such models are **hierarchical linear modeling** (HLM) and **structural equation modeling** (SEM). The former is basically a variation of MR that is especially well suited for analyzing **hierarchical (nested) data structures** where data points at a lower level are clustered into larger units, such as siblings within families. Repeated-measures datasets are also hierarchical in that multiple scores are clustered under each case, and these scores are probably not independent. The term "SEM" actually refers to a family of techniques for modeling presumed **covariance structures** and **mean structures**, which concern, respectively, patterns of presumed relations between variables (observed or latent) and their means.

If you work with longitudinal datasets in graduate school, you will hear more about HLM or SEM, especially about the latter. This is because the family of SEM techniques can be used to evaluate a wide range of hypotheses. Some of these hypotheses involve the estimation of direct or indirect causal effects among a set of variables. Indirect effects concern a **mediator effect** in which one variable is specified to affect another only through a third variable. For example, exercise could indirectly affect the experience of stress first by increasing fitness which then reduces stress (i.e., exercise → fitness → stress). In this example, fitness is a **mediator variable** that "passes on" beneficial effects of exercise that reduce stress. In contrast, a **moderator effect** refers to an interaction effect in which the association of one variable with another changes across the levels of a third variable, and vice versa. For the earlier example of a 2×2 factorial design, if the effect of instruction (compete, cooperate) on task performance depends on reward types (money, praise), then there is an interaction effect such that each of the instruction and praise factors acts as **moderator variable** in relation to the other. Moderator (interaction) effects can be estimated in ANOVA and standard MR with no special problem, but not so for mediator effects. It is also possible using SEM to explicitly model the distinction between observed variables and the latent variables presumed to underlie them, estimate group mean differences on latent variables instead of just observed variables, analyze repeated-measures data with fewer statistical assumptions compared with regression or ANOVA, estimate nonlinear effects of observed or latent variables, and analyze data from experimental, quasi-experimental, or nonexperimental designs, among others. However, both SEM and HLM may be too complex for undergraduate-level projects without extensive help from a supervisor.

Controlled Quasi-Experimental Designs

In these designs, cases are assigned to treatment or control groups using some method other than randomization. This implies that the groups may not be equivalent before the start of treatment. Accordingly, dealing with selection-related threats to internal validity in quasi-experimental designs is a major challenge. It is managed by (1) identifying plausible threats, which is a rational exercise guided by your substantive knowledge; and (2) adding appropriate design elements, such as additional measures (e.g., a pretest) or groups (conditions), that may reduce the seriousness of specific threats (Shadish et al., 2001). With sufficient controls, a quasi-experimental design can be a powerful tool for evaluating causal hypotheses. This is why a well-controlled quasi-experimental design should not be viewed as the shabby, dirt-poor cousin of an experimental design, especially when it is impossible to use randomization. Indeed, there has been a recent resurgence of interest in quasi-experimental designs across different fields, including child psychiatry (Morgan, Gliner, & Harmon, 2000) and clinical epidemiology (Schneeweiss, Maclure, Soumerai, Walker, & Glynn, 2002), among many others.

Considered next are two types of controlled quasi-experimental designs. In **nonequivalent-group** (NG) **designs**, the treatment and control groups are intact, or already formed. These groups may be self-selected, such as when patients volunteer for a new treatment, or formed by another means beyond the control of the researcher, such as grade 1 students enrolled in a particular school designated by their school board for a new reading program. Ideally, (1) the two groups should be as similar as possible, and (2) the choice of group that receives the treatment is made at random. However, these ideal conditions may not exist in practice. Intact groups may be different on any number of variables confounded with treatment effects. For example, patients who volunteer for a new treatment may be sicker or less well off financially than other patients. Without some of the design elements described later, the internal validity of NG designs may be quite weak due to selection-related threats.

In **regression-discontinuity** (RD) **designs**, cases are assigned to conditions based on a cutoff score from an **assignment variable**, which can be any variable measured before treatment. A continuous assignment variable is assumed, but the same basic logic applies to categorical assignment variables, too. Unlike a covariate, there is no requirement that the assignment variable should predict the outcome variable; that is, the two can be unrelated. Cases with scores on one side of the cutting score are assigned to one condition, and cases with scores on the other side are assigned to a different condition. The cutting score is often established based on merit or need. An example of merit-based assignment is a scholarship given only to students with high grades (e.g., > 3.5 on a 4-point scale), and an example of need-based assignment is a remedial (compensatory) program available only for students with low grades (e.g., < 1.0).

Assignment of cases to conditions based on a cutting score in RD designs implies that the treatment and control groups are not equivalent before treatment begins. The groups are also typically not equivalent before treatment begins in NG designs, too. However, RD designs are actually more similar to randomized experiments than NG designs. This is because the **selection process**—how cases wind up in treatment or control groups—is totally known in RD designs; that is, this design offers a complete model of selection. In experimental designs, the selection process is different (randomization), but it is also totally known. This means that the internal validity of RD designs is actually much closer to that of experimental designs than that of NG designs. In contrast, the selection process is almost never completely known in NG designs, and this is because we rarely know exactly how two intact groups differ before the start of treatment.

Nonequivalent-Group Designs

By substituting intact groups for randomized groups in any of the experimental designs represented in Table 4.1, the resulting design would be transformed into its quasi-experimental counterpart. Not all of these counterparts are discussed next. Instead, only major NG designs that highlight special challenges of dealing with selection-related threats to internal validity are emphasized. The structural elements of these designs are represented in the top part of Table 4.3 where *NR* refers to nonrandom assignment.

Posttest-Only Design

The most basic NG design has two groups measured at posttest only. The structural representation of this **posttest-only design** is diagrammed as follows:

$$NR \quad X \quad O$$
$$NR \quad \quad \ O$$

The absence of pretests makes it extremely difficult to separate treatment effects from initial group differences. Accordingly, the internal validity of this very weak design is threatened by basically all forms of selection-related bias (see Table 3.1). Shadish et al. (2001) suggested some ways to modestly strengthen this design. One is to administer a pretest within independent samples drawn randomly from the same population as the treatment and control groups. Another is to use matching or blocking to select comparable cases across the treatment and control groups. However, true random sampling is rarely possible in the behavioral sciences, and the use of matching or blocking as a way to try to equate very dissimilar groups is problematic.

Pretest–Posttest Design

A somewhat better NG design involves the administration of a pretest in both the treatment and control groups. The basic **pretest–posttest design** is represented as follows:

TABLE 4.3. Major Types of Controlled Quasi-Experimental Designs

Type	Representation					
Nonequivalent groups						
Weaker						
Basic (posttest only)	NR		X	O		
	NR			O		
Pretest–posttest	NR	O_1	X	O_2		
	NR	O_1		O_2		
Double pretest	NR	O_1		O_2	X	O_3
	NR	O_1		O_2		O_3
Stronger						
Switching replications	NR	O_1	X	O_2		O_3
	NR	O_1		O_2	X	O_3
Crossover	NR	O_1	X_A	O_2	X_B	O_3
	NR	O_1	X_B	O_2	X_A	O_3
Regression discontinuity						
Basic	O_A	C	X	O_2		
	O_A	C		O_2		

Note. NR, nonrandom assignment; O, observation; X, treatment; C, cutting score.

$$NR \quad O_1 \quad X \quad O_2$$
$$NR \quad O_1 \quad\quad O_2$$

Sometimes pretest data are collected after treatment begins, so the position of the O_1 in the structural diagram for the pretest–posttest design would accordingly vary. Possible types of pretests include proxy, repeated, and retrospective pretests. Of the three, a repeated pretest is best for gauging initial differences between the treatment and control groups. However, the basic pretest–posttest design is still subject to many selection-related threats even if the pretest and posttest are identical. For example, the threat of selection-regression bias is great if cases in one of the groups were selected because of extreme scores, such as when the sickest patients are selected for administration of a new treatment. The threat of selection-maturation concerns the possibility that the treatment and control groups are changing naturally at different rates in a way that mimics a treatment effect. A related concern is the threat of selection-history, or the possibility that events occurring between the pretest and posttest differentially affected the treatment and control groups. Basically all forms of internal validity threats for multiple-group studies apply to this design, too.

The basic pretest–posttest design can be extended by adding pretests, and multiple pretests can include any combination of proxy, repeated, or retrospective pretests. However, even multiple pretests may not measure all relevant dimensions along which the groups differ before treatment. Another extension involves the use of nonequivalent dependent variables administered at both pretest and posttest. The observation that posttest differences occurred only on dependent variables expected to show a treatment effect would bolster attribution of any posttest differences to treatment.

A covariate analysis that statistically controls for group differences on the pretest(s) would seem to be an obvious choice in pretest–posttest NG designs. One such technique is ANCOVA. The use of ANCOVA in experimental designs where the groups differ on pretests by chance only is not controversial, if its statistical requirements are satisfied. If so, then the only appreciable correction when ANCOVA is used in experimental designs is the reduction of error variance (Chapter 3). However, the use of ANCOVA to also adjust group mean differences on the dependent variable for group differences on pretests (see Figure 3.2) in NG designs is problematic. One reason is that unless the pretests measure all relevant dimensions along which intact groups differ that are also confounded with treatment, then any statistical correction may be inaccurate. As expressed by Cook and Campbell (1979):

> Since the ANCOVA introduces an adjustment for group pretest differences which can substantially alter the expected value of the treatment effect ... the critical question is whether this adjustment removes all bias due to selection differences. (p. 159)

The answer to this question would be "yes" assuming (1) scores on all pretests are perfectly reliable and (2) all appreciable confounding variables have been identified and measured with the pretests. In practice, though, it is extremely unlikely that both of these conditions would be met. A related problem is that the statistical assumptions of ANCOVA may be unlikely to hold in pretest–posttest NG designs. This is especially true concerning homogeneity of regression. That is, it could very well happen that the relation between the covariate and the dependent variable is not the same across intact groups (i.e., the slopes of the within-group regression lines are different). Given these problems, it is generally safer to assume that ANCOVA-adjusted estimates of treatment effects in NG designs are biased. Furthermore, the direction of this bias is generally unknown. That is, adjustment of means in ANCOVA could mask a true treatment effect or indicate one when treatment effects are actually nil. It could even make a beneficial compensatory program look harmful (e.g., D. T. Campbell & Erlebacher, 1975).

The discussion to this point has emphasized the reality that ANCOVA does not somehow magically equate nonequivalent groups when evaluating treatment effects through inspection of predicted means. This is especially true if (1) there is a single pretest, which may measure one facet of the selection process but not others; and (2) there are no other design elements that strengthen internal validity, such as the use of nonequivalent dependent measures. Two alternative statistical techniques are described next, but you should realize now that neither offers any magical "cure" for potential selection-related bias in pretest–posttest NG designs. Also, the first of these two ANCOVA alternatives is less complicated than the second, and thus may be more realistic to use in a student research project.

The more straightforward of the two alternatives is to conduct a covariate analysis using MR instead of ANCOVA. Recall that ANCOVA (or any type of ANOVA) is just a restricted form of MR. One of these restrictions is the homogeneity of regression assumption. However, this assumption can be relaxed when the data are analyzed in MR. This is because it is possible to represent in regression equations the inequality of slopes of within-group regression lines. In this way, what is a violation of a critical assumption in ANCOVA becomes an effect of interest in MR, or the finding that the capability of the covariate to predict the outcome variable depends on membership in either the treatment group or control group. Yes, it is somewhat more difficult to conduct a covariate analysis with relaxed assumptions in MR compared with ANCOVA, but with appropriate help from your supervisor, the MR approach may be feasible. A conceptual example follows. One of the exercises at the end of this chapter gives you a chance to experiment with these concepts using actual scores.

Suppose that the covariate in a basic pretest–posttest design is the continuous variable Z. The outcome variable, Y, is also continuous. Group membership is represented in the analysis with the dichotomous variable X, where a value of 0 indicates the control group and a value of 1 indicates the treatment group. In MR, a standard ANCOVA—one that assumes linearity and homogeneity of regression—is conducted by entering group membership and the covariate as the two predictors of the outcome variable. The specific form of this regression equation is

$$\hat{Y} = B_1X + B_2Z + A \qquad (4.1)$$

where $\hat{Y}$ is the predicted score on the outcome variable; B_1 is the unstandardized regression coefficient (weight) for the difference between treatment and control (X); B_2 is the unstandardized coefficient for the covariate (Z); and A is the intercept (constant) term of the equation. The latter equals the predicted value of Y when scores on both predictors are zero. Specifically, when $X = 0$, the control group is indicated, so the intercept, A, equals the predicted value on Y for cases in this group with scores of zero on the covariate, or $Z = 0$.

When the terms in the regression equation defined by Equation 4.1 are estimated in MR, the value of B_1, the unstandardized coefficient for group membership, equals the average difference between the treatment and control groups adjusted for the covariate (i.e., the predicted mean difference). Interpretation of this predicted mean difference assumes homogeneity of regression. However, suppose that the group scatterplots for the relation between the outcome variable and the covariate for this example are the ones presented in Figure 4.1. Now the slopes of the within-group regression lines are different, so the homogeneity of regression assumption is clearly violated. In a standard ANCOVA, there is really no way to fix this problem. In MR, however, it is not difficult to (1) add another

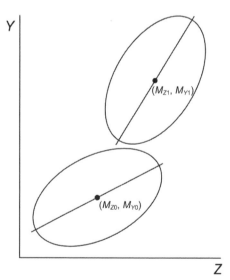

FIGURE 4.1. Heterogeneity of within-group regression lines for the dependent variable (Y) and the covariate (Z) across the control group (coded $X = 0$) and the treatment group (coded $X = 1$).

predictor to the regression equation that (2) allows for unequal slopes of within-group regression lines. Briefly, this term represents a group × covariate interaction, which indicates that the relation between the covariate and the outcome variable changes across the levels of group membership (i.e., control vs. treatment). In Figure 4.1, the covariation between Y and Z is greater in the treatment group than in the control group; thus, there is an interaction effect, or heterogeneity of regression. The type of analysis just described is a **moderated multiple regression** where the term "moderated" refers to the inclusion in the equation of terms that represent an interaction effect, in this case a group × covariate interaction.

For this example, the specific form of the regression equation estimated in MR that allows for a group × covariate interaction is

$$\hat{Y} = B_1X + B_2Z + B_3XZ + A \qquad (4.2)$$

where the new predictor is XZ, which is literally the product of scores on X for group membership (i.e., 0 or 1) and Z, the covariate, calculated for every case (compare Equations 4.1 and 4.2). This product term represents the interaction, and B_3 is the unstandardized regression coefficient (i.e., the numerical estimate) for this effect. In the MR approach to a covariate analysis represented by Equation 4.2, one studies the joint effect of the difference between treatment and control groups and the covariate on the outcome variable. Here, the simple adjusted mean difference between the two groups (i.e., B_1) is by itself of relatively little interest. This is because B_1 estimates the mean treatment effect, when we are controlling for the covariate. The more interesting question is: What is the predicted direction and size of the treatment effect at lower versus higher levels on the covariate? The question just stated refers to a conditional effect of treatment. This general analytical method can also accommodate multiple pretests or curvilinear relations between the covariate and the outcome variable. However, the analysis quickly becomes more complicated as terms that represent such effects are added to the regression equation, and the need for ever-larger samples to estimate equations with many predictors is a challenge.

A second alternative to ANCOVA is the more advanced technique of **propensity score analysis** (PSA). This technique is an increasingly important method for statistically matching cases from nonequivalent groups across multiple pretests. Unlike MR, the technique of PSA does not assume linear relations between the pretests and the outcome variable. There are generally two phases in a PSA. Estimated in the first phase are **propensity**

scores, which for each case is the probability of belonging to the treatment or control group, given the pattern of scores across the pretests. These scores can be estimated using **logistic regression** where (1) the pretests are treated as predictors of the dichotomous variable of being in the treatment versus control group, and (2) each case's scores across the pretests are reduced to a single propensity score. Standard matching can then be used to match treated cases with untreated based on similarity across all pretests. This includes both one-to-one matching and group matching. Another alternative is to stratify cases based on propensity scores (i.e., create a blocking factor) and then compare the treatment and control cases within each block across the outcome variable. In this approach, the design is treated as a quasi-experimental analogue of a randomized blocks design. There are other statistical methods to estimate propensity scores or match cases in PSA besides logistic regression, but the overall goal is the same: to yield comparable covariate distributions across nonequivalent groups. There are also ways in PSA to estimate **hidden bias**, which is the degree of undetected confounding that would be needed to appreciably change study outcome, such as from an apparent beneficial effect of treatment to none, or vice versa (Shadish et al., 2001). However, the technique of PSA offers no magic, too. This is because the accuracy of estimated propensity scores depends on whether the pretests measure in large part the selection process whereby treated versus untreated cases wound up in their respective groups.

In a large longitudinal sample of almost 4,000 households, Pagani, Larocque, Tremblay, and Lapointe (2003) evaluated whether students who attended junior kindergarten (i.e., preschool for 4-year-old children) in English Canada exhibited fewer behavior problems in later elementary school grades. Because junior kindergarten is voluntary, there may be differences between families in which parents elect to send a 4-year-old child to school versus not, and these differences may be confounded with effects of school. In an attempt to statistically control for these differences (i.e., the selection process), Pagani et al. collected scores on six proxy pretests, including household socioeconomic status, family size, quality of family functioning, geographic region, whether the birth mother graduated from high school, and whether the household was headed by one or two parents. The outcome variables were parent- and teacher-informant reports of problem behaviors, such as physical aggression. Because these data are hierarchical—children were clustered within households—Pagani et al. used the technique of HLM. Controlling for the proxy pretests and student age and gender, Pagani et al. found that attending junior kindergarten was not appreciably associated with fewer behavioral problems later on. However, the accuracy of this result depends on whether the particular mix of pretests and other predictors analyzed by Pagani et al. controlled for the major sources of selection bias.

Double-Pretest Design

The basic **double-pretest design** involves the administration of the same measure on three occasions, twice before treatment and again after. Its structural diagram is presented next:

$$NR \quad O_1 \quad O_2 \quad X \quad O_3$$
$$NR \quad O_1 \quad O_2 \quad \quad O_3$$

This design helps the researcher to assess the plausibility of certain kinds of internal validity threats. One is selection-maturation. With two pretests, one can compare the pretreatment growth rates of both groups before any treatment is administered. For example, presented in Figure 4.2 are means for treatment and control groups on an outcome variable where a higher score is a better result. Figure 4.2(a) corresponds to a pretest–posttest design with a single pretest. The means in Figure 4.2(a) indicate that both groups improved from pretest to posttest, but the treatment group did so at a greater rate. However, this group also started out at a higher level. Is the result at posttest due to the treatment or to selection-maturation bias? Presented in Figure 4.2(b) and Figure 4.2(c) are hypothetical results from a double-pretest design with the same groups. The pattern of means in Figure 4.2(b) suggests the absence of a treatment effect because the steeper grow rate of the treatment group continued despite treatment. However, the pattern of means in Figure 4.2(c) is more consistent with attribution of the posttest difference to treatment because the growth rates of the two groups were the same until treatment started. One of the exercises at the end of this chapter concerns how a double-pretest design is also useful for evaluating selection-regression bias. The internal validity of a double pretest design is still susceptible to other threats, however, including selection-history, selection-testing, and selection-instrumentation bias.

Stronger NG Designs

The internal validity of controlled NG designs with pretests can be strengthened further by adding the elements of switching treatments or

(a) Pretest–posttest outcome

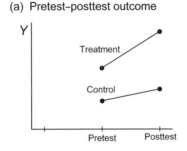

(b) Double pretest outcome 1

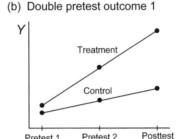

(c) Double pretest outcome 2

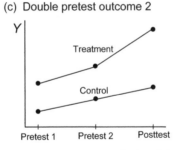

FIGURE 4.2. Results from a pretest–posttest design (a) and two alternative results from a double pretest design (b, c).

introducing a treatment and then removing it. An example follows. Bottge, Rueda, LaRoque, Serlin, and Kwon (2007) evaluated the effectiveness of a problem-based approach to teaching basic arithmetic skills to elementary and high school students with learning disabilities in math. All 100 students in the sample attended self-contained classrooms for math instruction at two different schools. In a switching-replications design, the classrooms were assigned to one of two different instructional orders where the control condition consisted of standard math instruction and the treatment condition consisted of a special problem-based program for teaching math. A content measure of math problem-solving skills (CP) was administered at all three occasions. Two standardized measures of math problem-solving skills (SP) and calculation skills (SC) were administered at pretest (O_1) and at the follow-up assessment (O_3). The diagram for the basic design is presented next:

$$NR \quad O_{1CP}, O_{1SP}, O_{1SC} \quad X \quad O_{2CP} \qquad\qquad O_{3CP}, O_{3SP}, O_{3SC}$$
$$NR \quad O_{1CP}, O_{1SP}, O_{1SC} \qquad\quad O_{2CP} \quad X \quad O_{3CP}, O_{3SP}, O_{3SC}$$

Assuming that treatment is correctly implemented at both times, this design controls for many threats to internal validity. An exception would be a pattern of historical events that just happens to match the sequence of the treatment introductions. Another is a selection-testing threat where the administration of a pretest has different effects on posttest scores across the two treatment orders. This design also permits the evaluation of whether any gains in CP observed in the first group after treatment (O_{2CP}) are maintained at follow-up (O_{3CP}). The readministration of SP and SC at follow-up (O_{3SP}, O_{3SC}) allows estimation of treatment effects in these areas since the pretest. In their analyses (repeated-measures ANOVA), Bottge et al. (2007) found that both treatment orders resulted in clear increases in math problem-solving skills but less so for calculation skills. Given these results, Bottge et al. suggested that it may not be necessary to delay the teaching of concepts for understanding until all related procedural skills are mastered.

Regression-Discontinuity Designs

The structural elements of basic RD designs are represented in the bottom part of Table 4.3 and next where the symbols O_A and C refer to, respectively, the assignment variable and the cutting score that determines membership in the treatment or control group. The notation for the basic RD design is written as follows:

$$O_A \quad C \quad X \quad O_2$$
$$O_A \quad C \qquad\quad O_2$$

The RD design is a type of pretest–posttest design where all participants are measured before treatment is administered and then again after. What distinguishes RD designs from NG designs is that cases in the former are assigned to treatment or control conditions based solely on a cutting score (C) on the pretest measure, the assignment variable (O_A). No other variable influences assignment of cases to groups, so the selection process is completely known. Furthermore, the selection process in RD designs is wholly quantified in the form of scores on the assignment variable, which permits statistical control of this variable in regression analyses. These two features partly explain why causal inferences from well-controlled RD designs have comparable internal validity to those from randomized experiments.

Presented in Figure 4.3 are graphical illustrations of two different outcomes in a basic RD design. Each outcome is represented using a scatterplot for the relation between the assignment variable (A) and posttest

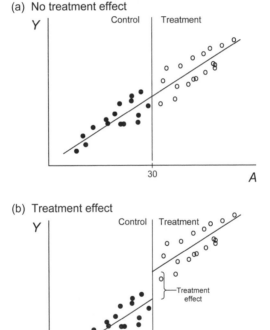

FIGURE 4.3. Outcomes in regression-discontinuity studies with a cutting score of 30 on the assignment variable (A) with (a) no treatment effect and (b) a treatment effect.

dependent variable (Y). The scatterplots in the figure indicate a positive correlation between A and Y, but there is no general requirement that the two should covary. Also represented in the figure is a cutting score of 30 on the assignment variable. Specifically, cases with scores above 30 are assigned to the treatment group, and cases with scores of 30 or less are assigned to the control group. Illustrated in Figure 4.3(a) is the expected outcome in an RD design when there is no treatment effect whatsoever. A treatment effect where scores of all treated cases increase by a constant amount is represented in Figure 4.3(b). This treatment effect is associated with a "break" or discontinuity in the regression line for the treatment group relative to the regression line for the control group. Also, this discontinuity begins exactly at the cutting score on the assignment variable (30).

In other designs for comparative studies, the mean difference (actual or predicted) between the treatment and control groups on the dependent variable estimates the treatment effect. In RD designs, however, it is the magnitude of the discontinuity between the regression lines at the cutting score that estimates the treatment effect. This discontinuity reflects the effect of assignment to the treatment condition where treated and untreated cases are most similar (Lesik, 2006). This characteristic in combination with other features of RD designs eliminates or reduces many threats to the internal validity of RD designs. For example, there is no selection bias because the selection process is known. Other threats, such as that of differential maturation or history, could bias the results only if their effects happen to coincide with the cutoff point, which may be unlikely. Even though the treatment and control groups were formed from the extremes of the assignment variable distribution, bias due to regression artifacts is not a problem because any such effects are already represented in the regression lines of both groups. Finally, measurement error in the assignment variable does not generally bias the treatment effect estimate in RD designs (Trochim, Cappelleri, & Reichardt, 1991). This all assumes that assignment to the treatment or control group is determined only on the basis of the cutting score on the assignment variable. This assumption precludes the use of discretion to override the cutoff, such as may be exercised by a selection committee in the case of "close calls," or cases with assignment variable scores that are close to the cutting score. One of the exercises for this chapter concerns the specification of a design to deal with "close-call" cases.

The technique of MR can be used to analyze data from a RD design.

Assuming linearity and homogeneity of regression (see Figure 4.3(b)), the predictors of the dependent variable are (1) the dichotomous variable of treatment versus control (X); and (2) the *difference* between the score on the assignment variable (O_A) and the cutting score (C) for each case, not just the assignment variable by itself. This subtraction has the effect of forcing the computer to estimate the treatment effect at the cutting score, which is also the point where the groups are the most similar (Shadish et al., 2001). The specific form of this regression equation is

$$\hat{Y} = B_1 X + B_2(O_A - C) + A \qquad (4.3)$$

where the unstandardized coefficient B_2 estimates the treatment effect, or the magnitude of the regression discontinuity at the cutoff point. However, if either the assumption of linearity or homogeneity is not tenable, then the analysis just described may not yield correct results. Nonparallel regression lines imply the presence of an interaction between the assignment variable and the outcome variable. Fortunately, it is possible to represent both interaction effects and curvilinear relations in MR, but failure to correctly model the functional form of the relation between the assignment variable and the outcome variable can seriously bias the results. The accuracy of the analysis also requires that the assignment of cases to treatment versus control by the cutting score is followed without exception.

Within a sample of 3,639 children in the United States enrolled in Medicaid for treatment of asthma, Zuckerman, Lee, Wutoh, Xue, and Stuart (2006) identified a total 333 (9.2%) cases whose prescriptions for short-acting β2-agonist inhalers (SAB) exceeded a national guideline of no more than an average of one prescription per month. The physicians treating these 333 children were sent letters explaining the problem (possible excessive SAB use) and giving the children's names. Zuckerman et al. evaluated in an RD analysis whether this letter intervention resulted in lower prescription rates for these children compared with the 3,306 control children over a 10-month period of time (5 months before intervention, 5 months after). Presented in Figure 4.4 are the scatterplots with fitted regression lines for SAB use in the pre- and postintervention periods for both the letter-intervention and control groups. Results of regression analyses indicated that children in the intervention group were prescribed on average about two-tenths (.2) of a canister less each month compared with children in the control condition.

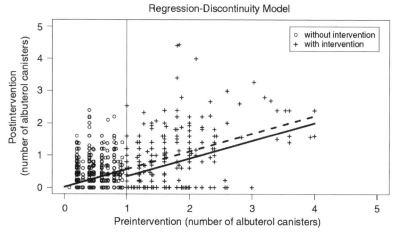

FIGURE 4.4. Scatterplots for short-acting β_2-agonist inhaler use in the pre- and postintervention periods with fitted regression lines. From Zuckerman, Lee, Wutoh, Xue, and Stuart (2006, p. 557). Copyright 2006 by Blackwell Publishing. Reprinted by permission.

Other Quasi-Experimental Designs

We consider in this section some other types of quasi-experimental designs. Unlike NG designs and RD designs, some of these designs lack control groups. However, there are ways to strengthen the internal validity of even uncontrolled quasi-experimental designs by adding the appropriate design elements.

Designs without Control Groups

The most primitive of quasi-experimental designs for evaluating treatment effects without control groups is what D. T. Campbell and Stanley (1963) referred to as the **one-shot case study** where a single group is measured once after an intervention, or:

$$X \qquad O$$

This extraordinarily weak design is subject to so many internal validity threats that it can hardly be considered a formal design at all. A slight improvement is the **one-group pretest–posttest design**, or:

$$O_1 \quad X \quad O_2$$

where a pretest and posttest are administered to one group. This design is also subject to many internal validity threats, so it is generally inadequate.

About the only way to appreciably strengthen the internal validity of a study without a control group is to use multiple pretests or posttests, especially in a **removed-treatment design** where an intervention is introduced and then later removed, or in a **repeated-treatment design** where an intervention is introduced, removed, and then reintroduced. The logic of the two designs just mentioned is analogous to that of, respectively, AB designs and ABA designs for single-case studies: Internal validity is bolstered if outcome rises or falls in a regular pattern following the introduction or removal of treatment. For example, Lesiuk (2005) evaluated the effect of listening to music on affect, work quality, and time on task in a sample of 56 software developers. In a removed- and repeated-treatment design, music listening was introduced, removed, and then reintroduced over a 5-week period. The tests were administered on a total of 10 occasions. In the following notation for this design, the symbol $\not{X}$ represents the removal of music listening. Also, only one observation is represented at each occasion even though three different tests were actually given:

$$O_1 \quad O_2 \quad O_3 \quad X \quad O_4 \quad O_5 \quad X \quad O_6 \quad O_7 \quad \not{X} \quad O_8 \quad O_9 \quad X \quad O_{10}$$

The results indicated that the introduction of music listening was associated with more positive affect and better work quality, but less time on task; the opposite occurred when music was removed. As noted by Shadish et al. (2001), threats to the attribution of changes to treatment in a repeated-treatment design would have to come and go on the same schedule as the introduction and removal of treatment.

Interrupted Time-Series Designs

A time series is a large number of observations made on a single variable over time. In an **interrupted time-series design**, the goal is to determine whether some discrete event—an interruption—affected subsequent observations in the series. Suppose that a new law which severely increases the penalties for drunk driving takes effect on a certain date. Time-series data in the form of the number of deaths each month due to alcohol-related car accidents are available for a 10-year period before the new law and for a 3-year period after the law took effect. Across the whole series, there is month-to-month variation in fatalities. There are also seasonal trends such that the number of deaths is higher in the summer, presumably because more people drive in good weather. The basic aims of a time-series analysis are threefold: (1) statistically model the nature of the time series before the intervention (the new law), taking account of seasonal variation; (2) determine whether the intervention had any appreciable impact on the series; and, if so, then (3) statistically model the intervention effect. The latter concerns whether the intervention had an immediate or delayed impact, whether this effect was persistent or decayed over time, and whether it altered the intercept or slope of the time series.

There are some specialized statistical techniques for time-series analysis that may require at least 50 observations or so. They are also generally advanced techniques that may be suitable in graduate-level research for students with strong quantitative skills. Perhaps the most widely used of these advanced methods is based on the **autoregressive integrative moving average** (ARIMA) **model**. This approach uses lags and shifts in a time series to uncover patterns, such as seasonal trends or various kinds of intervention effects. It is also used to develop forecasting models for a single time series or even multiple time series.

In July 2000, the state of Florida repealed the law that all motorcycle riders 21 years of age or older must wear helmets. After the law change, about 50% of motorcyclists in Florida stopped wearing helmets. Presented in Figure 4.5 is a diagram of the interrupted time series for the number of motorcycle fatalities in Florida analyzed by Ulmer and Northrup (2005). The trend in the figure seems to indicate a rather sharp increase in numbers of fatalities after the mandatory helmet law was repealed. For instance, the number of motorcycle fatalities in the 2 years following the law change (2001–2002) were about 70% greater than the number that occurred in 1998–1999. However, the total number of motorcycle registrations in Florida increased by about 35% during this time. Thus, the fact that there were more and more motorcyclists during the period 1998–2002 is confounded with the change in the helmet law in July 2000. In their analyses of ARIMA models for the time-series data in Figure 4.5, Ulmer and Northrup controlled for effects of the increase in motorcycle registrations. The results indicated that there was an average increase of 9.1 fatalities per month following the law change after taking increased registrations into account. That is, reduced helmet use may have contributed to the increase in motorcycle fatalities seen after repeal of the helmet law even after controlling for increasing numbers of motorcycle riders.

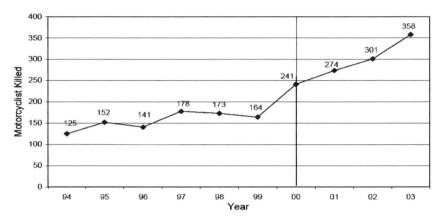

FIGURE 4.5. Number of motorcycle fatalities in Florida, 1994–2003. From Ulmer and Northrup (2005, p. 17). In the public domain.

Case-Control Designs

A **case-control design** is also referred to as a **case-referent design, case-history design**, or **retrospective design**. It is a type of comparative design, but not for directly evaluating treatment effects. Instead, cases are selected on the basis of an outcome variable that is typically dichotomous, such as ill versus healthy. In medical or epidemiological studies, one group consists of patients who already have a disease, but cases in the other group do not. It is also common to match cases across the two groups on relevant background variables. The two groups are then compared on other variables that concern possible risk factors for contracting the disease, such as exposure to secondhand smoke in studies of respiratory illness. Case-control designs are appropriate in situations where randomized longitudinal clinical trials are impossible or when infrequent outcomes are studied, such as death due to a rare form of cancer.

As you might expect, there are many possible threats to the internal validity of case-control studies. Shadish et al. (2001, pp. 131–133) listed a total of 56 such threats, many of which involve selection bias. For example, patients may have received treatment in the past due to their condition but not control cases. Differential attrition of cases across patient and nonpatient groups is another common threat to validity. In any one case-control study, it would be almost impossible to believe that all major internal validity threats were eliminated. Instead, the real value of case-control studies comes from review of replicated studies, that is, from a meta-analytic perspective. In this way, patterns of results that hold up over a series of studies may indicate true causes. There have also been some clear success stories concerning case-control designs, including the identification of smoking as a cause of lung cancer in humans.

Nonexperimental Designs

The typical nonexperimental study has no design elements that address requirements for inferring cause–effect relations, such as control groups or time precedence in measurement. If so, then all that remains to support causal inferences is statistical control when possible confounding variables are included in the analysis. That the accuracy of statistical control depends on the researcher's ability to identify and measure potential confounders was mentioned earlier. An implication is that without strong knowledge about which alternative explanations are plausible, causal inference in these designs breaks down right away.

There are statistical techniques that estimate direct and indirect causal effects among variables that were concurrently measured. An older technique in SEM that does so for observed variables only is **path analysis**, but more modern versions of path analysis estimate causal effects among observed or latent variables (i.e., constructs). Computer programs for SEM require researchers to provide a lot of information such as which variables are assumed to affect other variables and the directionalities of these effects. These a priori specifications reflect the researcher's hypotheses, and in total they make up the model to be evaluated in the analysis. But there is a *major* caveat: The results of an SEM analysis can be interpreted as evidence for causality, *but only if we can assume that the model is correct*. In other words, if the researcher knows in advance the true causal model, then he or she would input sample data to an SEM computer program in order to obtain numerical estimates of these effects.

However, behavioral science researchers almost never conduct SEM analyses in a context where the true causal model is already known. Instead, the researcher's model is at best a guess, and the accuracy of the statistical results that follow depends on the correctness of that initial guess. Also, it is very likely that there is at least one **equivalent model** that explains the data just as well as the researcher's preferred model, but it does so with a different configuration of hypothesized effects among the same variables. An equivalent model thus offers a competing account of the data. There are equivalent versions of perhaps most structural equation models described in the research literature. Unfortunately, too many authors do not even acknowledge the existence of equivalent models. This is in part why Wilkinson and the Task Force on Statistical Inference (1999) emphasized that the use of SEM computer programs "rarely yields any results that have any interpretation as causal effects" (p. 600). Put less formally: There is no Santa Claus, at least not one who brings the power to divine causal relations in studies with no inherent design elements that support causal inference.

The aim of this discussion is not to sow despair among students who expect to work with nonexperimental designs and wish to infer causality. It is just that given a single nonexperimental study, it would be extremely difficult to believe that all logical and statistical requirements for inferring causation with any confidence were met. It is only with the accumulation of the following types of evidence that the results of nonexperimental studies may eventually indicate causality: (1) replication of the study across independent samples; (2) elimination of plausible equivalent models; (3) the collection of corroborating evidence from experimental studies of variables in the model that are manipulable; and (4) the accurate prediction of effects of interventions. This proverb attributed to Saint Augustine is apropos for those who work with nonexperimental designs and wish to make causal inferences with any degree of certainty: Patience is the companion of wisdom.

Resources for Learning More

Listed in Table 4.4 are citations for selected works that provide more information about topics addressed in this chapter. Some works listed in the table are for more advanced (i.e., graduate-level) topics, such as ARIMA models, but many others are less technical and thus more accessible. As a set, the resources listed in the table represent many possibilities for learning even more about design and analysis. Use them wisely and well.

Summary

Major designs for comparative studies and options for analysis were considered in this chapter. When treatment effects are evaluated, experimental designs where cases are randomly assigned to conditions and RD designs

TABLE 4.4. Selected Works for Additional Study about Design and Analysis

Source	Topic
Breaugh and Arnold (2007)	Controlling nuisance variables in matched-groups designs
Ellis (1999)	Design issues in repeated-measures designs
Jones and Kenward (2003)	Design and analysis options for crossover studies
Bonate (2000)	Analysis options for pretest–posttest designs
Ciarleglio and Makuch (2007)	Introduction to hierarchical linear modeling (HLM)
Kline (2005)	Introduction to structural equation modeling (SEM)
Menard (2007)	Design and analysis options for longitudinal studies
Maxwell, Delaney, and Dill (1984)	Relative merits of blocking versus analysis of covariance
Aguinis (2004)	Moderated multiple regression
Luellen, Shadish, and Clark (2005)	Introduction to propensity score analysis (PSA)
Thompson (2006, Ch. 13)	Introduction to logistic regression
Chatfield (2004)	Introduction to autoregressive integrative moving average (ARIMA) models

where scores on an assignment variable determine group membership offer the greatest potential internal validity. This is because both designs just mentioned offer a complete model of selection. This is not true in NG designs where the treatment and control groups are intact groups. In this case, the selection process is typically unknown. In experimental designs, the administration of pretests offers a way to reduce the threat of attrition. When pretests are treated as covariates in the analysis, error variance may be reduced, too. However, covariate analyses in NG designs are much more problematic. This is because a particular set of pretests may measure some, but not all, aspects of the selection process, which means that any statistical correction may not be accurate (i.e., there is bias). This includes the standard technique of the ANCOVA, which does not somehow magically eliminate bias when intact groups are compared. If a design has no inherent features other than statistical control that support causal reasoning (e.g., switching replications and removed treatment), then internal validity is weak. In this case, data collected across many studies are needed before causal inferences can be made with any degree of certainty.

RECOMMENDED READINGS

Shadish (2002) provides an accessible description of recent advances and challenges when implementing quasi-experimental designs in field studies. Rausch et al. (2003) discuss various statistical options for analyzing data from PPF designs, including ANCOVA versus repeated-measures ANOVA. Lesik (2006) outlines conditions when the internal validity of RD designs is comparable to that of randomized experiments.

Lesik, S. A. (2006). Applying the regression-discontinuity design to infer causality with non-random assignment. *The Review of Higher Education, 30,* 1–19.

Rausch, J. R., Maxwell, S. E., & Kelly, K. (2003). Analytic methods for questions pertaining to a randomized pretest, posttest, follow-up design. *Journal of Clinical Child and Adolescent Psychology, 32,* 467–486.

Shadish, W. R. (2002). Revisiting field experimentation: Field notes for the future. *Psychological Methods, 7,* 3–18.

EXERCISES

1. What is the difference between counterbalancing and crossover?

2. Reported next are means from a randomized mixed within-subject factorial design where one group is rewarded with money and the other with praise across four trials on a difficult psychomotor task where a lower score indicates better performance:

	Trial 1	Trial 2	Trial 3	Trial 4
Money	38.00	30.00	20.00	15.00
Praise	52.00	32.00	16.00	12.00

    The researcher concludes that money is more effective than praise. Comment.

3. Students in grade 1 with high scores on an achievement test are placed in a special program for gifted children. When they are retested in grade 2, it is found that their average score does not differ appreciably from that of other grade 2 students in regular classrooms. It is concluded that the gifted program is ineffective. Comment.

4. For a 2×2 factorial design with factors A and B, specify a pattern of cell means that indicates (a) main effects only and (b) the presence of A and AB effects only.

5. Create a graphic like the one in Figure 4.2(b) but one that illustrates possible

selection-regression bias in a double-pretest design. Explain how sampling could explain this outcome.

6. There is a possible new drug treatment for a serious illness. In a basic randomized clinical trial, some patients would receive a pill–placebo but not treatment. Address through design specification the ethical problem that some patients are untreated in a basic trial.

7. Make up posttest cell means for a Solomon Four-Group Design that indicate a main effect of treatment and also a testing effect for the treatment group only.

8. Specify how to study the relation between anxiety and task performance (a continuous variable) in a nonexperimental design versus an experimental design.

9. Scientists monitor the pollution in a river for 3 months before a new, more strict water pollution law takes effect, and then again for 3 months after. Specify the design and threats to internal validity.

10. It is proposed that students with high grade-point averages (>3.50/4.00) be made eligible for an academic enrichment program. However, administrators are concerned about "close calls," or the possibility that students with relatively high grade-point averages that fall short of the cutoff (e.g., 3.00–3.50) could benefit from the program, too. Due to resource limitations, not all such students can be accommodated. Specify a design that evaluates the effectiveness of the program and also addresses this concern.

11. Presented next is a small dataset for two groups where membership is coded as $X = 0$ for the treatment group and $X = 1$ for the control group. For every case in each group, scores are reported as (Y, Z) where Y is the dependent variable and Z is the covariate:

```
X = 0:  (10,9),  (12,10),  (14,12),  (16,16),  (18,11)
X = 1:  (14,6),  (16,7),  (18,3),  (22,10),  (20,9)
```

Use a computer program for statistics and conduct a one-way ANOVA. Next, conduct an ANCOVA. Compare the two sets of results. Comment on the homogeneity of regression assumption.

12. This is an advanced exercise. Use the data for the previous exercise, but this time conduct an ANCOVA using a regression procedure. In this analysis, specify group membership X and the covariate Z as the two predictors of the dependent variable Y (i.e., Equation 4.1). Compare the regression output with the ANCOVA output from the previous exercise.

13. This is also an advanced exercise. Presented next is a small dataset for two

groups where membership is coded as $X = 0$ for the treatment group and $X = 1$ for the control group. For every case in each group, scores are reported as (Y, Z, XZ) where Y is the dependent variable, Z is the covariate, and XZ is the product of the score for group membership (i.e., 0 or 1) and the score on the covariate (i.e., $X \times Z$):

```
X = 0: (10,11,0), (12,16,0), (14,12,0), (16,10,0), (18,9,0)
X = 1: (14,6,6), (16,7,7), (18,3,3), (22,10,10), (20,9,9)
```

First, evaluate the homogeneity of regression assumption. Second, conduct a regression analysis for these data in which just X and Z are predictors of Y (i.e., Equation 4.1). Record from this analysis the total proportion of explained variance. Third, conduct a new regression analysis in which X, Z, and XZ are predictors of Y (i.e., Equation 4.2). Compare the proportion of total explained variance in this analysis with that in the previous analysis. Write the regression equation from this analysis, and then solve the equation for each group (i.e., plug appropriate values of X into the equation). Describe the resulting equations.

14. Presented next is a small dataset for an RD design where group membership is coded as $X = 0$ for the treatment group and $X = 1$ for the control group. For every case in each group, scores are reported as (Y, AS) where Y is the dependent variable and AS is the assignment variable with a cutting score of 8:

```
X = 0: (1,2), (4,3), (2,4), (5,5), (6,6)
X = 1: (10,9), (8,10), (12,11), (14,13), (15,16)
```

Calculate the observed mean difference on Y. Compare this result with the estimate of the treatment effect in an RD analysis (i.e., Equation 4.3).

CHAPTER 5

The Truth about Statistics

The social sciences have been led astray by significance tests. Scientific research can live without significance testing.

—J. SCOTT ARMSTRONG (2007b, p. 336)

Part of becoming a behavioral science researcher is recognizing that you need a higher level of sophistication about statistics. Part of this process involves realizing that some of what you learned in previous statistics courses may be dated or even incorrect. If so, then you are hardly alone, and it is not your fault. This is because many myths about statistical tests are unwittingly passed on from teachers and supervisors to students. Now is the best time, however, to see these myths for what they are so that you can clear your mind of them. Accordingly, the goals of this chapter are to (1) explain what results of statistical tests really mean, (2) outline the limitations of statistical tests, and (3) identify other ways to describe your results that are also part of statistics reform.

Study Strategy

Some suggestions are offered about how to most effectively study the material presented in this chapter. First, consider the question:

> What does it mean that a result is statistically
> significant at the .05 level (i.e., $p < .05$)?

and then read the eight statements listed in Table 5.1. Select the ones
that you think are correct interpretations for this outcome. The correct
answer(s) are given later. Do not worry about choosing a wrong statement
because the point of this exercise is to highlight the difference between
what many of us think statistical significance means versus what it actually
means. Next, skip to Appendix 5.1 at the end of this chapter for a review
of the concepts of standard errors, confidence intervals, and statistical
tests for means. This review will help prepare you to correctly interpret
the results of statistical tests and to better understand their limitations.
Because the exercises for this chapter follow the same general order in
which topics are covered in the appendix, it might help to complete the
exercises as you read the appendix. Resume reading here after you have
finished working with the appendix and exercises. Finally, take your time
with this chapter, especially if it has been a while since you took a statistics
course. It is important that you master the concepts discussed here, so be
patient and keep at it.

A Dozen Truths about Statistics

A total of 12 true things about statistics are listed next. You may already be
familiar with some of these points, but others you may find disconcerting.

TABLE 5.1. Statements for a Self-Quiz about the Meaning of Statistical Significance at the .05 Level

1. The null hypothesis (H_0) is disproved.
2. The probability that the null hypothesis is true is $< .05$.
3. The alternative hypothesis (H_1) is proved.
4. The probability that the alternative hypothesis is true is $> .95$.
5. The probability that a Type I error was made just in rejecting H_0 is $< .05$.
6. The probability that the same result will be found in a replication study is $> .95$.
7. The probability that the result is due to chance is $< .05$.
8. The probability of the data given the null hypothesis is $< .05$.

Note. These statements are based on ones described by Oakes (1986) and Haller and Krauss (2002).

Let us consider them in the spirit of this quotation attributed to Rabindranath Tagore, the Bengali poet and Nobel laureate: Let me not beg for the stilling of my pain, but for the heart to conquer it.

1. Behavioral science students are generally required to take at least one statistics course, but few relish the experience. Conners, Mccown, and Roskos-Ewoldson (1998) speculated that if "psychology students could choose to drop one required course from their curriculum, it would probably be statistics" (p. 40). This view is undoubtedly not unique to psychology students. However, the majority of undergraduate students in psychology and related disciplines do not go on to graduate school. If it is your aim to attend graduate school, you need strong knowledge about statistics, no matter how you feel about the subject.

2. There is no such thing as a shortcut or easy way to learn statistics. One sees many bogus claims about how particular products, especially books or computer programs, are supposed to make statistics easy. Well, it is not easy—it requires patience and careful, diligent study in order to master essential concepts. This is especially true for advanced students (i.e., you), who will not benefit from a dumbed-down presentation about statistics.

3. The mastery of statistical concepts is more important than being facile with computer programs for statistical analyses. One can always learn how to use a computer tool—it is just a matter of practice, even for programs with arcane, user-unfriendly interfaces. Without proper concept knowledge, though, use of a computer tool may not lead to worthwhile results. This is why Pedhazur and Schmelkin (1991) advised that "no amount of technical proficiency will do you any good, if you do not think" (p. 2).

4. Unfortunately, the basic statistics curriculum at both the undergraduate and graduate levels has not changed much in decades (e.g., Frederich et al., 2000). Specifically, today's students take about the same statistics course that students did in the 1970s. This stands in sharp contrast to rapid technological advances and progress in the natural sciences over the same period. It also raises the question about whether today's behavioral science students are learning what they will need tomorrow in this vital area.

5. One way in which our statistics curriculum is obsolete is that statistical tests are often presented as the pinnacle in many undergraduate-level courses. Graduate courses often do little more than cover additional statistical tests or strategies for their use. This narrow perspective gives the false

impression that (1) statistical tests are the only way to evaluate hypotheses, and (2) whether or not results are "significant" is the most important thing to know. This near-exclusive focus on statistical tests prevents students from learning about alternatives. It may also distract them from learning more about measurement.

6. Our statistics curriculum has also generally failed to keep pace with recent developments concerning statistics reform. Part of this reform emphasizes the use of alternative kinds of statistics, especially effect sizes and confidence intervals. Indeed, about two dozen research journals in education and psychology now *require* the reporting of effect sizes, when it is possible to do so (and it usually is).

7. At the end of a conventional statistics course, most students cannot correctly interpret the results of statistical tests. That is, students learn how to calculate these tests, but they do not typically understand what the results mean. In my experience, nearly all students who have taken even several statistics courses nevertheless hold false beliefs about the outcomes of statistical tests.

8. Many—perhaps most—professional educators and researchers in the behavioral sciences hold false beliefs about statistical tests, too. For example, about 80% of psychology professors—including those who teach statistics or research methods courses (i.e., they should know better)—endorse one or more incorrect interpretations of statistical tests (Haller & Krauss, 2002; Oakes, 1986). It is also easy to find similar misinterpretations in books and articles (J. Cohen, 1994). Thus, it seems that students get their false beliefs from teachers and also from what students read.

9. Most misunderstandings about statistical tests involve overinterpretation, or the tendency to see too much meaning in results that are statistically significant or not. Specifically, we tend to believe that statistical tests tell us what we really want to know, but, unfortunately, this is wishful thinking. Also, these overinterpretations are so pervasive that one could argue that much of our practice of data analysis is based on myth.

10. The use of statistical tests as the sole way to evaluate hypotheses is becoming increasingly controversial not just in education and psychology (e.g., Kehle, Bray, Chafouleas, & Kawano, 2007) but also in other disciplines, such as forecasting and empirical economics (e.g., Armstrong, 2007a, 2007b; Ziliak & McCloskey, 2008). Some authors in various fields have even called for a ban on the use of statistical tests. This suggestion is actually not as radical as it may sound, and it reflects the concern about

how overreliance on statistical tests has hindered progress in the behavioral sciences.

11. The developments just described point to a smaller and smaller role for statistical tests in the behavioral sciences. In their place, we will (a) report the directions and magnitudes of our effects, (b) determine whether they replicate, and (c) evaluate them for their theoretical, clinical, or practical significance, not just their statistical significance (e.g., Kirk, 1996; Kline, 2004). Students can better prepare for this future by learning now about alternatives to statistical tests.

12. However—and this is very important—statistical tests are not about to disappear overnight. This means that you will still be expected to report results of statistical tests in written reports. This is because, to be frank, your supervisor may reject a manuscript with no statistical tests; so too would most journals. Even so, you should give much less interpretive weight to outcomes of statistical tests. Specifically, you should:

a. Not view a statistically significant result as particularly informative. For example, do not automatically conclude that such results are noteworthy. Give your readers more information, especially about effect size.

b. *Never* describe a result as "significant" without the preceding qualifier "statistically." Doing so reminds us that statistically significant results are not necessarily meaningful or interesting.

c. Not discount results that fail to reach statistical significance, especially if power is low. Also, results that are not statistically significant can still be important, depending on the context. One example is when artifactual results from one study are not replicated across other studies.

What Statistical Significance Really Means

The most widely used test statistics include t, F, and χ^2, but there are many others. Although different in their applications and assumptions, most work basically the same way:

1. A result is summarized with a sample statistic, such as $M_1 - M_2 = 7.50$ for a mean contrast between two independent samples.

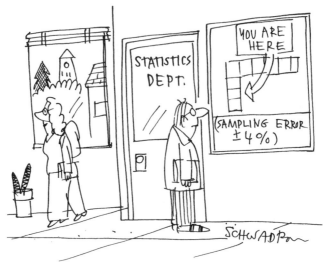

Good statisticians always estimate sampling error. Copyright 1999 by Harley
Schwadron. Reprinted with permission of CartoonStock.

2. The amount of sampling error associated with that statistic is esti-
    mated, such as $SE_{M_1 - M_2}$ = 3.50 (the standard error) for the statistic
    $M_1 - M_2$ = 7.50 when the group size is, say, $n_1 = n_2 = 15$.

3. The difference between the statistic and the value of the corre-
    sponding population parameter in the null hypothesis is evaluated
    against estimated sampling error. If we are referring to the t-test
    and to the null hypothesis H_0: $\mu_1 - \mu_2 = 0$, then the ratio $t(28) =$
    $(7.50 - 0)/3.50$, or 2.14, summarizes the result of this evaluation
    for the hypothetical data presented so far.

4. A computer program for statistical analyses will convert the ob-
    served (sample) value of a test statistic to a probability, or p value,
    based on the appropriate theoretical sampling distribution and
    whether the alternative hypothesis is directional (one-tailed) or
    nondirectional (two-tailed). This probability is the **exact level of
    statistical significance**. For the present example, the probability
    associated with $t(28) = 2.14$ for a two-tailed test (i.e., H_1: $\mu_1 - \mu_2 \neq 0$)
    is $p = .0406$.

5. The value of exact level of statistical significance p is compared
    with that of alpha (α), the **a priori level of statistical significance**

selected by the researcher. In practice, the value of α is usually either .05 or .01, but it is theoretically possible to specify different values (e.g., α = .001). If it is observed that $p < \alpha$, then the null hypothesis is rejected at that level of statistical significance. For example, given α = .05 and p = .0406, the null hypothesis would be rejected at the .05 level, but not at the .01 level.

It is important to realize that p values from statistical tests are actually conditional probabilities that should be interpreted from a frequentist or "in-the-long-run" perspective (see Appendix 5.1). The general form of this conditional probability is

$$p \, (\text{Data} \mid H_0 \text{ true})$$

which stands for the likelihood of a result even more extreme than that observed across all possible random samples assuming that the null hypothesis is true and all assumptions of that test statistic (e.g., independence, normality, and homogeneity of variance) are satisfied. Some correct interpretations for the specific case α = .05 and $p < .05$ are listed next:

1. Assuming that H_0 is true and the study is repeated many times by drawing random samples from the same population(s), less than 5% of these results will be even more inconsistent with H_0 than the actual result.

2. Less than 5% of test statistics from random samples are further away from the mean of the sampling distribution under H_0 than the one for the observed result.

3. The odds are less than 1 to 19 of getting a result from a random sample even more extreme than the observed one when H_0 is true.

That is about it. Other correct definitions may be just variations of those just listed. The range of correct interpretations of p is thus actually quite narrow. Let us refer to any correct definition as $p \, (D \mid H_0)$, which emphasizes p values from statistical tests as conditional probabilities of the data (D) under the null hypothesis. Note that of the various statements listed in Table 5.1 regarding the meaning of statistical significance at $p < .05$, only the last one (no. 8) is true. In the survey by Oakes (1986), only about 10% of academic psychologists selected this alternative, so do not feel bad if your own performance on this self-quiz was no better.

We should also even more clearly distinguish between p values from statistical tests, or conditional probabilities of data under H_0, and α, the a priori level of statistical significance. Even though both p and α are defined in the same sampling distribution, they are not identical. Specifically, α is the conditional probability of making a Type I error, or rejecting H_0 when it is actually true. In other words:

$$\alpha = p \ (\text{Reject } H_0 \mid H_0 \text{ true})$$

Thus, α can also be understood as the probability of getting a result across all possible random samples that leads to the incorrect decision to reject the null hypothesis. All of these descriptions of α are frequentist or in-the-long-run probability statements about the risk of a Type I error across theoretical replications of the study.

Misinterpretations of Statistical Significance[1]

There are many incorrect interpretations of p values that are also very common in the behavioral sciences. Listed in Table 5.2 are what I refer to as the "Big Five" false beliefs about p values. As mentioned, it seems that the large majority of professionals, near professionals, and students hold at least one of these false beliefs. Three concern misinterpretation of p values themselves, but two concern misinterpretations of $1 - p$, the complements of p values. Also reported in Table 5.2 are base rates for specific misinterpretations found in samples of psychology professors or psychology students by Oakes (1986) and Haller and Krauss (2002). Overall, psychology students are no worse than psychology professors concerning incorrect interpretation of p values. These poor results are probably not specific to psychology. That is, I believe that the misinterpretation of p values is just as pervasive in other disciplines where statistical significance tests are used. This speculation is supported by numerous works in other disciplines about misinterpretation of statistical tests, such as Banasiewicz (2005) in the area of marketing.

What I believe is the biggest of the Big Five is what Carver (1978) referred to as the **odds-against-chance fallacy** (Table 5.2). This is the false belief that p indicates the probability that a result happened by chance or

[1]Part of this discussion is based on Kline (2004, Ch. 3).

sampling error (e.g., if $p < .05$, then the likelihood that the result is due to chance is $< 5\%$). There are three reasons why this belief is wrong:

1. When p is calculated, it is already assumed that the null hypothesis is true, so the probability that chance is the only explanation of the result is already taken to be 1.0. Thus, it is illogical to view p as somehow measuring the probability of chance.

2. Recall that p values are best seen as in-the-long-run probabilities that apply to theoretical replications but not to a specific sample result. Yes, it is true that $p < .05$ means that less than 5% of results from all random samples are expected to be even more extreme than the observed result under the null hypothesis, but this statement does not apply to a particular result as the probability that chance was the sole cause.

3. In general, there is no such thing as a statistical technique that determines the probability that various causal agents, including chance, acted on a particular result. It would be great to have such a technique but, unfortunately, no such thing exists. Instead, the inference of causality is a rational exercise that takes into account results within the context of design, measurement, and analysis (Chapter 3); it is never solely a statistical one.

TABLE 5.2. The "Big Five" Misinterpretations of Statistical Significance at the .05 Level ($p < .05$) and Base Rates among Psychology Professors and Students

Type	Fallacy	Description	Base rate (%)	
			Professors[a]	Students[b]
p				
	Odds against chance	Likelihood that result is due to chance is $< 5\%$	—	—
	Local Type I error	Likelihood that Type I error was just committed is $< 5\%$	67–73	68
	Inverse probability	Likelihood that null hypothesis is true is $< 5\%$	17–36	32
$1 - p$				
	Replicability	Likelihood that result will be replicated is $> 95\%$	37–60	41
	Validity	Likelihood that alternative hypothesis is true is $> 95\%$	33–66	59

[a]Haller and Krauss (2002); Oakes (1986).
[b]Haller and Krauss (2002).

The odds-against-chance fallacy seems to be a short-cut version of the correct interpretation of p values that omits the part about the likelihood of a range of results across all random samples. I am not aware of an estimate of the base rate of the odds-against-chance fallacy, but I think that it is nearly universal (close to 100%) in the behavioral sciences. This is because one can find this misinterpretation just about everywhere, including textbooks and Web pages devoted to statistical issues.[2] One also hears the odds-against-chance fallacy a lot in casual conversations with professionals or students about what statistical significance means.

The rest of the Big Five misinterpretations of p values are listed in Table 5.2. One of these is what I refer to as the **local Type I error fallacy**. For the case $\alpha = .05$ and $p < .05$, it can be expressed as follows: I just rejected the null hypothesis at the .05 level; therefore, the probability that this particular (local) decision is wrong (i.e., a Type I error) is less than 5%. This false belief seems to be held by the majority of psychology professors and students (Table 5.2). Nevertheless, it is wrong for these reasons:

1. The decision to reject H_0 based on a particular result is either correct or incorrect, so no probability (either than 0 or 1.0) is associated with it. It is only with sufficient replication that we could determine whether this specific decision was correct or not.

2. This fallacy confuses the correct definition of α as the conditional probability of rejecting the null hypothesis given that the null hypothesis is true, or

$$\checkmark \quad \alpha = p \text{ (Reject } H_0 \mid H_0 \text{ true)}$$

with its inverse, or the conditional probability of a Type I error given that the null hypothesis has been rejected:

$$\text{✗} \quad \alpha = p \text{ (}H_0 \text{ true } \mid \text{ Reject } H_0\text{)}$$

The third of the Big Five is the **inverse probability error** (J. Cohen, 1994), and it goes like this: Given $p < .05$; therefore, the likelihood that the

---

[2]For example, on July 3, 2007, I entered the term "define: statistical significance" in the search dialog box of Google. Virtually all of the 21 definitions returned by Google contained the odds-against-chance fallacy. Here is one from the Centers for Disease Control and Prevention website (*www.cdc.gov/niosh/2001-133o.html*): "The likelihood that an association between exposure and disease risk could have occurred by chance alone."

null hypothesis is true is < 5%, or $p\,(H_0 \mid D) < .05$. This misinterpretation seems to be made by about one-third of psychology professors and students (Table 5.2). This error stems from forgetting that p values are conditional probabilities of the data under the null hypothesis, or $p\,(D \mid H_0)$, not the other way around. Although the probability of some hypothesis in light of the data is what most of us would really like to know, this is not what p tells us. There are ways to estimate conditional probabilities of hypotheses given the data in **Bayesian statistics**, which are widely used in medicine, engineering, and computer science, but not in our disciplines. Bayesian statistics can be seen as a method for orderly expression and revision of belief about hypotheses as new evidence is gathered; see Kline (2004, Ch. 9) for more information. In this method, there are ways to estimate conditional probabilities of hypotheses, given the data, or $p\,(H \mid D)$. However, this estimation process works best when conducted over a series of replications.

Two of the Big Five false beliefs concern $1 - p$ (Table 5.2). One is the **replicability fallacy** (Carver, 1978), which for the case of $p < .05$ says that the probability of finding the same result in a replication sample exceeds .95. This view seems to be held by near majorities of psychology professors and students. If this fallacy were true, knowing the probability of replication would be very useful. Unfortunately, a p value is just the probability of a range of results in a particular sample under a specific null hypothesis. In general, replication is a matter of experimental design and whether some effect actually exists in the population. It is thus an empirical question and one that cannot be directly addressed by statistical tests in a single study.

However, you should know that there is a way that p values *indirectly* concern replication. Greenwald, Gonzalez, Harris, and Guthrie (1996) noted there is generally a curvilinear relation between p values and the average statistical power of hypothetical replications. But without special graphs like ones presented by these authors, one cannot directly convert p to the power of a replication. And it is only in the very specific case when effect size is exactly the same in both the sample and the population that $1 - p$ will equal the average power of a replication. The population effect size is almost never known, however, nor do we usually know how far away the sample effect size falls from the population effect size. Killeen (2005) made a similar point concerning the statistic p_{rep}, which refers to the average probability of getting a result of the same sign (direction) in both an original study and in a hypothetical replication: The relation between p and p_{rep} is curvilinear. Killeen described a method to estimate p_{rep} and also suggested that p_{rep} may be less subject to misinterpretation than standard

p values from statistical tests, but not everyone agrees with this assessment (Cumming, 2005). Also, p_{rep} is based on the same unrealistic assumption of random sampling as p values. Finally, p_{rep} is just a sample statistic and as such is subject to sampling error, too. It remains to be seen whether p_{rep} is a useful alternative to p. In the meantime, it is better to actually conduct replication studies than rely on statistical prediction.

The last of the Big Five is the **validity fallacy** (Mulaik, Raju, & Harshman, 1997), and it refers to the false belief that the probability that the alternative hypothesis is true is greater than .95, given $p < .05$ (Table 5.2). The complement of p, or $1 - p$, is also a probability, but it is just the probability of getting a result even *less* extreme under the null hypothesis than the one actually found. Again, p refers to the probability of the data, not to that of any particular hypothesis, null or alternative.

Listed in Table 5.3 are other common misinterpretations of the outcomes of statistical tests. Those presented in the top part of the table describe false beliefs about what rejecting the null hypothesis means. One is the **magnitude fallacy**, or the belief that statistical significance implies a large effect size. The value of a test statistic summarizes the influence of both effect size and sample size together (see Appendix 5.1), so a small effect size together with a large sample size could yield a statistically significant effect. The **meaningfulness fallacy** is the view that rejection of the null hypothesis confirms both the alternative hypothesis and the research hypothesis behind it. Statistical significance does not "prove" any hypothesis, and there are times when the same numerical result is consistent with more than one substantive hypothesis. The only way to differentiate competing explanations of the same observation is to devise an experiment that would yield different results depending on which explanation is correct. For the same reason, the **causality fallacy** that statistical significance means that the underlying causal mechanism is identified is just that. The **quality fallacy** and the **success fallacy** concern the false views that statistical significance confirms, respectively, the quality of the experimental design and the success of the study. These related myths are equally false. Poor study design or just plain old sampling error can lead to the incorrect rejection of the null hypothesis. Failure to reject the null hypothesis can also be the product of good science, especially when a counterfeit claim is not substantiated by other researchers. In an article about the warning signs of bogus science, Park (2003) noted that there is "no scientific claim so preposterous that a scientist cannot be found to vouch for it" (p. B20). When this happens, the lack of positive results from replication studies is highly informative.

Misunderstandings listed in the middle part of Table 5.3 concern false beliefs about what failing to reject the null hypothesis (i.e., the results are not statistically significant) means. The **failure fallacy** is the mirror image of the success fallacy, or the mistaken belief that lack of statistical significance brands the study as a failure. The **zero fallacy** is the mistaken conclusion that the failure to reject a null hypothesis that specifies a zero effect (e.g., H_0: $\mu_1 - \mu_2 = 0$) means that the population effect size must be zero. Maybe it is, but you cannot tell based on a single result in one sample, especially if power is low. A related misunderstanding for the same type of null hypothesis is the **equivalence fallacy**, or the false belief that failure to reject H_0: $\mu_1 - \mu_2 = 0$ implies that the two populations are equivalent. This view is wrong because this particular hypothesis concerns only means, and distributions can differ in other ways besides central tendency, such as variability or shape. There are special methods for **equivalence testing** that evaluate whether two different treatments are equivalent, but they are better known in other areas such as biology and psychopharmacology; see Rogers, Howard, and Vessey (1993) for more information.

Two of the last three false beliefs listed at the bottom of Table 5.3 include the **reification fallacy** and the **sanctification fallacy**. The former refers to the wrong idea that a result is considered not replicated if the

TABLE 5.3. Other Common Misinterpretations of Statistical Significance

Type	Description
H_0 rejected	
Magnitude	Statistical significance → large effect size
Meaningfulness	Statistical significance → theory behind alternative hypothesis is correct
Causality	Statistical significance → causal mechanism is known
Quality	Statistical significance → good design quality
Success	Statistical significance → study is successful
H_0 not rejected	
Failure	Lack of statistical significance → study is a failure
Zero	Lack of statistical significance → zero population effect size
Equivalence	Failure to reject H_0: $\mu_1 - \mu_2 = 0$ → two populations are equivalent
Other	
Reification	H_0 rejected in first study but not in second → no evidence for replication
Sanctification	$p < .05$ is very meaningful, but $p = .06$ is not
Objectivity	Statistical tests are objective; all other methods are subjective

Note. →, implies.

null hypothesis is rejected in the first study but not in the second (Dixon & O'Reilly, 1999). However, this view ignores the sample size, effect size and direction, and power of the statistical test in a second study. The latter fallacy refers to dichotomous thinking about p values which are actually continuous. If $\alpha = .05$, for instance, then a result where $p = .049$ versus one where $p = .051$ is practically identical in terms of statistical test outcomes. However, a researcher may make a big deal about the first (it's significant!) but ignore the second. This type of black-and-white thinking along a sanctified level of statistical significance is out of proportion with continuous changes in p values. The **objectivity fallacy** is the false belief that statistical tests somehow make up a technical, essentially objective process of decision making, but all other kinds of data analysis are subjective (Gorard, 2006). On the contrary, there are several decisions to be made in using statistical tests that are not entirely objective, some of which can directly affect the results. For example, one is supposed to specify the level of statistical significance before the data are collected. If $\alpha = .01$ but the result from a statistical test is $p = .03$, then one is supposed to fail to reject the null hypothesis. However, the temptation to increase α based on the data (i.e., from .01 to .05) in order to reject the null hypothesis may be strong here.

Considering all these misinterpretations, it seems that most researchers may believe for the case $\alpha = .01$ and $p < .01$ that the result is very unlikely to be due to sampling error, and also that the likelihood that a Type I error was committed is just as unlikely ($< 1\%$ chance for both). Many researchers might also conclude that the alternative hypothesis is very likely to be true and that the result is very likely to replicate ($> 99\%$ chance for both). The next (il)logical step would be to conclude that the result must be important. Why? Because it's *significant!* Of course, none of these things are true. But if we believed them, it is easy to see how we could become overly confident about our results, perhaps so much so that we do not bother to replicate. Many of the same false beliefs could also facilitate research about fad topics with little scientific value (Meehl, 1990). Does this sound familiar (Chapter 2)?

Why Are There So Many Myths?

It is striking that myth pervades so much of our thinking about statistical tests, especially considering that virtually all who use them have science backgrounds. Why, then, is there so much misunderstanding about statistical tests? Three possible explanations are briefly considered.

First, the whole framework of null hypothesis significance testing is hardly the most transparent of inference systems (but you know that already). Indeed, it is hard to explain the convoluted logic of null hypothesis significance testing and dispel confusion about it. The very unfortunate decision to use the word "significant" in regard to rejection of the null hypothesis is a related problem. This is because this word in everyday language means "important," "noteworthy," or "meaningful," but not in the framework of statistical tests. When we forget the latter, we may falsely believe that our results are important, noteworthy, or meaningful by virtue of their statistical significance.

Second, people in general are just not very good at intuitive reasoning about probabilities. That is, many people—even very educated ones—readily make judgment errors based on perceived probabilities of events. For example, there are many cognitive errors about probabilities in the areas of gambling and investing in the stock market that lead to disastrous outcomes for many people. Dawes (2001) described many examples in everyday life of the failure to think rationally about a wide range of issues when probabilities are involved. In general, people are much better at pattern recognition and making decisions based on frequencies of events, not their probabilities. The fact that the main outcomes of statistical tests are probabilities—and conditional probabilities at that—just invites misunderstanding.

Third, I believe that myths about statistical significance are maintained in part by a fundamental cognitive error known as **illusory correlation**, which is the expectation that two things should be correlated when in fact they are not. When this expectation is based on an apparently logical or semantic association between the two things, the false belief that they go together may be very resistant to disconfirmation, even in the face of evidence to the contrary. For example, many psychotherapists believe that with greater experience comes better client outcomes, but much evidence supports the conclusion that the two are in fact unrelated (Dawes, 1994). Illusory correlation can be seen as a kind of conformation bias that can affect the judgment of even highly educated professionals. In the behavioral sciences, semantic associations between the concept of "probability" and other ideas related to statistical tests, such as those of "chance" or "hypothesis," combined with poor inherent probabilistic reasoning may engender illusory correlations in this area. Once engrained, such false beliefs are hard to change.

Other Drawbacks of Statistical Tests

Some other potential problems with the overuse of statistical tests in the behavioral sciences are considered next. Some of these problems are related to the misinterpretations outlined earlier.

The Power Problem

Recall that power is the probability of getting a statistically significant result when there is a real effect in the population (i.e., H_0 is false). Its mirror image is Type II error, which occurs when there is no statistical significance in the sample but the null hypothesis is false. The probability of making a Type II error is often designated by the symbol β. Because power and Type II error are complementary (i.e., power + β = 1.0), whatever increases power decreases β, and vice versa.

Power is affected by some factors more or less under control of the researcher, including study design, level of statistical significance, directionality of the alternative hypothesis, the test statistic used, score reliability, and sample size. It is also affected by a property of nature, the magnitude of the real effect in the population (Chapter 3). In an **a priori power analysis**, the researcher uses a computer tool to estimate power before the data are collected. A variation is to specify a desired minimum power (e.g., .80) and then estimate the minimum sample size needed to obtain it. There are commercial computer programs that estimate power, and some programs for general statistical analyses have power analysis modules. There are also some power calculators that are freely available over the Internet.[3] In contrast, a **retrospective (post hoc) power analysis** is conducted after the data are collected. The effect size observed in the sample is treated as the population effect size, and the probability of rejecting the null hypothesis given the study's other characteristics is estimated. However, a retrospective analysis is not generally acceptable (Wilkinson & the Task Force on Statistical Inference, 1999). This is in part because a retrospective analysis power is more like an autopsy conducted after things go wrong rather than a diagnostic procedure (i.e., a priori power analysis).

There is a serious problem if the estimated power is .50 or less. If power is only .50, then the researcher is just as likely to correctly guess the outcome of a series of coin tosses as he or she is to get statistically signifi-

---

[3]See Russell Lenth's Java applets for power analysis; note that this Web address is case sensitive: *www.stat.uiowa.edu/~rlenth/Power/*

cant results across a series of replications. In this case, tossing a coin to determine whether to reject the null hypothesis or not instead of actually conducting the study would save both time and money (Schmidt & Hunter, 1997). That is, if power is so low, why bother to carry out the study? This is why some funding agencies require an a priori power analysis as part of the application. Otherwise, funds may be wasted if power is not at least equal to some minimally acceptable value, such as .80.

The results of several reviews from the 1970s and 1980s indicated that the typical power of behavioral science research is only about .50 (e.g., Sedlmeier & Gigerenzer, 1989), and similarly low levels of power remain a problem in some research areas (e.g., Dybå, Kampenes, & Sjøberg, 2006). Low power is probably more characteristic of studies based on nonexperimental designs conducted with people than of experimental studies conducted with either people or animals. Increasing sample size is one way to increase power, but the number of additional cases necessary to reach even a power level of .80 when studying small- or medium-size effects may be so great as to be practically impossible (Schmidt & Hunter, 1997). This is a critical limitation of relying solely on statistical tests to evaluate hypotheses: Some studies will be doomed to have low statistical power. One consequence in health-related research is that potentially beneficial treatments for relatively rare disorders (i.e., small group sizes are expected) may be overlooked.

Another consequence of low power is that the research literature may be difficult to interpret. Specifically, if there is a real effect but power is only .50, then about half the studies will yield positive results (H_0 rejected) and the rest, negative results (H_0 not rejected). If all these studies were somehow published, then the numbers of positive and negative results would appear roughly equal. In an old-fashioned, narrative literature review (i.e., not a meta-analysis), the research literature would appear to be ambiguous given this balance. It may be concluded that "more research is needed" to resolve the ambiguity. However, any new results will probably just reinforce the ambiguity, if power remains low. Researchers may lose interest in the topic and move on to study something else, but this pattern may repeat itself if power in the new research area is also low. Again, does this sound familiar?

The Replication Problem

Replication is a critical scientific activity. In the natural sciences, it is rightly viewed as the gold standard for establishing generalizability (external validity). Replication is also the ultimate way to deal with the problem of sampling error. Although sampling error is estimated in individual studies by statistical tests, sufficient replication makes the use of such tests unnecessary. As Robinson and Levin (1997) succinctly put it, "A replication is worth a thousandth p value" (p. 25). Unfortunately, little of our research literature is devoted to replication. For instance, proportions of articles published in psychology, education, or business research journals specifically described as replications are very low, sometimes < 1% of the literature (e.g., Evanschitzky, Baumgarth, Hubbard, & Armstrong, 2007). Pervasive cognitive errors related to statistical tests may be part of the problem. That is, if one believes either that (1) $p < .01$ means that a result is likely to be repeated 99 times out of 100, or (2) $p > .05$ means that the population effect size is zero, then why bother to replicate? To be fair, there are probably other factors that work against developing a stronger tradition of replication in the behavioral sciences. One is the clear editorial preference to publish studies with statistically significant results. Another is the editorial preference for novelty, or for work seen as original or unique. Sometimes even students are discouraged by their supervisors or instructors from conducting replications of published studies. This unfortunate advice sends the wrong message.

The Assumptions Problem

There are two types of problems about assumptions of statistical tests. First, p values for test statistics are estimated in sampling distributions that assume random sampling from known populations. However, very few samples in the behavioral sciences are true random (probability) samples—most are probably convenience samples (Chapter 3). Thus, outcomes of statistical tests are interpreted in reference to ideas about sampling that have little connection with reality. Second, it happens too often that no evidence about whether distributional or other assumptions are met is provided in journal articles (e.g., Keselman et al., 1998). If certain key assumptions are violated (e.g., sphericity for repeated-measures ANOVA), then p values may be quite inaccurate. If so, then decisions based on p values could be wrong, too.

The Null Hypothesis Problem

The most common type of null hypothesis tested in the behavioral sciences is a **nil hypothesis**, which is usually a statement that some effect, difference, or association is zero. For example, the typical null hypothesis for the *t*-test is the nil hypothesis H_0: $\mu_1 - \mu_2 = 0$. It is possible to specify a non-nil hypothesis for the *t*-test, such as H_0: $\mu_1 - \mu_2 = 5.00$, but this is rarely done in practice. However, it is more difficult to specify and test non-nil hypotheses for other types of statistical tests, including the *F*-test. One reason is that computer programs for statistics almost always assume a nil hypothesis. Nil hypotheses may be appropriate when it is unknown whether effects exist at all, such as in new research areas where studies are mostly exploratory. However, nil hypotheses are less suitable when it is already known that an effect is probably not zero, which is more likely in established research areas. When a nil hypothesis is implausible, then (1) it is a "strawman" argument that is easily rejected, and (2) estimated probabilities of the data under that hypothesis are too low. This also means that the risk of a Type I error is basically zero and a Type II error is the only kind possible when the null hypothesis is known in advance to be false.

In Defense of Statistical Tests

Statistical tests are not inherently evil, and their continued use is defended by some. Krantz (1999) argued that misinterpretations of outcomes of statistical tests are the fault of those who use them; that is, a tool should not be blamed for its misuse. That over 50 years of debate has failed to dispel myths about statistical tests is unsettling, though. Even if we could correctly interpret *p* values, statistical tests just may be the wrong tool for our needs. For example, most behavioral scientists do not study large probability samples with distributional characteristics that clearly meet the assumptions of statistical tests. Although a small minority, there are behavioral science researchers who study probability samples and who can also precisely estimate sampling error and the relative costs of different types of decision errors (e.g., Type I vs. Type II). There are also times when a null hypothesis of a zero effect is theoretically justified.

Abelson (1997a) noted that other kinds of statistics suggested as alternatives to traditional statistical tests, such as effect sizes and confidence intervals, are not immune to misinterpretation (see Appendix 5.1). Harris (1997) described a variation of standard hypothesis testing that may be useful in evaluating ordinal effects where just the direction of the effect (positive or negative) is critical. In this approach, two directional alternative hypotheses are simultaneously tested. The logic of this test of ordinal effects is similar to that of equivalence testing in the biological sciences. Chow (1998) argued that some research questions require a yes/no answer, including, for instance, should this treatment be implemented? Statistical tests provide a yes/no answer regarding the decision to reject the null hypothesis or not. However, one must be careful not to accept false inferences after making either decision (e.g., Table 5.3). There is also a role for statistical tests in data screening, such as in the identification of outlier scores (Chapter 8). This is how statistical tests are generally used in the natural sciences, but not for testing hypotheses.

Recommendations for Changing Times

The last time of marked change in data analysis practices in the behavioral sciences occurred in the 20-year period from roughly 1940 to 1960. Gigerenzer (1993) referred to this period as the **probabilistic revolution** in psychology where the inference process about hypotheses was standardized based on the logic of null hypothesis significance testing. During that time, the use of statistical tests became increasingly universal so that by about 1970 almost all journal articles for empirical studies in the behavioral science literature contained references to statistical tests. However, this was true in just a minority of empirical studies published before about 1940, so behavioral scientists have not always relied on statistical tests to the degree they do now.

I and others who advocate statistics reform believe that now is another period of transition, one that will see a decreasing role for statistical tests and a deemphasis on statistical significance as meaningful. In their place, we should emphasize effect size; confidence intervals; practical, clinical, or theoretical significance; and, most important, replication. Many of these attributes are now part of most meta-analytic studies, and I believe that meta-analytic thinking will become the standard bearer for the inference process in the behavioral sciences. However, this new transition may take at least a generation (20 years) to unfold, as did the previous one from about 1940 to 1960. Also, I expect that students will play a critical role in statistics reform because they are the future behavioral scientists. It also helps that students are probably not as set in their ways as the rest of us.

Elsewhere I gave the nine recommendations listed in Table 5.4 for data analysis practices in this time of transition (Kline, 2004). These recommendations acknowledge the reality that today's students and researchers will still be expected to report results of statistical tests and, at the same time, provide additional information, especially about effect sizes. These suggestions are now briefly summarized. Statistical tests may have a primary role only in exploratory research where it is unknown whether effects exist. The use of statistical tests in this case should be supported by the

TABLE 5.4. Recommendations Regarding Data Analysis Practices in the Behavioral Sciences

1. A primary role for statistical tests may be appropriate only in new research areas where it is unknown whether effects exist.

2. Report a priori power estimates whenever statistical tests are used.

3. It is unacceptable to describe results solely in terms of statistical significance.

4. Use the word "significant" without the qualifier "statistically" only to describe results that are truly noteworthy.

5. Effect sizes and confidence intervals must be reported whenever possible.

6. It is the researcher's responsibility to explain why the results have substantive significance. Statistical tests are inadequate for this purpose.

7. Replication is the best way to deal with sampling error.

8. Reform statistics education by deemphasizing statistical tests and emphasizing how to evaluate substantive significance and replicate effects.

9. Computer programs for statistical analyses should be able to calculate effect sizes and confidential intervals.

Note. These recommendations are based on those presented in Kline (2004, pp. 86–90).

results of an a priori power analysis. Power estimates would help readers to better understand the implications of results that are not statistically significant, especially if estimated power is low. Statistical significance should *never* be the sole criterion for claiming that a result is important. This is instead a matter of relating the results to a particular theoretical context or translating them into a metric, such as effect size, that more directly says something about practical import. At the end of the day, there is no substitute for replication as a way to verify claims, and it is time for us to "grow up" as scientists and walk the walk of replication, not just talk the talk. In methods and statistics courses, students should learn more than just about statistical tests and classical methods for statistical hypothesis testing. More emphasis should be placed on measurement, effect size estimation, and expressing results in terms of their substantive significance. Less emphasis on statistical tests may also encourage students to select simpler statistical techniques that are closer to the level of the data. We also need better computer tools for statistics, ones that automatically calculate effect sizes and confidence intervals instead of just statistical tests.

Finally, you can prepare now for changing times by developing this skill: You should be able to describe your results *without reference to statistical tests at all.* In their place, refer to descriptive statistics and effect sizes instead. Doing so will seem strange at first—perhaps even heretical—but it is critical to realize that statistical tests are not generally necessary to detect meaningful or noteworthy effects, which should be obvious to visual inspection of relatively simple kinds of graphical displays (Cohen, 1994). The description of results at a level closer to the data may also help you to develop better communication skills.

Summary

Data analysis practices are slowly but surely changing in the behavioral sciences. Part of these changes concern statistics reform, which has five basic elements: (1) the recognition that most of us incorrectly interpret the results of statistical tests; (2) the presumption that these cognitive distortions explain in part the overall poor state of behavioral science research; (3) the emphasis on meta-analytic thinking, which emphasizes replication; (4) the reporting of information about effect sizes and confidence intervals; and (5) the interpretation of results in terms of their substantive significance, not just statistical significance. In the near future, you will undoubtedly still be required to report the results of statistical tests. Given what you know now, however, you should try hard not to make the types of interpretive errors described earlier. There is also nothing incompatible about using statistical tests and a reform perspective, if those tests are properly applied to plausible null hypotheses in large, representative samples in which distributional assumptions of the tests are clearly met and where estimated statistical power is reasonably high. Otherwise, there is great potential for misuse of statistical tests. The next chapter deals with how to estimate effect size for different types of outcome variables and how to construct confidence intervals for population effect sizes.

RECOMMENDED READINGS

Nickerson (2000) reviewed in detail the history and specific arguments of the debate about the use of statistical tests in psychology. The third chapter in Kline (2004) considers what is wrong with statistical tests but also addresses some legitimate uses. Schmidt and Hunter (1997) reviewed eight common but false objections among researchers to discontinuing the use of statistical tests.

Kline, R. B. (2004). *Beyond significance testing: Reforming data analysis methods in behavioral research* (Chap. 3). Washington, DC: American Psychological Association.
Nickerson, R. S. (2000). Null hypothesis significance testing: A review of an old and continuing controversy. *Psychological Methods, 5*, 241–301.

Schmidt, F. L., & Hunter, J. E. (1997). Eight common but false objections to the discontinuation of significance testing in the analysis of research data. In L. L. Harlow, S. A. Mulaik, & J. H. Steiger (Eds.), *What if there were no significance tests?* (pp. 37–64). Mahwah, NJ: Erlbaum.

EXERCISES

1. Comment: A larger sample is always better than a smaller sample.

2. What is the difference between SD and SE_M?

3. Given: $M = 115.00$ and $SE_M = 3.00$. Explain why this statement is probably false: The sample mean is within 3 points away from the population mean.

4. Comment: If $M_1 - M_2 = 0$, then $SE_{M_1 - M_2} = 0$.

5. Presented next is a small dataset for two independent groups. Construct and interpret the 95% confidence interval for $\mu_1 - \mu_2$:

   ```
   Condition 1: 9, 12, 13, 15, 16
   Condition 2: 8, 12, 11, 10, 14
   ```

6. Use the same dataset as in the previous exercise, but now assume a repeated-measures design where each pair of cross-condition scores (e.g., 9 and 8) come from the same case. Construct the 95% confidence interval for μ_D. Compare your result with that for the previous exercise.

7. Given: $M_1 - M_2 = 2.00$, $s_1^2 = 7.50$, and $s_2^2 = 5.00$ for a balanced design with independent samples. Calculate s_p^2, $SE_{M_1 - M_2}$, and the t-test for a two-tailed alternative hypothesis at $\alpha = .05$ for three different group sizes (n), 5, 15, and 30. Explain the pattern of results.

8. Given: $t = 25.00$, p < .0001. Explain what the "25.00" means. A researcher concludes that a large mean difference is indicated because the p value is so small. Comment.

9. Given: $M_1 = 13.00$, $M_2 = 11.00$, $M_3 = 12.00$, $s_1^2 = 7.50$, $s_2^2 = 5.00$, and $s_3^2 = 7.50$ for a balanced one-way design with independent samples. Calculate the ANOVA source tables for two different group sizes, $n = 15$ and $n = 30$. Explain the pattern of results.

10. Given: $F = 200.00$, $p < .0001$. Explain what the "200.00" means and why we cannot conclude that there are large differences among the means.

11. Find three incorrect definitions of statistical significance. Explain what is wrong with each.

APPENDIX 5.1.

Review of Statistics Fundamentals[4]

Reviewed here are essential concepts about standard errors, confidence intervals, and basic statistical tests for means. This review is condensed because most of these concepts are dealt with in introductory-level statistics courses, but a few others may be new. If something looks unfamiliar, you can review it in your statistics book. Another good resource is Thompson (2006), which offers a modern, reform-minded perspective on statistics.

Standard Errors for Means

A **standard error** is the standard deviation of a **sampling distribution**, which is a probability distribution of a statistic across all random samples drawn from the same population(s) and each based on the same number of cases (N). A standard error estimates **sampling error**, the difference between a statistic and the corresponding population parameter. These differences arise because values of sample statistics tend to vary around that of the population parameter. Some of these statistics will be too high and others too low, and only a handful will exactly equal the population value, but most should cluster around the population value. Given constant variability among population cases, sampling error varies inversely with sample size. That is, distributions of statistics from larger samples are generally narrower than distributions of the same statistic from smaller samples. This implies that statistics in large samples tend to be closer on average to the population parameter than in smaller samples. This is why larger samples are preferred over smaller ones, given equally representative sampling of cases across both.

An estimate of the population standard error in a distribution of means from random samples, or σ_M, is the statistic

$$SE_M = \sqrt{\frac{s^2}{N}} \qquad (5.1)$$

where s^2 is the sample variance, which estimates σ^2, the population variance. The denominator of s^2 equals the degrees of freedom, or $df = N - 1$,

[4]This presentation is based in part on Kline (2004, Ch. 2).

and its square root is *SD*, the sample standard deviation. Suppose in a sample of 25 cases that $M = 80.00$ and $s^2 = 81.00$. The estimated standard error of the mean is calculated as follows:

$$SE_M = (81.00/25)^{1/2} = 1.80$$

This result says that the estimated standard deviation among all random means each based on 25 cases selected from the same population is 1.80. How this information can be used to construct a confidence interval for μ, the parameter estimated by M, is considered later.

The population standard error for a distribution of random differences (contrasts) between the means of two independent samples, or $M_1 - M_2$, each based on, respectively, n_1 and n_2 cases is represented with the symbol $\sigma_{M_1 - M_2}$. It is estimated by the statistic

$$SE_{M_1 - M_2} = \sqrt{s_P^2 \left(\frac{1}{n_1} + \frac{1}{n_2} \right)} \qquad (5.2)$$

where s_P^2 is the pooled within-group variance. The latter is the average of the two variances from each group, s_1^2 and s_2^2, each weighted by their corresponding degrees of freedom, $df_1 = n_1 - 1$ and $df_2 = n_2 - 1$, as follows:

$$s_P^2 = \frac{df_1 (s_1^2) + df_2 (s_2^2)}{df_1 + df_2} = \frac{SS_W}{df_W} \qquad (5.3)$$

The numerator in the ratio to the far right in Equation 5.3, SS_W, is the pooled within-group sum of squares, and the denominator, df_W, is the pooled within-group degrees of freedom. The latter can also be expressed as $df_W = N - 2$. If the group sizes are equal ($n_1 = n_2$), then s_P^2 is just the arithmetic average of the two within-group variances, or $(s_1^2 + s_2^2)/2$. Suppose that the following data are from a between-subject design where $n_1 = n_2 = 10$:

$$M_1 - M_2 = 2.00, s_2^2 = 7.50, s_2^2 = 6.00$$

The pooled within-group variance is calculated as

$$s_p^2 = [9 \, (7.50) + 9 \, (6.00)]/(9 + 9) = (7.50 + 6.00)/2 = 6.75$$

which implies that the estimated standard error of the mean difference for this example equals:

$$SE_{M_1 - M_2} = [6.75 \, (1/10 + 1/10)]^{1/2} = 1.16$$

In words, the estimated standard deviation in the distribution of mean differences, where the first mean in each pair is based on 10 cases randomly drawn from one population and the second mean is based on 10 cases randomly drawn from a different population, equals 1.16. The next section describes how to use this information to construct a confidence for $\mu_1 - \mu_2$, the parameter estimated by $M_1 - M_2$.

Equation 5.2 applies only when the two means are from independent samples. When the means are dependent—that is, the design is within subject—then a different method must be used to estimate standard error. Below, the symbol M_D refers to the average difference score when two dependent samples are compared, and it estimates μ_D, the population mean difference score. A **difference score** is computed as $D = Y_1 - Y_2$ for each of the n cases in a repeated-measures design or for each of the n pairs of cases in a matched-groups design (assuming one-to-one matching). If $D = 0$, there is no difference; any other value indicates a higher score in one condition than in the other. The average of all D scores equals the dependent mean contrast in a within-subject design, or $M_D = M_1 - M_2$. The population standard error of mean difference scores across is σ_{M_D}, and it is estimated by

$$SE_{M_D} = \sqrt{\frac{s_D^2}{n}} \qquad (5.4)$$

where s_D^2 is the sample variance of the difference scores. This variance is calculated as

$$s_D^2 = s_1^2 + s_2^2 - 2cov_{12} \qquad (5.5)$$

where cov_{12} is the covariance of the observed scores across the two conditions. It is the product of the cross-condition correlation and the two within-condition standard deviations, or:

$$cov_{12} = r_{12}\, SD_1\, SD_2 \qquad (5.6)$$

When there is a stronger **subject effect**—the tendency for cases to maintain their relative positions (ranks) across levels of a within-subject factor—the value of r_{12} approaches 1.00.[5] This makes the variance s_D^2 get smaller, which in turn decreases the estimated standard error of the dependent mean contrast (Equations 5.4–5.5). However, the standard error for a dependent mean contrast is larger for $r_{12} \leq 0$ (i.e., cases do not maintain their rank order). Suppose that the following data are observed in a repeated-measures design where $n = 10$ cases are each tested across two different conditions:

$$M_D = 2.00,\ s_1^2 = 7.50,\ s_2^2 = 6.00,\ r_{12} = .60$$

[5]In a between-subject design, r_{12} is assumed to be zero.

Given this information, we calculate:

$$s_D^2 = 7.50 + 6.00 - 2\,(.60)\,(7.50^{1/2})\,(6.00^{1/2}) = 5.45$$

$$SE_{M_D} = (5.45/10)^{1/2} = .738$$

Note that the value of the standard error for $M_D = 2.00$ in the present example, or .738, is smaller than that of the standard error for $M_1 - M_2 = 2.00$ in the previous example, or 1.16, for the same group size and within-condition variances. This is because the value of r_{12} is positive and relatively large in the present example; that is, there is a strong subject effect. How to construct a confidence interval for μ_D is considered in the next section.

Confidence Intervals for Means

The general form of a traditional $100\,(1 - \alpha)\%$ confidence interval based on a sample statistic is

$$\text{Statistic} \pm SE_{\text{Statistic}}\,(TS_{H_0 \text{ versus two-tail } H_1,\ \alpha,\ df}) \tag{5.7}$$

where $SE_{\text{Statistic}}$ is the standard error of the statistic and the term in parentheses is the positive critical value of the relevant test statistic under the null hypothesis tested against a two-tailed (nondirectional) alternative hypothesis (H_0 vs. two-tailed H_1) at the level of statistical significance (α) and degrees of freedom for that study. The specific form of a $100\,(1 - \alpha)\%$ **confidence interval for μ** based on the mean from a single random sample is

$$M \pm SE_M\,[t_{\text{two-tail},\,\alpha}\,(N - 1)] \tag{5.8}$$

where the relevant test statistic is central t with $N - 1$ degrees of freedom. A **central-t distribution** assumes that the null hypothesis is true. Tables of critical values of t found in most books for introductory statistics are based on central-t distributions. There are also **noncentral-t distributions** that allow for the null hypothesis to be false. Noncentral-t distributions are required for confidence intervals based on effect sizes and for power analysis, too, but we will deal with this issue in the next chapter.

Because the most common levels of statistical significance are either $\alpha = .05$ or $\alpha = .01$, one usually sees in the literature either

$$100\,(1 - .05)\% = 95\% \text{ or } 100\,(1 - .01)\% = 99\%$$

confidence intervals. In general, the width of a 95% confidence interval on either side of a statistic is approximately two standard errors wide in large samples. It is also possible to construct confidence intervals that correspond to other levels of statistical significance. For example, **standard error bars** around points that represent means in graphs are sometimes each one standard error wide, which corresponds roughly to $\alpha = .32$ and a 68% confidence interval.

Suppose we find in a sample of 25 cases that $M = 80.00$ and $s^2 = 81.00$. Earlier we calculated the standard error as $SE_M = 1.80$. For a 95% confidence interval, the relevant test statistic is central t with $N - 1$ degrees of freedom, and the positive two-tailed critical value at the $\alpha = .05$ level of statistical significance is $t_{\text{two-tail}, .05}(24) = 2.064$.[6] The 95% confidence for μ is

$$80.00 \pm 1.80\,(2.064)$$

or 80.00 ± 3.72, which defines the interval 76.28–83.72. Listed next are variations on correct interpretations of this result:

1. The interval 76.28–83.72 defines a range of outcomes that should be considered equivalent to the observed result ($M = 80.00$) within the margin of expected sampling error at the 95% confidence level.

2. The interval 76.28–83.72 provides a reasonable estimate of the population mean; that is, μ could be as low as 76.28 or μ could be as high as 83.72, at the 95% confidence level. Of course, there is no guarantee that μ is actually included in this particular confidence interval. We could construct a 95% confidence interval around the mean in another sample, but the center (i.e., the mean) or endpoints of this new interval will probably be different compared with those of the original. This is because confidence intervals are subject to sampling error, too.

3. However, if 95% confidence intervals are constructed around the means of all random samples drawn from the same population, then 95/100 of them will include μ.

The last point just listed is critical for the correction interpretation of confidence intervals. It refers to a **frequentist approach to probability** as the likelihood of an outcome over repeatable events under constant conditions except for random error. That is, an event's probability is based on its expected relative frequency over a large number of trials, or "in the long run." From this perspective, it is *incorrect* to say that there is a .95 probability (95% chance) that the interval 76.28–83.72 contains μ. This is

[6]There are several freely available Web probability calculators that calculate critical values of central test distributions, including z (i.e., a normal curve), t, F, and χ^2, for user-specified levels of α; for example, see *statpages.org/#Tables*

because this particular interval either contains μ or it does not. That is, the probability is either 0 or 1.0 that the value of μ falls somewhere between 76.28 and 83.72. The numerals ".95" or "95%" associated with this interval apply as a probability or chance statement only across a set of confidence intervals each constructed the same way in random samples with the same number of cases.[7]

There is a related error for confidence intervals known as the **confidence-level misconception** (Cumming & Maillardet, 2006). In the case of the 95% confidence interval for μ we just calculated, this false belief would be stated as follows: The interval 76.28–83.72 contains 95% of all replications. This view is wrong because although this interval will contain some proportion of replication means, the actual proportion is typically much less than 95%. This is because two types of sampling error are operating here, including (1) the difference between the original mean ($M = 80.00$) and μ, and (2) the variability of replication means around μ. For example, a particular confidence interval will contain more of the replication means if both the original mean and replication means fall close to μ, and it will contain fewer if neither condition holds. Although a particular 95% confidence interval for μ *may* contain the majority of replication means, the actual percentage is usually less than .95. See Thompson (2006, pp. 203–207) for more information on misconceptions about confidence intervals.

The general form of a $100 \, (1 - \alpha)\%$ **confidence interval for $\mu_1 - \mu_2$** based on the difference between two independent means is

$$(M_1 - M_2) \pm [t_{\text{two-tail}, \, \alpha} \, (N - 2)] \tag{5.9}$$

where the relevant test statistic is central t with $N - 2$ degrees of freedom (i.e., df_W). Suppose that the following data are from a two-group design where $n_1 = n_2 = 10$:

$$M_1 - M_2 = 2.00, \, s_1^2 = 7.50, \, s_2^2 = 6.00, \, s_P^2 = 6.75, \, SE_{M_1 - M_2} = 1.16$$

The relevant test statistic for the 95% confidence interval for $\mu_1 - \mu_2$ is central t with 18 degrees of freedom, and the positive two-tailed critical value is $t_{\text{two-tail}, \, .05} \, (18) = 2.101$. The 95% confidence interval for this example is computed as:

$$2.00 \pm 1.16 \, (2.101)$$

---

[7]Here is a simple example: Flip a coin in the air, catch it, and slap it down on your wrist without looking at the outcome. Now guess heads or tails. What is the probability that your guess is correct? It is *not* .50 because your guess is either right or wrong. (Now you can look.) The ".50" applies only in the long run over a series of guesses: You should be right about half the time across all trials.

or 2.00 ± 2.44, which defines the interval $-.44$–4.44. Based on these results, we can say that $\mu_1 - \mu_2$ could be as low as $-.44$ or $\mu_1 - \mu_2$ could be as high as 4.44, with 95% confidence. Note that this interval includes zero as a reasonable estimate of $\mu_1 - \mu_2$. This fact is subject to misinterpretation. For example, it would be *wrong* to conclude that $\mu_1 - \mu_2 = 0$ just because zero falls between the lower and upper bounds of this particular confidence interval. This is because zero is only one value within a range of estimates, so in this sense it has no special status. Besides, the interval $-.44$–4.44 is itself subject to sampling error, and zero may not be included within the 95% confidence interval for $\mu_1 - \mu_2$ in a replication.

The general form of a $100(1 - \alpha)\%$ **confidence interval for μ_D** based on the difference between two dependent means is

$$M_D \pm SE_{M_D} [t_{\text{two-tail}, \alpha} (n - 1)] \tag{5.10}$$

Suppose that these data are from a two-condition repeated-measures design where $n = 10$:

$$M_D = 2.00, s_1^2 = 7.50, s_2^2 = 6.00, r_{12} = .60, s_D^2 = 5.45, SE_{M_D} = .738$$

The relevant test statistic here is central t with 9 degrees of freedom, and the positive two-tailed critical value is $t_{\text{two-tail}, .05}(9) = 2.262$. Thus, the 95% confidence interval for this example is

$$2.00 \pm .738 (2.262)$$

which defines the interval 2.00 ± 1.67, or $.33$–3.67. Note that the 95% confidence interval assuming a within-subject design is narrower than the 95% confidence interval calculated earlier for a between-subject design with the same mean contrast, within-condition variances, and group size ($-.44$–4.44). This result is expected due to the strong subject in the repeated-measures data.

Statistical Tests for Comparing Means

Reviewed next are characteristics of t-tests and F-tests for comparing means. The basic principles generalize to other kinds of statistical tests.

t-Tests

The t-tests described here compare two means from either independent or dependent samples. Both are special cases of the F-test for means. Specifically, $t^2 = F$ when both test statistics are calculated for the same mean contrast. The general form of the independent-samples t-test is

$$t(N-2) = \frac{(M_1 - M_2) - (\mu_1 - \mu_2)}{SE_{M_1 - M_2}} \qquad (5.11)$$

where $N-2$ is df_W, the pooled within-group degrees of freedom, and $\mu_1 - \mu_2$ is the population mean difference specified in the null hypothesis. If the latter is predicted to be zero (e.g., H_0: $\mu_1 - \mu_2 = 0$), then this expression drops out of the equation. The general form of the dependent-samples t-test is

$$t(n-1) = \frac{M_D - \mu_D}{SE_{M_D}} \qquad (5.12)$$

where n is the number of pairs of scores and μ_D is the population average difference score specified in the null hypothesis. For the null hypothesis H_0: $\mu_D = 0$, the latter term drops out of the equation. Both versions of the t-test are a kind of **critical ratio**, which is the ratio of a statistic over its standard error. A critical ratio is perhaps the most basic form of a statistical test. Critical ratios for means follow t-distributions when the population variance is unknown, but critical ratios for other kinds of statistics may be distributed as other kinds of test statistics, such as z in a normal curve. (Means are distributed as z when the population standard deviation is known.) The statistical assumptions of the t-test for either independent or dependent samples are the same as those for the independent-samples F-test (independence, normality, homogeneity of variance).

Both t-tests just defined express a mean difference as the proportion of its standard error. For example, $t = 2.50$ says that the observed mean contrast is two and a half times greater than its standard error. It also says that the first mean (M_1) is two and a half standard errors higher than the second mean (M_2). The standard error metric of t is affected by the sample size and whether the means are independent or dependent. Specifically, this standard error is less (1) when the sample size is larger or (2) the means are dependent *and* the cross-condition correlation is positive ($r_{12} > 0$), holding all else constant. As the standard error gets smaller, the value of t increases in absolute value when the mean contrast is not zero. This explains the relative power advantage of the t-test for dependent samples over that of the t-test for independent samples.

There is a special relation between confidence intervals for means and the t-test for means: Whether a $100(1 - \alpha)\%$ confidence interval includes zero always yields an outcome equivalent to either rejecting or not rejecting the corresponding null hypothesis (Thompson, 2006), assuming a two-tailed alternative hypothesis. For example, these data are from independent samples each with 10 cases:

$$M_1 - M_2 = 2.00, \; s_1^2 = 7.50, \; s_2^2 = 6.00, \; s_p^2 = 6.75, \; SE_{M_1 - M_2} = 1.16$$

Earlier we calculated for these data the 95% confidence interval for $\mu_1 - \mu_2$, which is –.44–4.44. Because zero falls within this interval, we can predict that the outcome of the independent-samples t-test for these data will not be statistically significant at the .05 level. Let us confirm this prediction: For these data, the value of t for the observed mean contrast is:

$$t\,(18) = 2.00/1.16 = 1.721$$

The positive critical value at the .05 level for the two-tailed alternative hypothesis H_1: $\mu_1 - \mu_2 \neq 0$ is $t_{\text{two-tail, .05}}\,(18) = 2.101$. Because the empirical (calculated) value of t is less than the positive critical value (i.e., $1.721 < 2.101$), we fail to reject the null hypothesis for these data.

As noted by Thompson (2006), do not falsely believe that confidence intervals are just statistical tests in a different guise. One reason is that a null hypothesis is required for a statistical test, but it is not for a confidence interval. Another is that the particular null hypothesis associated with a statistical test may have no substantive scientific value. For example, men and women differ on several cognitive, personality, and health-related variables. In the study of these variables, the null hypothesis of equal population means by gender, such as H_0: $\mu_W - \mu_M = 0$, may be so implausible that it could be dismissed even before the data are collected. Confidence intervals have the additional advantage that the degree of imprecision associated with a statistic is plain for all to see. Information about sampling error also contributes to a statistical test, but it winds up "hidden" when just values of test statistics and associated probabilities are reported.

There is a common rule of thumb which says that the difference between two independent means is statistically significant at the α level if there is no overlap of the two $100\,(1 - \alpha)\%$ confidence intervals for μ. It also maintains that overlap of the two intervals indicates that the mean contrast is not statistically significant at the corresponding level of α. This rule is often applied to diagrams where confidence intervals for μ are represented as error bars extending outward from dots that represent group means. Although widely believed, this rule is actually false. For the specific case of $\alpha = .05$, (1) nonoverlap of two 95% confidence intervals for μ does indicate a statistically significant contrast, but with a probability quite a bit less than .05; and (2) overlap of the two intervals does not automatically indicate that the contrast is not statistically significant (Belia, Fidler, Williams, & Cumming, 2005).

F-Tests

The t-test compares only two means; that is, it analyzes contrasts (focused comparisons) only. The F-test can analyze contrasts, too, but only the F-test can also analyze omnibus comparisons, in which three or more means are compared for equality. Suppose that factor A has $a = 3$ levels. The F-test for the omnibus effect evaluates the null hypothesis H_0: $\mu_1 = \mu_2 = \mu_3$. Rejecting this null hypothesis implies only that differences among the observed means, M_1, M_2, and M_3, are unlikely assuming equal population means. This result alone may not be very informative. This is why researchers often choose to analyze contrasts after analyzing the omnibus effect, or they may ignore the omnibus effect and analyze contrasts only.

The general form of the F-test for the omnibus effect in designs with a single fixed-effects factor and independent samples is

$$F\,(df_A, df_W) = \frac{MS_A}{MS_W} \tag{5.13}$$

where df_A and df_W are, respectively, the degrees of freedom for the numerator and denominator of F. The former equals the number of levels of factor A minus one, or $df_A = (a - 1)$, and the latter is the pooled within-group degrees of freedom, which can be calculated as $df_W = N - a$.

The numerator of F is the between-group (condition) mean square. Its equation is

$$MS_A = \frac{SS_A}{df_A} = \frac{\sum_{i=1}^{a} n_i\,(M_i - M_T)^2}{a - 1} \tag{5.14}$$

where SS_A is the between-group sum of squares; n_i and M_i are, respectively, the size and mean of the ith condition; and M_T is the grand mean for the total dataset, or the average of all N scores. The term MS_A reflects group size and sources of variability that give rise to unequal group means, such as a systematic effect of factor A or sampling error. It is the denominator of F, the pooled within-group mean square, or MS_W, that measures only unexplained variance. This is because cases within the same group are treated alike, such as when patients in a treatment group are all given the same medication. Because a drug is a constant for these patients, it cannot explain individual differences among them. For this reason, the denominator of F is often referred to as the **error term**. The equation is

$$MS_W = \frac{\sum_{i=1}^{a} df_i\,\left(s_i^2\right)}{N - a} = \frac{SS_W}{df_W} \tag{5.15}$$

where df_i and s_i^2 are, respectively, the degrees of freedom (i.e., $n_i - 1$) and the variance of the ith group. Note in Equation 5.15 that group size contributes to both the numerator (SS_W) and denominator (df_W), which effectively cancels out its impact on the error term. The total sum of squares, SS_T, reflects the amount of variability in the total dataset. It is the sum of squared deviations of the individual scores from the grand mean; it also equals $SS_A + SS_W$. We will see in the next chapter that SS_T is important for effect size estimation with descriptive measures of association in studies where ANOVA is used.

In one-way designs with three or more groups, it is common practice for researchers to first test the omnibus effect and, if it is statistically significant, then test all possible pairwise comparisons for statistical significance. These post hoc tests are often conducted using a method that controls for inflation of Type I error due to multiple testing, such as the Newman–Keuls procedure or the Scheffé procedure. However, Wilkinson and the Task Force on Statistical Inference (1999) noted that this tactic is typically *wrong*. Not only does this approach make the individual comparisons unnecessarily conservative when a post hoc method is used, but it is rare that all such contrasts are interesting. The cost for reducing Type I error across all comparisons is reduced power for the specific tests the researcher really cares about. It is better to evaluate just the contrasts of substantive interest.

In within-subject designs with a single fixed-effects factor, the between-condition variance, MS_A, and the within-condition variance, MS_W, are calculated the same way as in a between-subject design (see Equations 5.14–5.15). However, the latter no longer reflects just unexplained variance when the samples are dependent, so it is not the error term in the F-test for dependent samples. This is because of the subject effect, which in a single-factor design is manifested in positive covariances between every pair of conditions (see Equation 5.6). For within-subject factors with three or more levels, the average covariance across all pairs of conditions, M_{cov}, estimates the subject effect. Removing this effect from the pooled within-condition variance (literally, $MS_W - M_{cov}$) generates the error term for the dependent-samples F-test. The resulting error term reflects inconsistent performance across the conditions, or the degree to which cases do not maintain their relative positions. Such inconsistency could be due to random error or an effect of factor A that is not the same for all cases. The latter could occur due to an interaction between the independent variable and some *unmeasured* characteristic of cases. If the effects of a drug depend on age, for example, then the performance of younger versus older cases may not be consistent across different dosages of the drug. A conditional effect of factor A is referred to here as the **A × subject (S) interaction**.

We can now define the general form of the dependent-samples F-test:

$$F\,(df_A,\,df_{A \times S}) = \frac{MS_A}{MS_{A \times S}} \tag{5.16}$$

where $df_{A \times S} = (a - 1)(n - 1)$ and $MS_{A \times S} = MS_W - M_{cov}$. The error term can also be expressed as

$$MS_{A \times S} = \frac{SS_{A \times S}}{df_{A \times S}} = \frac{SS_W - SS_S}{df_W - df_S} \tag{5.17}$$

where SS_S is the sum of squares for the subject effect with $df_S = (n - 1)$ degrees of freedom. Equation 5.17 shows the removal of the subject effect from the pooled within-condition variance in a dependent-samples design. If the subject effect is large, then the value of $MS_{A \times S}$ may be small relative to that of MS_W. This accounts for the generally greater power of the dependent-samples F-test compared with the independent-samples F-test. When there are at least three levels of a within-subject factor, the F-test for the omnibus effect assumes sphericity.

Statistical Tests and Effect Size

It can be shown that many test statistics can be expressed as the product

$$\text{Test statistic} = f(N) \times \text{ES} \tag{5.18}$$

where $f(N)$ is a function of sample size for a particular test statistic and ES is an effect size index that expresses the degree of discrepancy between the data and the null hypothesis in a standardized metric. Specific effect size statistics are introduced in the next chapter, but for now consider these implications of Equation 5.18:

1. Holding sample size constant, absolute values of test statistics increase with no upper bound and their associated probabilities approach zero as the effect size increases.

2. Holding constant a nonzero effect size, increasing the sample size causes the same change in test statistics and their associated probabilities.

These implications explain how it is possible for even trivial effects to be statistically significant in large samples. They also explain how even large effects may not be statistically significant in small samples. That is, statistical significance by itself says very little about effect size.

CHAPTER 6

Effect Size Estimation

The way psychologists report and interpret research is changing. More and more, they are considering effect sizes as critical for effective research interpretation, and single *p* values are often of little value in the grand research scheme.

—Robin K. Henson (2006, p. 604)

This chapter deals with an important aspect of statistics reform, the estimation of effect size. In experimental studies, effect size refers to the magnitude of the impact of the independent variable on the dependent variable. It can also be described as the degree of covariation between variables of interest in nonexperimental designs. Three types of parametric effect size indexes for continuous outcome variables are described, standardized mean differences, measures of association, and proportion effect sizes for case-level analyses. Nonparametric effect sizes for categorical outcomes, such as relapsed–not relapsed, are also described. The kinds of effect sizes just mentioned are among the most widely reported in the literature. Also dealt with here is how to construct confidence intervals for effect sizes. Effect sizes are subject to sampling error, too, and reporting them as both point estimates and interval estimates directly conveys this reality. Examples of effect size estimation in actual empirical studies are also presented.

Contexts for Estimating Effect Size

Effect size estimation is an increasingly important topic in several different research areas, including counseling psychology (Henson, 2006) and biological psychiatry (Kraemer & Kupfer, 2005), among others. It offers a way to offset some of the limitations of statistical tests. One is the fact that statistical tests measure the contribution of both sample size and effect size together (Chapter 5). The assessment of the magnitude of an effect apart from the influence of sample size distinguishes effect size estimation. Both effect size estimation and interval estimation are also described as better ways to communicate results of empirical studies to social policymakers than through use of statistical tests (McCartney & Rosenthal, 2000). This is in part because some effect size statistics are nothing more than proportions, which need little background in statistics in order to understand. Other effect size indexes, though, are basically standard deviations or correlations, so an understanding of these kinds of descriptive statistics is required.

The most recent edition (fifth) of the *Publication Manual* of the American Psychological Association (APA; 2005) cited the absence of effect size information as a study defect (p. 5); it also noted that effect sizes should "almost always" be reported (p. 23).[1] An exception would be in some complex repeated-measures or multivariate designs where it is difficult or impossible to compute effect sizes (Fidler, 2002). However, such cases are relatively rare, and effect size can be estimated in most behavioral studies. Earlier editions of the *Publication Manual* also called for the reporting of effect size, but there was little indication in the 1980s–1990s that authors actually heeded this call (Kirk, 1996). However, it seems that more authors are doing so now, especially in applied psychology journals (Dunleavy, Barr, Glenn, & Miller, 2006). An even stronger statement is apparent in the editorial policies of about a dozen research journals that now *require* the reporting of effect sizes (e.g., Trusty, Thompson, & Petrocelli, 2004).

The idea of effect size is crucial in an a priori power analysis, which requires specification of the expected population effect size (Chapter 5). These estimates are often expressed as population parameters of the statistics described here. A related context is that of meta-analysis, in which a common problem is that results about the same basic outcome are of-

---

[1]Likewise, the International Committee of Medical Journal Editors (2006) advised authors to "avoid relying solely on statistical hypothesis testing, such as the use of p values, which fails to convey important information about effect size" (pp. 27–28).

ten reported in different metrics across a set of studies. Some effect size indexes are standardized or metric-free statistics, which allows for direct comparison of results originally measured on different scales. This is why both the central tendency and variability of standardized effect sizes are estimated in perhaps most meta-analytic studies.

Families of Parametric Effect Sizes[2]

Presentations about effect size are often chock full of equations. This is because there are typically different methods to calculate the same effect size statistic. Some methods require complete descriptive statistics from the groups, but other methods require only test statistics and group sizes. However, these different methods generate the same value of a particular effect size statistic for the same data. Also, there are just a handful of various effect size indexes that are reported most often, and these essential statistics are emphasized next.

There are three general kinds of parametric effect sizes for comparative studies with continuous outcomes. Two of these are for analysis at the level of groups or variables, and they include **standardized mean differences** and **measures of association**. These two categories are also referred to as, respectively, *d*-**family effect sizes** and *r*-**family effect sizes** (Rosenthal, Rosnow, & Rubin, 2000) and also as, respectively, **group difference indexes** and **relationship indexes** (Huberty, 2002). The third kind is for analysis at the case level. This type of analysis involves the comparison of the proportions of scores from two different groups that fall above or below certain reference points, such as the median of one group. These statistics are referred to as **group overlap indexes** (Huberty, 2002), and they are usually suitable for communication with audiences with little background in statistics. In contrast, one needs to know about standard deviations and correlations in order to understand *d*-family or *r*-family effect sizes.

Standardized Mean Differences

A population standardized mean difference is represented by the lower-case Greek letter delta (δ), and its general form is

$$\delta = \frac{\mu_1 - \mu_2}{\sigma *} \qquad (6.1)$$

[2]Part of this presentation is based on Kline (2004, pp. 95–101).

where the numerator is the population mean contrast and the denominator is a population standard deviation. There is more than one possible population standard deviation for a comparative study. For instance, σ^* could be the standard deviation in just one of the populations (e.g., $\sigma^* = \sigma_1$) or, assuming homogeneity of variance, it could be the common population standard deviation (i.e., $\sigma^* = \sigma_1 = \sigma_2 = \sigma$). The general form of a sample standardized mean difference is

$$d = \frac{M_1 - M_2}{SD^*} \qquad (6.2)$$

where the numerator is the observed mean contrast and the denominator SD^* is an estimate of σ^* that is not the same in all kinds of d statistics.[3] Because d compares just two means at a time, it is most useful in the analysis of focused comparisons, such as treatment versus no treatment. Measures of association are generally more useful for omnibus comparisons in which means from three or more conditions or groups are simultaneously compared.

A d statistic expresses a mean contrast as the proportion of a standard deviation on the variable along which it is measured. If $d = .60$, for instance, then M_1 is .6 standard deviations higher than M_2. The sign of d is arbitrary because it is determined by the direction of the subtraction, which is itself arbitrary. Always indicate the meaning of its sign when reporting d. Note that d can exceed 1.0 in absolute value. For example, $d = 1.5$ says that the mean contrast is 1½ standard deviations large. The standard deviation metric of d makes it generally insensitive to group size, keeping all else constant. In contrast, the standard error metric of the t-test is affected by group size (Chapter 5). This means that d measures just the magnitude of a mean contrast, not also the sizes of the groups on which it is based.

Measures of Association

A measure of association describes the degree of covariation between two variables. It is usually expressed in either an unsquared metric or a squared metric. (The metric of d is unsquared.) In samples, an unsquared measure of association is typically a correlation coefficient. For example, the Pearson correlation r indicates the strength of the relation between

---

[3]Note that some authors use the term "Cohen's d" to refer to sample standardized mean differences. This is not technically correct because J. Cohen (1988) used the symbol d to represent a population standardized mean difference.

two continuous variables, and its square, r^2, is the observed proportion of explained (shared) variance. The parameter estimated by r^2 is rho-squared (ρ^2), the population proportion of explained variance. A squared measure of association is also referred to as a **variance-accounted-for effect size**. Unless a correlation is zero, its square is less than its original (unsquared) absolute value (e.g., if $r = .10$, then $r^2 = .01$). Squared correlations can make some effects look smaller than they really are in terms of their substantive significance. For example, it may not seem impressive to explain only 1% of the variance, but effects so "small" can actually be important. Rutledge and Loh (2004) described several studies in medicine considered as landmark investigations where variance-accounted-for effect sizes were only about 1%.

In comparative studies in which ANOVA is used, the square of the sample multiple correlation R, or R^2, is often called the **correlation ratio**. (Recall that ANOVA is just a special case of multiple regression.) Another name for the same statistic is **estimated eta-squared**, or $\hat{\eta}^2$. The symbol $\hat{\eta}^2$ is used here instead of R^2 because the former is seen more often in the ANOVA literature than the latter. The parameter estimated by $\hat{\eta}^2$ is η^2, the population proportion of explained variance when all factors are fixed, not random (d is also for fixed-effects factors). The general form of η^2 is

$$\eta^2 = \frac{\sigma^2_{\text{effect}}}{\sigma^2_{\text{total}}} \tag{6.3}$$

where the numerator is the variance due to the effect of interest and the denominator is the variance of the dependent variable computed about the population grand mean.

The most general form of a sample measure of association for comparative studies is

$$\hat{\eta}^2 = \frac{SS_{\text{effect}}}{SS_T} \tag{6.4}$$

where the numerator is the sum of squares for the effect of interest and the denominator is the total sum of squares for the whole design. The value of $\hat{\eta}^2$ is the proportion of total observed variance explained by the effect, and its square root, $\hat{\eta}$, is the correlation between that effect and the outcome variable. If the degrees of freedom for the effect are greater than one ($df > 1$), then $\hat{\eta}$ is just a multiple correlation (R); otherwise, $\hat{\eta}$ is a bivariate correlation (r) between the effect and the dependent variable. An example follows.

Suppose that in a design with a single factor A there are two treatment groups and two control groups. It is found for the omnibus effect with three degrees of freedom ($df_A = 3$) that the between-group sum of squares is $SS_A = 30.00$ and the within-group sum of squares is $SS_W = 175.00$. Here

$$\hat{\eta}_A^2 = 30.00/(30.00 + 175.00) = 30.00/205.00 = .146$$

which says that factor A explains about 14.6% of the total variance, and the multiple correlation between this factor and the dependent variable is about $\hat{\eta}_A = .146^{1/2}$, or .383. The statistic $\hat{\eta}^2$ can be calculated in basically *any* design with fixed factors where ANOVA is conducted. This flexibility of application makes $\hat{\eta}^2$ perhaps the most universal of all the effect size indexes described here. And $\hat{\eta}^2$ is so easy to calculate that it is remarkable that researchers do not always report it for each and every use of ANOVA in comparative studies.

Because of **capitalization on chance**, $\hat{\eta}^2$ is generally a positively biased estimator of η^2, which means that the expected value of $\hat{\eta}^2$ across all random samples is greater than that of η^2. This happens because when a correlation is calculated, its value reflects all possible predictive power. In doing so, it takes advantage of variability that may be idiosyncratic in the sample. This is a greater problem when the sample size is small. There are various methods that generate corrected estimates of η^2 that are generally functions of $\hat{\eta}^2$, the number of groups or their variances, and group size. The best known of these bias-adjusted estimators for designs with fixed-factors is **estimated omega-squared** ($\hat{\omega}^2$). In general, the value of $\hat{\omega}^2$ is lower than that of $\hat{\eta}^2$ for the same result. However, the difference between $\hat{\omega}^2$ and $\hat{\eta}^2$ gets smaller as the sample size increases. In large samples, their values are practically the same; that is, bias correction is unnecessary in large samples. We will deal with the $\hat{\omega}^2$ statistic later.

Estimating Effect Size When Comparing Two Samples[4]

This section deals with effect size estimation when two independent samples, such as treatment group and a control group, are compared on a continuous outcome variable. These methods also apply to the comparison of two dependent samples, such as when each case is tested under two different conditions. If so, then effect sizes when studying some phe-

---

[4]Part of this presentation is based on Kline (2004, pp. 101–104, 114–116).

nomenon using a between-subject design are comparable with effect sizes when studying the same phenomenon using a within-subject design. Some special methods for dependent samples are not covered here, but see Kline (2004, pp. 104–107) or Morris (2000). However, these special methods are not used as often as the ones described next.

Group-Level Indexes

The particular d statistic reported most often in the literature is probably **Hedges's g**. It estimates the parameter $\delta = (\mu_1 - \mu_2)/\sigma$ where σ is the common population standard deviation; that is, it is assumed that $\sigma_1 = \sigma_2 = \sigma$. The equation for g is

$$g = \frac{M_1 - M_2}{\sqrt{s_P^2}} \tag{6.5}$$

where the denominator is the square root of the pooled within-group variance. This statistic (s_P^2) estimates σ^2 and assumes homogeneity of population variance. Its equation is

$$s_P^2 = \frac{df_1 \left(s_1^2\right) + df_2 \left(s_2^2\right)}{df_1 + df_2} = \frac{SS_W}{df_W} \tag{6.6}$$

where $df_1 = n_1 - 1$, $df_2 = n_2 - 1$, and SS_W and df_W are, respectively, the pooled within-group sum of squares and degrees of freedom. The latter can also be expressed as $df_W = N - 2$. Another way to calculate g requires only the group sizes and the value of the independent-samples t $(N - 2)$ statistic for the test of the nil hypothesis H_0: $\mu_1 - \mu_2 = 0$, or:

$$g = t \sqrt{\frac{1}{n_1} + \frac{1}{n_2}} \tag{6.7}$$

Equation 6.7 is useful when working with secondary sources, such as journal articles, that do not report sufficient group descriptive statistics to use Equations 6.5–6.6. Solving Equation 6.7 for t represents this test statistic as a function of effect size (g) and group size (n_1, n_2).

Hedges's g is a positively biased estimator of the population standardized mean difference δ, but the degree of this bias is slight unless the group size is small, such as $n < 20$. The following statistic is an approximate unbiased estimator of δ:

$$\hat{\delta} = \left(1 - \frac{3}{4df_W - 1}\right) g \tag{6.8}$$

where the term in parentheses is a correction factor applied to g. For $n = 10$, the correction factor equals .9578, but for $n = 20$ it is .9801. For even larger group sizes, the correction factor is close to 1.0, which implies little adjustment for bias.

Suppose for a two-group design that

$$M_1 - M_2 = 7.50, n_1 = 20, n_2 = 25, s_1^2 = 100.00, s_2^2 = 110.00$$

which implies $s_P^2 = 105.58$ and $t\,(43) = 2.43$. (You should verify these facts.) Hedges's g for these data is calculated as:

$$g = 7.50/105.58^{1/2} = 2.43\,(1/20 + 1/25)^{1/2} = .73$$

In other words, the size of the mean contrast is about .73 standard deviations. As an exercise, show that the value of the approximate unbiased estimator of δ is very similar for these data ($\hat{\delta} = .72$).

A second standardized mean difference is **Glass's delta**, which is often represented with the symbol Δ even though it is a sample statistic. The parameter estimated by Δ is the ratio of the population mean contrast over the standard deviation of just one of the populations, usually that for the control condition. In this case, Δ estimates $\delta = (\mu_1 - \mu_2)/\sigma_C$, and the equation for Δ is

$$\Delta = \frac{M_1 - M_2}{SD_C} \tag{6.9}$$

where the denominator is the control group standard deviation. Because SD_C comes from just one group, homogeneity of variance is not assumed. Accordingly, Δ may be preferred over g when treatment affects both central tendency and variability. Suppose that most treated cases improve, others show no change, but some get worse, perhaps due to treatment itself. This pattern may increase the variability of treated cases compared with untreated cases. In this case, Δ based on the control group standard deviation describes the effect of treatment on central tendency only. Otherwise, g is generally preferred over Δ because the denominator of g is based on more information, the variances of the two groups instead of just one. In a study where

$$M_1 - M_2 = 7.50, n_1 = 20, n_2 = 25, s_1^2 = 100.00, s_2^2 = 110.00$$

and the control condition corresponds to the first group, then

$$\Delta = 7.50/100.00^{1/2} = .75$$

Recall for the same data that $g = .73$. The two d statistics have different values here because Δ reflects the variability of just the control group.

A correlation effect size for two-group designs is the **point-biserial correlation,** r_{pb}. It can be derived using the standard equation for the Pearson correlation r if group membership is coded as 0 or 1. Its value indicates the correlation between membership in one of two different groups and a continuous outcome variable. A more conceptual equation is

$$r_{pb} = \left(\frac{M_1 - M_2}{\sqrt{s_T^2}} \right) \sqrt{pq} \qquad (6.10)$$

where s_T^2 is the variance of the total dataset (i.e., scores from both groups combined) computed as SS_T/N, and p and q are the proportions of cases in each group ($p + q = 1.0$). Note that the expression in parentheses in Equation 6.10 is actually a d statistic where the denominator estimates the full range of variability. It is the multiplication of this d statistic by the standard deviation of the dichotomous factor, $(pq)^{1/2}$, that transforms the whole expression to correlation units. This correlation can also be computed from the value of the independent-samples t ($N - 2$) statistic and the pooled within-group degrees of freedom as follows:

$$r_{pb} = \frac{t}{\sqrt{t^2 + df_W}} \qquad (6.11)$$

Another variation involves the independent-samples F (1, df_W) statistic for the mean contrast:

$$| \, r_{pb} \, | = \sqrt{\frac{F}{F + df_W}} = \sqrt{\frac{SS_A}{SS_T}} = \hat{\eta} \qquad (6.12)$$

Equation 6.12 shows the absolute value of r_{pb} as a special case of $\hat{\eta}$, the square root of the correlation ratio. Unlike r_{pb}, however, $\hat{\eta}$ is an **unsigned correlation**, so it is insensitive to the direction of the mean difference. The correlation r_{pb} is a **signed correlation**, so always explain the meaning of its sign when reporting r_{pb}.

Suppose that these data are from a two-group design:

$M_1 - M_2 = 7.50$, $n_1 = 20$, $n_2 = 25$, $s_1^2 = 100.00$, $s_2^2 = 110.00$, t (43) = 2.43, $g = .73$

There are a few ways to calculate r_{pb} for these data:

$$r_{pb} = 2.43/(2.43^2 + 43)^{1/2} = .73/[.73^2 + 43 \, (1/20 + 1/25)]^{1/2} = .35$$

This result says that the correlation between group membership and the outcome variable is about .35; thus, the former explains about $.35^2 = .123$, or 12.3% of the variance in the latter. This effect size expressed in correlation units is equivalent to the effect size expressed in standard deviation units for the same data. That is, $r_{pb} = .35$ and $g = .73$ both describe the magnitude of the same effect but on different scales.

For the same data, it is possible to transform a standard deviation effect size to a correlation effect size, and vice versa. The following equation transforms r_{pb} to g:

$$g = r_{pb}^2 \sqrt{\left(\frac{df_W}{1 - r_{pb}^2}\right)\left(\frac{1}{n_1} + \frac{1}{n_2}\right)} \tag{6.13}$$

Likewise, this next equation transforms g to r_{pb}:

$$r_{pb} = \frac{g}{\sqrt{g^2 + df_W\left(\frac{1}{n_1} + \frac{1}{n_2}\right)}} \tag{6.14}$$

Equations 6.13–6.14 are handy when effect size is measured in one metric, but the researcher wishes to describe results in the other metric.

The value of r_{pb} is affected by the proportion of cases in one group or the other, p and q (see Equation 6.10), but g is not. It (r_{pb}) tends to be highest in balanced designs with equal group sizes, or $p = q = .50$. As the group sizes become more unequal, holding all else constant, r_{pb} approaches zero. For this reason, r_{pb} is described as **margin bound** because its value is affected by changes in relative group size. This implies that values of r_{pb} may not be directly comparable across studies with dissimilar relative group sizes. In this case, g may be preferred over r_{pb}. The value of r_{pb} is also affected by group size when the latter is small, such as $n < 20$. This reflects a general characteristic of correlations: They approach their maximum absolute values in very small samples. In the extreme case where the group size is $n = 1$ and the two scores are not equal, $r_{pb} = \pm 1.00$. This happens for mathematical reasons and is not real evidence for a perfect association.

The statistic r_{pb}^2 is a positively biased estimator of the population proportion of explained variance, and the degree of this bias is greater in smaller samples. But estimated omega-squared, $\hat{\omega}^2$, is a bias-corrected estimate that takes account of sample size. The value of $\hat{\omega}^2$ may be substantially less than that of r_{pb}^2 for the same data when the group sizes are small, such as $n < 10$. For much larger group sizes, the values of r_{pb}^2 and $\hat{\omega}^2$ are generally more similar. The statistic $\hat{\omega}^2$ assumes a balanced design, but r_{pb}^2 does not. An equation for $\hat{\omega}^2$ that is good for any effect in a completely between-subject design with fixed factors is presented next:

$$\hat{\omega}_{\text{effect}}^2 = \frac{df_{\text{effect}}(MS_{\text{effect}} + MS_W)}{SS_T + MS_W} \quad (6.15)$$

where df_{effect} and MS_{effect} are, respectively, the degrees of freedom and the mean square for the effect of interest, and MS_W is the total within-group mean square. In two-group designs, the mean contrast is the sole effect (i.e., $df_{\text{effect}} = 1$), and $\hat{\omega}^2$ can be computed from the independent-samples $t\ (N - 2)$ statistic as follows:

$$\hat{\omega}^2 = \frac{t^2}{t^2 + N - 1} \quad (6.16)$$

These data are from a balanced two-group design:

$$M_1 - M_2 = 7.50,\ n_1 = n_2 = 10,\ s_1^2 = 100.00,\ s_2^2 = 110.00$$

which implies $t\ (18) = 1.64$, $r_{pb} = .36$, and $r_{pb}^2 = .130$. (Verify these results.) Thus, the observed proportion of explained variance is about 13.0%. We calculate $\hat{\omega}^2$ for these data as follows:

$$\hat{\omega}^2 = (1.64^2 - 1)/(1.64^2 + 20 - 1) = .078$$

which indicates only about 7.8% explained variance taking account of group size, which is here quite small ($n = 10$). The statistic $\hat{\omega}^2$ may be preferred over r_{pb}^2 when the group size is not large.

Case-Level Indexes[5]

Standardized mean differences and measures of association describe effect size at the group level. Consequently, they do not directly reflect the status of individual cases, and there are times when group-level effects do not tell the whole story. However, it is possible to also evaluate group differences at the case level. The two group overlap indexes described next do so through the comparison of proportions of scores from two different

---

[5]Part of this presentation is based on Kline (2004, pp. 122–132).

groups that fall above or below certain reference points. These proportions also describe the relative amounts of the overlap of two distributions. If the overlap is small, the two distributions are relatively distinct at the case level. If overlap is substantial, though, then the groups are not distinct at the case level.

Presented in Figure 6.1 are two pairs of frequency distributions that each illustrate one of J. Cohen's (1988) measures of overlap, U_1 and U_3. Both pairs of distributions show a higher mean in one group than in the other, normal distributions, and equal group sizes and variances. The shaded regions in Figure 6.1(a) represent areas where the two distributions do *not* overlap, and U_1 is the proportion of scores across both groups that fall within these areas. The difference $1 - U_1$ is thus the proportion of scores within the area of overlap. If the group mean contrast is zero, then $U_1 = 0$, but if the mean difference is so great that no scores overlap, then $U_1 = 1.00$. The range of U_1 is thus 0–1.00. Figure 6.1(b) illustrates U_3, the proportion of scores in the lower group exceeded by a typical score, such as the median, in the upper group. If the two distributions are identical, then $U_3 = .50$; if $U_3 = 1.00$, however, the medians are so different that the typical score in the upper group exceeds all scores in the lower group. In actual datasets, U_1 and U_3 are derived by inspecting group frequency

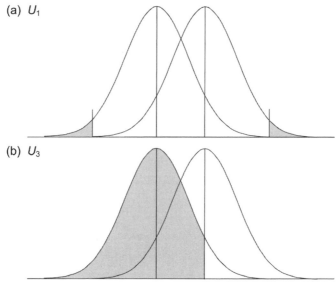

(a) U_1

(b) U_3

FIGURE 6.1. Measures of distribution overlap, U_1 and U_3.

distributions. For U_1, count the total number of scores from each group outside the range of the other and divide this number by N. For U_3, locate the typical score from the upper group in the frequency distribution of the lower group and then find the proportion of scores below that point (i.e., the percentile).

Relation of Group-Level to Case-Level Effect Size

Under the assumptions of normality, homogeneity of variance, and large and equal group sizes, the case-level proportions U_1 and U_3 are functions of effect size magnitude at the group level. Presented in the first column of Table 6.1 are selected absolute values of g in the range 0–3.00. Listed in the remaining columns of the table are absolute values of r_{pb} (i.e., $\hat{\eta}$), U_1, and U_3. Reading each row of Table 6.1 gives a case-level perspective on a group mean difference of a particular magnitude. For example, if $g = .70$, then the corresponding value of r_{pb} is .33 (i.e., 10.9% explained variance). For the same effect size, we expect at the case level that:

1. About 43% of the cases are *not* in the area of overlap between the two frequency distributions ($U_1 = .430$).

TABLE 6.1. Relation of Selected Values of the Standardized Mean Difference to the Point-Biserial Correlation and Case-Level Proportions of Distribution Overlap

Group level		Case level	
g	r_{pb}	U_1	U_3
0	0	0	.500
.10	.05	.007	.540
.20	.10	.148	.579
.30	.15	.213	.618
.40	.20	.274	.655
.50	.24	.330	.691
.60	.29	.382	.726
.70	.33	.430	.758
.80	.37	.474	.788
.90	.41	.516	.816
1.00	.45	.554	.841
1.25	.53	.638	.894
1.50	.60	.707	.933
1.75	.66	.764	.960
2.00	.71	.811	.977
2.50	.78	.882	.994
3.00	.83	.928	.999

2. The typical score in the upper group is higher than about 76% of all scores in the lower group ($U_3 = .758$).

If $g = .70$ referred to a treatment effect, then we could say that the typical treated case does better than about three-quarters of the untreated cases. This result may be quite meaningful even though group membership explains only about 10% of the variability in outcome. Remember that the relations summarized in Table 6.1 hold only under the assumptions stated at the beginning of this paragraph. In actual datasets, all these assumptions are unlikely to hold, so it is almost always necessary to calculate g, r_{pb}, U_1, and U_3 from the observed distributions. See Huberty (2002) and Kline (2004) for descriptions of other indexes of group overlap, some of which are used in the context of selection and classification of applicants.

Measures of Association for More Complex Designs

In more complex designs, such as single-factor designs with three or more conditions or designs with multiple factors, the use of standardized mean differences or bivariate correlations as effect size indexes can be awkward. This is because such statistics compare only two means as a time. However, the correlation ratio $\hat{\eta}^2 = SS_{effect}/SS_T$ can be calculated for any individual effect or combination of effects in designs where ANOVA is conducted and all factors are fixed. This makes $\hat{\eta}^2$ an efficient way to summarize effect size across the whole design. Two examples follow.

Suppose in a between-subject design with a single factor A that there are three treatment groups and three control groups (i.e., $df_A = 5$). The results of a one-way ANOVA indicate that $SS_A = 300.00$ and $SS_W = 1,500.00$. With no other information, we can say that the omnibus effect of factor A explains $\hat{\eta}_A^2 = 300.00/1,800.00 = .167$, or about 16.7% of the variance. It is also true that the correlation between factor A and the dependent variable equals $.167^{1/2}$, or about $.41$. However, the omnibus effect size index $\hat{\eta}_A^2$ does not indicate which focused comparisons (contrasts) account for the overall effect. This presents no special problem because $\hat{\eta}^2$ can also be calculated for any contrast (i.e., a single-df effect) in the design. For example, if $SS_{\hat{\psi}}$ represents the sum of squares for a particular contrast $\hat{\psi}$, such as all three treatment groups combined versus all three control groups combined, then $\hat{\eta}_{\hat{\psi}}^2$ would be calculated as $SS_{\hat{\psi}}/SS_T$. Because a contrast is just one facet of the omnibus effect, it is true that $\hat{\eta}_{\hat{\psi}}^2 \le \hat{\eta}_A^2$. From this perspective, the estimation of the effect sizes for a series of contrasts provides a way to break down the omnibus effect into more specific, directional effects.

In factorial designs, it is possible to calculate $\hat{\eta}^2$ for any individual effect, including contrasts, main effects, interaction effects, or any combination of effects. Suppose that ANOVA results for a balanced, completely between-subject 2×3 factorial design with $n = 10$ cases per cell (i.e., $N = 60$) are as follows:

$$SS_A = 75.00, \; SS_B = 25.00, \; SS_{AB} = 350.00, \; SS_W = 2{,}250.00, \; SS_T = 2{,}700.00$$

Values of $\hat{\eta}^2$ for each of the main effects and interaction effects are calculated next:

$$\hat{\eta}^2_A = 75.00/2{,}700.00 = .027$$
$$\hat{\eta}^2_B = 25.00/2{,}700.00 = .009$$
$$\hat{\eta}^2_{AB} = 350.00/2{,}700.00 = .130$$

In other words, the A main effect explains about 2.7% of the total variance, the B main effect just less than about 1%, and the AB interaction effect about 13%. It is clear that the magnitude of the interaction effect is greater than those of both main effects. Because this design is balanced, we can also estimate the total predictive power across the whole design as follows:

$$\hat{\eta}^2_{A, B, AB} = SS_{A, B, AB}/SS_T = (75.00 + 25.00 + 350.00)/2{,}700.00 = .167$$

where $SS_{A, B, AB}$ is the sum of squares for the total effects, or both main effects and the interaction effect. That is, all effects estimated together explain about 16.7% of the total variance. A different method may be required to compute $SS_{A, B, AB}$ in unbalanced factorial designs, but it is still possible to estimate size magnitude for the total effects in such designs. See Olejnik and Algina (2000) for more examples of effect size estimation in designs with multiple factors.

You should know about **partial eta-squared** (partial $\hat{\eta}^2$), which is based on $\hat{\eta}^2$ but estimates the proportion of variance explained controlling for all other systematic effects in the design. It does so by removing those other effects from the total observed variance. That is, partial $\hat{\eta}^2$ indicates the proportion of explained variance relative to an *adjusted* total variance. Its general form is:

$$\text{partial } \hat{\eta}_{\text{effect}}^2 = \frac{SS_{\text{effect}}}{SS_{\text{effect}} + SS_{\text{error}}} \qquad (6.17)$$

where SS_{error} is the sum of squares for that effect's ANOVA error term. In contrast, the denominator of $\hat{\eta}^2$ is SS_T, which includes not only the sums of squares for the effect and its error term but also those for all other effects or error terms in the whole design. Suppose that these data are from a two-way factorial design with independent samples:

$$SS_A = 75.00, \; SS_B = 25.00, \; SS_{AB} = 350.00, \; SS_W = 2{,}250.00, \; SS_T = 2{,}700.00$$

Earlier we computed for the same data the value of $\hat{\eta}_A^2$ for the A main effect as $75.00/2{,}700.00$, or $.027$. The error term for all effects in this design is MS_W, the pooled within-group mean square. Accordingly, the partial proportion of explained variance for the A effect is calculated as

$$\text{partial } \hat{\eta}_A^2 = 75.00/(75.00 + 2{,}250.00) = 75.00/2{,}325.00 = .032$$

That is, the A main effect explains about 3.2% of the residual variance controlling for the B and AB effects. The square root of this value, or $.032^{1/2} = .179$, equals the partial correlation of factor A effect with the dependent variable, again controlling for the effects of B and AB.

In some cases, the value of partial $\hat{\eta}^2$ can be substantially higher than that of $\hat{\eta}^2$ for the same effect. This is not contradictory because the two statistics estimate the proportion of explained variance relative to two different variances, total observed variance $(\hat{\eta}^2)$ versus an adjusted total variance (partial $\hat{\eta}^2$). It is fairly common practice in factorial designs to report $\hat{\eta}^2$ for the total effects, such as $\hat{\eta}_{A, B, AB}^2$ in a two-way design, and partial $\hat{\eta}^2$ for individual effects, including the main and interaction effects. But note that values of partial $\hat{\eta}^2$ for different effects are not directly comparable because they each refer to different adjusted total variances (i.e., their denominators may be different). For the same reason, values of partial $\hat{\eta}^2$ are not generally additive. For example, you cannot sum the separate values of partial $\hat{\eta}^2$ for the A, B, and AB effects in a balanced factorial design as you can corresponding values of $\hat{\eta}^2$ for the same effects. Of the two proportions of explained variance, it is generally more straightforward to report $\hat{\eta}^2$ only for each effect. If you choose to report values of both $\hat{\eta}^2$ and partial $\hat{\eta}^2$, however, then clearly distinguish between the two in written summaries of the results.

Effect Sizes for Dichotomous Outcomes[6]

Many studies in medicine, epidemiology, and related areas compare groups on dichotomous (binary) outcomes, such as relapsed versus not relapsed or survived versus died. When two groups are compared on a dichotomy, the data are frequencies that are represented in a 2 × 2 contingency table, also called a **fourfold table**. Presented in Table 6.2 is a fourfold table for the contrast of treatment and control groups on the dichotomy relapsed–not relapsed. The letters in the table represent observed frequencies in each cell. For example, there are $n_C = A + B$ cases in the control group where A and B stand for, respectively, the number of untreated cases that relapsed or did not relapse. The size of the treatment group is $n_T = C + D$, where C and D stand for, respectively, the number of treated cases that relapsed or not. The total sample size is thus $N = A + B + C + D$.

Three of the most widely used effect size indexes in comparative studies of dichotomous outcomes are described next. They all measure the degree of relative risk for an adverse outcome across different groups. These same statistics can be used when neither level of the dichotomy corresponds to something undesirable, such as agree–disagree. The idea of "risk" is just replaced by that of comparing relative frequencies for two different outcomes. Suppose that treatment and control groups are to be compared on the dichotomy relapsed–not relapsed. Referring to Table 6.2, the proportion of cases that relapsed in the control group is $p_C = A/(A + B)$, and the corresponding proportion in the treatment group is $p_T = C/(C + D)$. The simple difference between the two probabilities just described is the **risk difference** (RD), or:

TABLE 6.2. A Fourfold (2 × 2) Table for a Group Contrast on a Dichotomous Outcome

Group	Relapsed	Not relapsed
Control	A	B
Treatment	C	D

Note. The letters $A–D$ represent observed cell frequencies.

[6]Part of this presentation is based on Kline (2004, pp. 143–152).

$$RD = p_C - p_T \tag{6.18}$$

So defined, RD = .10 indicates a relapse rate 10% higher in the control group than in the treatment group. Likewise, RD = –.20 indicates a higher relapse rate in the treatment group by 20%. The parameter estimated by RD is the population risk difference $\pi_C - \pi_T$.

The **risk ratio** (RR) is the ratio of the proportions for the adverse outcome, in this case relapse. It is defined as follows:

$$RR = \frac{p_C}{p_T} \tag{6.19}$$

If RR = 1.50, for example, the risk for relapse is 1.5 times higher in the control group than in the treatment group. Likewise, if RR = .70, the relapse among untreated cases is only 70% as great as that among treated cases. The statistic RR thus estimates the proportionate difference in risk across the two groups. The parameter estimated by RR is π_C/π_T, the population risk ratio.

The **odds ratio** (OR) is the ratio of the within-group odds for relapse. Referring to Table 6.2, the odds for relapse in the control group equals

$$o_C = \frac{p_C}{1 - p_C} = \frac{A}{B} \tag{6.20}$$

and the corresponding odds in the treatment group equals

$$o_T = \frac{p_T}{1 - p_T} = \frac{C}{D} \tag{6.21}$$

The statistic OR is thus defined as follows:

$$OR = \frac{o_C}{o_T} = \frac{A/B}{C/D} = \frac{AD}{BC} \tag{6.22}$$

Suppose that p_C = .60 and p_T = .40. The odds for relapse in the control group are o_C = .60/.40 = 1.50; that is, the chances of relapsing are 1½ times greater than not relapsing. The odds for relapse in the treatment group are o_T = .40/.60 = .67; that is, the chances of relapsing are two-thirds that of not relapsing. The odds ratio is OR = 1.50/.67, or 2.25, which says that the odds of relapse are $2\frac{1}{4}$ times higher among untreated cases than treated cases. The parameter estimated by OR is the population odds ratio $\omega = \Omega_C/\Omega_T$. Note that the symbol ω^2 stands for the parameter estimated by $\hat{\omega}^2$ for a continuous outcome (see Equation 6.15).

The statistics RD, RR, and OR all describe relative risk but on different scales. Of the three, OR is analyzed the most often. This is true even though OR may be the least intuitive among these comparative risk indexes. The statistics RD and RR have some problematic mathematical properties that render them useful mainly as descriptive statistics. For example, the range of RD depends on the values of the population proportions π_C and π_T. Specifically, the theoretical range of RD is greater when both π_C and π_T are closer to .50 than when they are closer to zero. The theoretical range of RR varies according to its denominator. Suppose that p_T is .40 in one sample but .60 in another sample. The theoretical range of RR = p_C/p_T in the first sample is 0–2.50, but in the second sample it is 0–1.67. The characteristics just described limit the value of RD and RR as standardized indexes for comparing results across different samples. In contrast, it is possible to analyze OR in a way that avoids these problems, but this may require the analysis of logarithmic (log) transformations of OR before the results are converted back to their original units for interpretation.

A special property of OR is that it can be converted to a kind of standardized mean difference known as a **logit** d. A **logit** is the natural log (base $e \cong 2.7183$) of OR, designated here as ln (OR). The logistic distribution is used in statistical analyses to model distributions of binary variables, and it is approximately normal with a standard deviation that equals pi/$3^{1/2}$, which is about 1.8138. The ratio of ln (OR) over pi/$3^{1/2}$ is a logit d that is directly comparable with a standardized mean difference for a contrast of two groups on a continuous outcome. Suppose that the odds of relapse in a control group relative to a treatment group equals OR = 2.25. The logit d for this result is

$$\text{logit } d = \ln (2.25)/(\text{pi}/3^{1/2}) = .8109/1.8138 = .45$$

Thus, the result OR = 2.25 is roughly comparable to a treatment effect size of about half a standard deviation on a continuous outcome variable.

You may already know that the primary test statistic for a fourfold table like the one presented in Table 6.2 is χ^2 (1), or chi square with a single degree of freedom. There is a Pearson correlation known as the **phi coefficient** and designated here as $\hat{\phi}$ that is closely related to χ^2 for fourfold tables. The correlation $\hat{\phi}$ indicates the degree of association between two dichotomous variables, such as treatment–control and relapsed–not relapsed. The unsigned value of $\hat{\phi}$ can be computed from the χ^2 statistic for the fourfold table and the sample size as follows:

$$| \hat{\varphi} | = \sqrt{\frac{\chi^2}{N}} \qquad (6.23)$$

For example, if the χ^2 (1) = 10.50 and N = 300, then the unsigned Pearson correlation between the two dichotomous variables is $\hat{\varphi}$ = $(10.50/300)^{1/2}$ = .187. Unfortunately, the mathematical properties of $\hat{\varphi}$ as a standardized effect size index are poor. For example, it is a margin-bound index because its value will change if the cell frequencies in any row or column in a fourfold table are multiplied by an arbitrary constant. This reduces the usefulness of $\hat{\varphi}$ as a standardized measure of comparative risk when relative group sizes or rates of the negative outcome vary across studies. Consequently, we will not consider the phi coefficient further.

T-Shirt Effect Sizes, Importance, and Cautions[7]

T-shirts come in basic sizes including "small," "medium," and "large," among others. These are more or less standard size categories, and different T-shirts of the same size should all theoretically fit the same person just as well. It seems that some researchers tend to think about effect size magnitude in terms of categories that resemble T-shirt sizes. For instance, it is natural to pose the questions, What is a large effect? a small effect? and what is in between, or a medium-size effect? J. Cohen (1988) devised what are the best-known guidelines for describing effect sizes in these terms. The descriptor *medium* in these guidelines corresponds to a subjective average effect size magnitude in the behavioral science literature. The other two descriptors are intended for situations where neither theory nor previous empirical results help us to differentiate between small versus large effects. However, it is quite rare in practice when there is no basis for hazarding a reasonable guess about anticipated effect size magnitude. These interpretive guidelines are laden with the potential problems clearly noted by J. Cohen and others since then. They are summarized next for absolute values of the statistics g and r_{pb} and discussed afterward. These guidelines assume normality, homogeneity of variance, and large and equal group sizes:

1. A "small" effect size corresponds to about g = .20 or r_{pb} = .10 (1% explained variance).

[7]Part of this presentation is based on Kline (2004, pp. 132–136).

2. A "medium" effect size corresponds to about $g = .50$ or $r_{pb} = .25$ (6% explained variance).

3. A "large" effect size corresponds to about $g = .80$ or $r_{pb} = .25$ (16% explained variance).

Now let us consider some of the many limitations of the interpretive guidelines just listed: These guidelines are *not* empirically based. That is, the interpretation of an effect size as "smaller" versus "larger" should be made relative to other results in that research area. Meta-analytic studies are some of the best sources of information about the range of effect sizes found in a particular area. Typical effect size magnitudes vary greatly across different research areas. Not surprisingly, they tend to be larger in controlled laboratory studies and smaller in uncontrolled field studies. For example, a mean difference that corresponds to $g = .80$ may be considered too small to be of much interest in experimental studies in one area, but effect sizes so large may almost never be found in nonexperimental studies in another. T-shirt sizes are generally standard, but the same effect size category does not fit all research areas.

J. Cohen never intended anyone to rigidly apply the descriptors small, medium, or large. For instance, it would be silly to refer to $g = .81$ as a large effect size in one study but to $g = .79$ as a medium effect size in another. This is the same type of flawed dichotomous reasoning that has character-ized our misinterpretations of p values from statistical tests (specifically, the sanctification fallacy; Chap. 5). As noted by Thompson (2001), we should avoid "merely being stupid in another metric" (pp. 82–83) by in-terpreting effect sizes with the same rigidity that $\alpha = .05$ has been applied to statistical tests. If the group sizes are unequal or the distributions have very different shapes, the general relation between g and r_{pb} implied in the qualitative descriptions of effect size magnitude (and in Table 6.1, too) may not hold. For instance, it is possible to find $g = .50$ and $r_{pb} = .10$ for the same mean contrast. The former corresponds to a "medium" effect size in these guidelines but the latter to a "small" effect size. Both statistics de-scribe the same result, however, and thus are *not* contradictory. In general, it is best to avoid using generic, T-shirt-size categories to describe effect size magnitude. Look to the research literature—and to your supervisor—for guidance.

It is critical to realize that T-shirt effect sizes do not say much about the importance of an effect. That is, an effect described in qualitative terms as "large" is not necessarily also an important result. Likewise, a "small" effect size may not be unimportant or trivial. This is because the assessment of the importance or substantive significance of a result depends on several factors, including the particular research question, the status of extant theory or previous empirical results, the researcher's personal values, societal concerns, and, yes, the size of the effect, too. That is, the evaluation of the importance of a result is ultimately a matter of judgment, and this judgment is not wholly objective (Kirk, 1996). This is just as true in the natural sciences as in the behavioral sciences. Also, it is better to be open about this role for judgment, however, than to base such decisions solely on techniques such as statistical tests, which give the appearance of objectivity when such is not really true (Gorard, 2006).

Prentice and Miller (1992) described several circumstances where "small" effect sizes are nevertheless important. These include situations in which (1) minimal manipulation of the independent variable results in an appreciable change in the outcome variable; and (2) an effect is found when, according to theory, none is expected at all. Other ways to fool yourself with effect size estimation are listed in Table 6.3. An important one is forgetting that low score reliability tends to truncate (reduce) observed

TABLE 6.3. How to Fool Yourself with Effect Size Estimation

1. Ignore effect size at the case level (i.e., estimate it at the group level only).

2. Apply T-shirt size categories to effect sizes without first consulting the empirical literature.

3. Believe that a T-shirt effect size of "large" indicates an important result and that a "small" effect does not.

4. Ignore other considerations in your research area for judging substantive significance, including theory and results of meta-analytic studies.

5. Estimate effect size magnitude only for statistically significant results.

6. Believe that effect size estimation is a substitute for replication.

7. Fail to report confidence intervals for effect sizes, when it is feasible to do so. That is, forget that effect sizes are subject to sampling error, too.`

8. Forget that effect size reflects characteristics of your study, such as the design, variability of participants, and how variables are measured.

9. Blindly substitute effect size magnitude for statistical significance as the criterion for judging scientific merit.

Note. These points are based on those presented in Kline (2004, p. 136).

effect size. Other detrimental effects of low score reliability on the analysis were mentioned in earlier chapters.

Effect size estimation is an important part of a specific set of methods for evaluating the clinical significance of treatments. **Clinical significance** refers to whether a particular intervention makes a *meaningful* difference in an applied setting, not just whether the difference between a treatment group and a control group is statistically significant. Clinical significance is evaluated at both the group and case levels. At the group level, the magnitude of a treatment effect is often described with standardized mean differences that compare treated with untreated cases or groups with different levels of illness severity (e.g., mild vs. severe). At the case level, proportion effect sizes are used to describe the overlap of the distributions between treated and untreated groups. The latter type of analysis indicates whether a treatment that results in a group mean difference also has distinct effects for the majority of patients. Effect size magnitude is one consideration in the evaluation of clinical significance, but it is not the only one. See T. C. Campbell (2005) for more information about clinical significance.

Approximate Confidence Intervals

Distributions of effect size statistics are typically complex because their shapes vary as a function of the parameter they estimate. And some effect sizes estimate two different parameters, such as g, which estimates the ratio of the population mean contrast over a population standard deviation (see Equation 6.1). One method to construct confidence intervals for some effect sizes is to approximate. The approximate method is also amenable to hand calculation, so a specialized computer tool is not necessary. This is because it uses the same basic method for constructing confidence intervals based on statistics with simple distributions, such as means (Chapter 5). For effect sizes, the width of an approximate confidence interval is the product of the two-tailed critical value of the appropriate central test statistic and an approximate standard error. Recall that central test distributions assume that the null hypothesis is true. An approximate standard error is also referred to as an **asymptotic standard error**, and it is the estimated value one would expect to find in a large sample.

The approximate method is suitable for the standardized mean differences g and Δ and also for the indexes of comparative risk RD, RR, and OR. However, there is no approximate method amenable to hand calculation that constructs confidence intervals for measures of association. This is because the distributions of $\hat{\eta}^2$, partial $\hat{\eta}^2$, and related statistics are generally so complex that one needs a computer in order to construct reasonably accurate confidence intervals. One such method is called **noncentrality interval estimation**, and it deals with situations for statistics with complex distributions that cannot be handled by approximate methods. It is also the basis for correction estimation in a priori power analysis. This method uses noncentral test statistics that do not assume a true null hypothesis. Noncentrality interval estimation is impractical without relatively sophisticated computer programs. Until recently, such programs have not been widely available to researchers. However, there are now a few different stand-alone programs or scripts (macros) for noncentrality interval estimation, some freely available over the Internet. This chapter's appendix deals with noncentrality interval estimation for effect sizes and related computer tools (i.e., it is an advanced topic). Next we consider how to construct approximate confidence intervals based on some types of effect sizes.

The general form of an approximate $100 (1 - \alpha)\%$ confidence interval is

$$ES \pm est.\ SE_{ES}\ (z_{\text{two-tail},\ \alpha}) \tag{6.24}$$

where ES is one of the effect sizes (1) g, Δ, or RD or (2) the natural logarithm RR or OR; est. SE_{ES} is the estimated (asymptotic) standard error of ES; and $z_{\text{two-tail},\ \alpha}$ is the positive two-tailed critical value of z in a normal curve at the α level of statistical significance. Presented in Table 6.4 are formulas for the estimated standard errors of the effect sizes just mentioned. Two examples follow.

Suppose in a two-group design we observe that

$$M_1 - M_2 = 7.50,\ n_1 = 20,\ n_2 = 25,\ s_1^2 = 100.00,\ s_2^2 = 110.00$$

We determined earlier for these same data that $g = .73$. We estimate the standard error of g with the first equation in Table 6.4 as:

$$est.\ SE_g = [.73^2/(2 \times 43) + 45/(20 \times 25)]^{1/2} = .3102$$

The value of $z_{\text{two-tail},\ .05}$ is 1.96, so the approximate 95% **confidence interval for δ** is:

TABLE 6.4. Estimated Standard Errors for Standard Mean Differences and Comparative Risk Indexes

Parameter	Statistic	Estimated standard error
$\delta = (\mu_1 - \mu_2)/\sigma$	g	$\sqrt{\dfrac{g^2}{2\,df_W} + \dfrac{N}{n_1\,n_2}}$
$\delta = (\mu_1 - \mu_2)/\sigma_C$	Δ	$\sqrt{\dfrac{\Delta^2}{2(n_C - 1)} + \dfrac{N}{n_1\,n_2}}$
$\pi_C - \pi_T$	RD	$\sqrt{\dfrac{p_C(1 - p_C)}{n_C} + \dfrac{p_T(1 - p_T)}{n_T}}$
π_C / π_T	ln (RR)	$\sqrt{\dfrac{1 - p_C}{n_C\,p_C} + \dfrac{1 - p_T}{n_T\,p_T}}$
$\omega = \Omega_C / \Omega_T$	ln (OR)	$\sqrt{\dfrac{1}{n_C\,p_C(1 - p_C)} + \dfrac{1}{n_T\,p_T(1 - p_T)}}$

Note. RD, risk difference; RR, risk ratio; OR, odds ratio; ln, natural log; n_C, number of control cases; p_C, proportion of control cases with outcome of interest; n_T, number of treated cases; p_T, proportion of treated cases with outcome of interest.

$$.73 \pm .3102\,(1.96) \text{ or } .73 \pm .61$$

which defines the interval .12–1.34. Thus, the data (i.e., $g = .73$) are just as consistent with a population effect size as low as $\delta = .12$ or as high as $\delta = 1.34$, with 95% confidence. This wide range of imprecision is mainly due to the relatively small sample size ($N = 45$). Approximate confidence intervals for δ based on Δ are constructed in a similar way.

Now let's construct an approximate 95% **confidence interval for ω** based on the sample odds ratio. Suppose that relapse rates among $n_C = n_T = 100$ control and treated case are, respectively, $p_C = .60$ and $p_T = .40$. That is, the relapse rate is 20% higher in the control group (RD = .60 – .40 = .20), which corresponds to a risk that is 1½ times higher among untreated cases (RR = .60/.40 = 1.50). The odds of relapse in the control groups are 1.50 ($o_C = .60/.40$) and the odds in the treatment group are .67 ($o_T = .40/.60$); thus, the odds ratio for data equals OR = 1.50/.67, or 2.25. Using a hand calculator (or one on your computer) with log and inverse log capabilities,[8] follow these steps:

[8]The standard calculator in Microsoft Windows, but set to scientific view, has these capabilities.

1. Convert OR to its natural log, or ln (OR).

2. Calculate the estimated standard error of ln (OR) using the equation in Table 6.4.

3. Construct the 100 (1 – α)% confidence interval about ln (OR) and find its lower bound and upper bound.

4. Convert the lower bound and the upper bound back to their original metric by taking their antilogs (i.e., find their inverse logs).

The natural log transformation of the odds ratio is ln (2.25) = .8109. The estimated standard error of this log-transformed odds ratio, calculated using the last equation in Table 6.4, equals

$$\text{est. } SE_{\ln(OR)} = \{1/[100 \times .60(1 - .60)] + 1/[100 \times .40(1 - .40)]\}^{1/2} = .2887$$

The approximate 95% confidence interval based on the transformed odds ratio is

$$.8109 \pm .2887(1.96) \text{ or } .8109 \pm .5659$$

which defines the interval .2450–1.3768 in log units. To convert the lower and upper bounds of this interval back to the original metric, we take their antilogs:

$$\ln^{-1}(.2450) = e^{.2450} = 1.2776$$
$$\ln^{-1}(1.3768) = e^{1.3768} = 3.9622$$

The approximate 95% confidence interval for ω is thus 1.28–3.96 at two-decimal accuracy. We can say that the observed result OR = 2.25 is just as consistent with a population odds ratio as low as ω = 1.28 as it is with a population odds ratio as high as ω = 3.96, with 95% confidence.

Research Examples

Examples of effect size estimation in three actual empirical studies are described next.

Markers for Schizophrenia

A **marker** is an objective biological or behavioral indication of an illness. It is not necessarily a symptom, such as hallucinations during a psychotic episode. Instead, a marker is presumably related to the underlying pathology or dysfunction. Unlike symptoms, which may wax and wane over time, a marker is thought to be a more permanent characteristic. If a marker is associated with a genetic contribution to the disease, then it should be found in blood relatives who may exhibit no overt symptoms, albeit at a lower level than among affected family members. An example of a biological marker for Alzheimer's disease is neurofibrillary tangles in brain cells, and for Down syndrome it is Trisomy 21, the presence of an extra 21st chromosome.

Several different variables have been studied as possible markers for schizophrenia, including performance on tasks of attention, eye tracking or backward visual masking, evoked brain potentials, and concentrations of polypeptide patterns in cerebrospinal fluid, to name a few. Heinrichs (2000) noted that statistical tests are practically useless in the analysis of candidate marker variables. One reason is that schizophrenia is a relatively rare disorder—the base rate is only about 1%—so group sizes are often small, which reduces power. Another reason is that whether a comparison of schizophrenia patients and normal controls on a potential marker is statistically significant or not says very little about distribution overlap. Heinrichs argued that the latter is a key criterion. Specifically, an ideal marker variable should discriminate at least 90% of patients and controls. Another way to express this requirement is to say that the value of U_1 should be $\geq .90$. Recall that U_1 indicates the proportion of scores that are *not* in the area of overlap between two distributions (see Figure 6.1a). It is also related to the value of the standardized mean difference for the contrast. Specifically, the result $U_1 = .90$ at the case level corresponds to about $g = 3.00$ at the group level (see Table 6.1), assuming normality and homogeneity of variance. Thus, a more informative benchmark than a statistically significant group mean difference for a potential marker variable is the observation of $g \geq 3.00$ and $U_1 \geq .90$.

Heinrichs conducted a series of "mini" meta-analyses by converting the results from several different studies in which schizophrenia patients were compared with control cases on possible markers to standardized mean differences. He then averaged these effect sizes and estimated their ranges for each dependent variable. Markers with the best overall results included the P50 (gating) component of evoked brain potentials with an average effect size (and range) of 1.55 (1.21–1.89) over 20 different studies and backward visual masking with an average effect size of 1.27 (.78–1.76) over 18 studies (Heinrichs, 2000, p. 60). Briefly, P50 reflects the degree of habituation or reduction in electrical brain activity when exposed to a repeating stimulus, such as a brief tone that sounds at regular intervals. Schizophrenia patients tend to show less habituation. In backward visual masking, a visual target stimulus is presented, followed after a brief interval by a masking stimulus that interferes with recognition of the target stimulus. Schizophrenia patients tend to show greater interference effects. These effect size results are not ideal, but a standardized mean difference of about 1.50 corresponds to a U_1 value of about .70 (see Table 6.1). Although short of ideal (i.e., $g \geq 3.00$), these "best" markers to date nevertheless discriminate the majority of schizophrenia patients from control cases.

Depression and Functional Outcomes in Long-Term Treatment of Schizophrenia

In a study of long-term treatment outcomes, Conley, Ascher-Svanum, Zhu, Faries, and Kinon (2007) classified schizophrenia patients as either depressed or nondepressed at an initial evaluation. Three years later, outcomes for both groups were measured across several domains. Reported in the first through third columns of Table 6.5 are group descriptive statistics reported by Conley et al. (2007) for the areas of substance abuse and resource utilization. Some of these outcomes are dichotomous, such as the proportions of depressed or nondepressed patients with schizophrenia who were hospitalized in the past 6 months. Other outcomes are continuous, such as the number of psychiatric contacts over the last 6 months. Conley et al. (2007) also reported test statistics for each outcome listed in Table 6.5—basically all were statistically significant at the .001 level controlling for age, gender, and ethnicity—but they did not also report effect sizes.

Reported in the fourth column in Table 6.5 are values of Hedges's g calculated from the group descriptive statistics for the continuous outcomes. Also reported for each g statistic in the table is the approximate 95% confidence for δ. For example, the depressed patients with schizophrenia reported higher mean levels of alcohol- and drug-related problems than nondepressed patients with schizophrenia by, respectively, .14 and .17 standard deviations. They also had more recent psychiatric contacts than did their nondepressed counterparts by about the same magnitude (g = .18). These effect sizes are not large, but they are associated with serious

TABLE 6.5. Three-Year Substance Resource Utilization Abuse and Outcomes for Depressed and Nondepressed Patients with Schizophrenia

Outcome 3 years later	Initial status		Effect sizes[a]		
	Depressed	Nondepressed	g^a	OR^a	logit d
n	461	702			
Substance abuse[b]					
Alcohol problems, M (SD)	.3 (.9)	.2 (.6)	.14 (.02–.26)	—	—
Drug problems, M (SD)	.2 (.7)	.1 (.5)	.17 (.05–.29)	—	—
Substance use, %	28.8	21.4	—	1.49 (1.14–1.95)	.22
Resource utilization					
Hospitalizations, %[c]	22.4	14.9	—	1.65 (1.22–2.23)	.28
Emergency psychiatric services, %[b]	12.4	4.1	—	3.31 (2.08–5.27)	.66
Emergency room visit, %[c]	14.5	7.4	—	2.12 (1.44–3.11)	.41
Number of psychiatric contacts, M $(SD)^c$	4.0 (3.3)	3.3 (4.3)	.18 (.06–.30)	—	—

Note. From Conley, Ascher-Svanum, Zhu, Faries, & Kinon (2007, p. 191). Copyright 2007 Elsevier Ltd. Reprinted by permission.
[a]Effect size (approximate 95% confidence interval).
[b]Past 4 weeks.
[c]Past 6 months.

problems. These same effect sizes are also generally consistent with population effect sizes as large as approximately $\delta = .30$, with 95% confidence (but they are also just as consistent with population effect sizes as small as about $\delta = .05$). Reported in the fifth column of Table 6.5 are values of OR calculated for the dichotomous outcomes and corresponding approximate 95% confidence intervals for ω. For example, the odds of substance abuse were 1.49 times higher among depressed patients with schizophrenia than among nondepressed patients with schizophrenia. Also, the odds that emergency psychiatric services were needed over the last 4 weeks were 3.31 times higher among the depressed patients. Reported in the last column of Table 6.5 are logit d values for each dichotomous outcome. These statistics are comparable with g for continuous outcomes. For instance, OR = 3.31 for the emergency psychiatric services (yes–no) outcome is comparable to an effect size magnitude of about .66 standard deviations on a continuous outcome (Table 6.5). These and other results reported by Conley et al. (2007) indicate that patients with schizophrenia with concurrent depression have poorer long-term outcomes.

Perceptions of Women and Men as Entrepreneurs

Women who aspire to become entrepreneurs face greater obstacles to doing so than men. These include negative traditional gender stereotypes of women as less bold or assertive than men and the relative lack of same-gender business mentors for women, among others. Baron, Markman, and Hirsa (2001) evaluated the hypothesis that perceptions of women who become entrepreneurs are enhanced by attributional augmenting because they assume this role despite major barriers. However, Baron et al. (2001) expected that this augmenting effect would be less for men who become entrepreneurs because they face fewer obstacles compared with women. In a 2 × 2 factorial design, Baron et al. presented to adult raters photographs of women and men (gender of stimulus person) described as either entrepreneurs or managers (position type). The participants rated the photograph of each stimulus person in terms of several different perceived personality characteristics, including decisiveness, assertiveness, and so on.

Presented in the top part of Table 6.6 are descriptive statistics on the perceived assertiveness variable for the four possible conditions. A balanced design is assumed here ($n = 13$ in each of four cells), but the original design was slightly unbalanced. Also, the gender factor was treated in the analysis as a repeated-measures variable by Baron et al. (2001). For the sake of simplicity, the data in Table 6.6 were treated here as though

TABLE 6.6. Descriptive Statistics, ANOVA Results, and Effect Sizes for Ratings of Assertiveness as a Function of Gender of Stimulus Person and Position Type

	Gender of stimulus person	
Position	Female	Male
Managers	3.08 (.34)[a]	3.44 (.50)
Entrepreneurs	3.33 (.44)	3.30 (.16)

Source	SS	df	MS	F	$\hat{\eta}^2$
Total effects	.8876	3	.2959	2.02[b]	.112
Gender	.3539	1	.3539	2.42[c]	.045
Position	.0393	1	.0393	.27[d]	.005
Gender × Position	.4943	1	.4943	3.38[e]	.063
Within cells (error)	7.0176	48	.1462		
Total	7.9052	51			

Note. Cell descriptive statistics are from Baron, Markman, and Hirsa (2001, p. 927). Copyright 2001 by the American Psychological Association. Reprinted with permission of Robert A. Baron (personal communication, October 20, 2007) and the American Psychological Association.
[a]Cell mean (standard deviation); n = 13 for all cells.
[b]p = .124; [c]p = .126; [d]p = .072; [e]p = .221.

the whole design were a completely between-subject design. However, the results assuming equal cell sizes and no repeated measures are similar to those reported by Baron et al. for the same dependent variable. Baron et al. did not report a complete ANOVA source table. These results were estimated for a 2 × 2 factorial design from the study's descriptive statistics, and they are reported in the bottom part of Table 6.6 along with values of variance-accounted-for effect sizes.

The observed proportion of total variance of assertiveness ratings explained by the main effects of gender and position and the two-way interaction between these factors altogether is $\hat{\eta}^2$ = .112, or about 11.2% (see the bottom part of Table 6.6). Of this overall explanatory power for the total effects, it is clear the largest single effect size is associated with the interaction, which by itself explains about 6.3% of the total observed variance. The main effect of gender of stimulus person explains about 4.5% of the total variance, and the main effect of position (entrepreneur vs. manager) accounts for a smaller proportion of total variance, specifically, only about .5%. Because these data were analyzed assuming a balanced design, the variance-accounted-for values for the individual main and interaction effects sum within slight rounding error to that of $\hat{\eta}^2$ for the total effects, or about .112. Inspections of the means for the whole design reported in the top part of Table 6.6 indicate that women presented as entrepreneurs were rated as more assertive ($M = 3.33$) than women presented as managers ($M = 3.08$). However, the reverse was true for men presented as entrepreneurs ($M = 3.30$) versus managers ($M = 3.44$). Thus, these results and others described by Baron et al. (2001) are consistent with the hypothesis of differential attributional augmentation.

Summary

Effect size estimation is an important part of statistics reform; therefore, today's students need to know something about it. When means from two groups or conditions are compared, a standardized mean difference describes the contrast as the proportion of a standard deviation on the outcome variable, which takes the scale of that variable into account. When ANOVA is used to compare means in comparative studies with one or more fixed-effects factors, a measure of association in a squared metric indicates the proportion of explained variance and in an unsquared metric it indicates the correlation. It is also possible to estimate effect size at the case level using quite simple statistics (proportions) that reflect the degree of overlap between two frequency distributions. This type of analysis is especially useful for describing treatment effects at the case level. Effect size estimation is not a magical alternative to statistical tests, and there are ways to misinterpret effect sizes, too. One of these involves the blind application of T-shirt size categories to describe effect sizes as small, medium, or large. Reporting effect sizes with proper interpretive caution can be much more informative to those who read your work than reporting just outcomes of statistical tests.

RECOMMENDED READINGS

The book about effect size estimation by Grissom and Kim (2005) is intended for applied researchers and describes many examples. More detail about the effect size statistics introduced in this chapter and additional indexes for group- or case-level estimation is available in Kline (2004). Henson (2006) describes the close relation between meta-analytic thinking and effect size estimation in the context of counseling psychology.

Grissom, R. J., & Kim, J. J. (2005). *Effect sizes for research: A broad practical approach*. Mahwah, NJ: Erlbaum.

Henson, R. K. (2006). Effect-size measures and meta-analytic thinking in counseling psychology research. *Counseling Psychologist, 34*, 601–629.

Kline, R. B. (2004). *Beyond significance testing: Reforming data analysis methods in behavioral research* (Chaps. 4–7). Washington, DC: American Psychological Association.

EXERCISES

1. What is measured by the independent-samples t-test for a nil hypothesis versus Hedges's g?

2. Given: $M_1 - M_2 = 2.00$, $s_1^2 = 7.50$, and $s_2^2 = 5.00$ for a balanced design with independent samples. Calculate the t-test for a nil hypothesis, g, and r_{pb} for three different group sizes (n), 5, 15, and 30. Describe the pattern of results. (Note that you already calculated t for the same data in exercise no. 6 in Chapter 5.)

3. A treatment effect is estimated to be .50 standard deviations in magnitude. Use Table 6.1 to describe expected results at the case level assuming normal distributions and homogeneity of variance.

4. Comment: A researcher finds $g = .85$ and claims that there is a large effect because $g > .80$.

5. Comment: A researcher finds $g = 0$ and concludes that there is no difference between the groups.

6. For the alcohol problem outcome variable listed in Table 6.5, show how $g = .14$ and the corresponding approximate 95% confidence interval of .02–.26 were calculated.

7. For the substance use outcome variable listed in Table 6.5, show how OR = 1.49, the corresponding approximate 95% confidence interval of 1.14–1.95, and logit $d = .22$ were calculated.

8. For the data in Table 6.6, calculate partial $\hat{\eta}^2$ for the main and interaction effects. Compare these results with those for $\hat{\eta}^2$ that are listed in the table.

APPENDIX 6.1

Noncentrality Interval Estimation for Effect Sizes[9]

The discussion about this advanced topic concerns how to construct non-central confidence intervals based on the effect sizes g or $\hat{\eta}^2$. Compared with central distributions of test statistics, noncentral distributions have an additional parameter called the **noncentrality parameter** (NCP). The NCP basically indicates the degree to which the null hypothesis is false. For example, central t-distributions are described by a single parameter, the degrees of freedom df, but noncentral t-distributions are described by both df and NCP. If NCP = 0, then the resulting distribution is the familiar and symmetrical t-distribution. That is, central t is just a special case of noncentral t. As the value of NCP is increasingly positive, the noncentral t-distributions described by it become increasingly positively skewed. For example, presented in Figure 6.2 are two t-distributions each where $df = 10$. For the central t-distribution in the left part of the figure, NCP = 0. However, NCP = 4.17 for the noncentral t distribution in the right side of the figure. Note that the latter distribution in Figure 6.2 is positively skewed. The same thing happens but in the opposite direction for negative values of NCP for t-distributions. The value of NCP is related to the population effect size δ and the group sizes as follows:

$$\text{NCP} = \delta \sqrt{\frac{n_1 n_2}{n_1 + n_2}} \qquad (6.25)$$

where δ is the population standardized mean difference. When the null hypothesis is true, $\delta = 0$ and NCP = 0; otherwise, $\delta \neq 0$ and NCP has the same sign as δ.

In practice, we almost never know the real population effect size. Thus, it is generally necessary to use a special computer tool to both estimate NCP and find the appropriate noncentral distributions for the corresponding effect size statistic. There are some commercial computer tools that calculate confidence intervals for δ using noncentral t-distributions. These include Exploratory Software for Confidence Intervals (ECSI) by

---

[9]Part of this presentation is based on Kline (2004, pp. 34–35, 109–112, 118–121, 190–191).

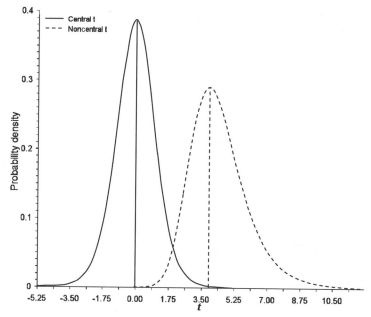

FIGURE 6.2. Distributions of central t and noncentral t for 10 degrees of freedom and where the noncentrality parameter equals 4.17 for noncentral t.

Cumming,[10] which runs under Microsoft Excel—I used ESCI to create Figure 6.2—and the Power Analysis module of STATISTICA, a program for general statistical analyses. There are also some freely available scripts (macros) by M. J. Smithson[11] that calculate noncentral confidence intervals for δ when Hedges's g is the effect size index. These scripts run under the SPSS, SAS, or SPlus/R computer programs for general statistical analyses. Wuensch (2006)[12] gave clear instructions for using Smithson's scripts in SPSS. See also Kline (2004, p. 120) for SAS syntax that computes noncentral confidence intervals for δ based on g in two-group designs. An example follows.

Suppose in a two-group design that

$$M_1 - M_2 = 7.50, \; n_1 = 20, \; n_2 = 25, \; s_1^2 = 100.00, \; s_2^2 = 110.00,$$
$$t\,(43) = 2.43, \; g = .73$$

[10] *www.latrobe.edu.au/psy/esci/*
[11] *psychology.anu.edu.au/people/smithson/details/CIstuff/CI.html*
[12] *core.ecu.edu/psyc/wuenschk/SPSS/CI-d-SPSS.doc*

Earlier we calculated for these same data the approximate 95% confidence interval for δ, which is .12–1.34. This approximation is based on a central t (43)-distribution. Following Wuensch's instructions, I used Smithson's script to compute in SPSS for the same data the noncentral 95% confidence interval for δ based on noncentral t (43, NCP)-distributions. The results of this analysis indicated that the noncentral 95% confidence is .12–1.33, which is practically identical to the approximate 95% confidence interval for the same data. In this case, the approximate method was quite accurate.

Noncentral confidence intervals for η^2 when $\hat{\eta}^2$ measures effect size use noncentral F-distributions. These confidence intervals may be asymmetrical around the value of $\hat{\eta}^2$; that is, $\hat{\eta}^2$ may not fall exactly in the middle of the interval. (The same thing can happen with noncentral confidence intervals for δ, too.) In designs with two or more independent samples and a single fixed factor, a script for SAS listed in Kline (2004, p. 120) calculates noncentral 95% confidence intervals for η^2 when the omnibus effect is analyzed or for partial η^2 when any other effect, such as a contrast, is analyzed. There are also freely available scripts for SPSS, SAS, or SPlus/R by Smithson that calculate noncentral confidence intervals for η^2 for the total effects (e.g., the A, B, and AB effects together in a two-way factorial design) and for partial η^2 for all other effects (e.g., just the A effect) in completely between-subject designs with one or more fixed factors. (The website address for these Smithson scripts is given in footnote 11.) An example follows.

Suppose that the sums of squares and F-statistics for the main, interaction, and total effects in an ANOVA for a balanced 2×3 factorial design with independent samples ($n = 10$) and fixed factors are as follows:

$$SS_A = 75.00, \; SS_B = 25.00, \; SS_{AB} = 350.00,$$
$$SS_{A, B, AB} = 450.00, \; SS_W = 2{,}250.00, \; SS_T = 2{,}700.00$$

$$F_A \,(1, 54) = 1.80, \; F_B \,(2, 54) = .30, \; F_{AB} \,(2, 54) = 4.20, \; F_{A, B, AB} \,(5, 54) = 2.16$$

Earlier for these same data we determined that the proportion of total variance explained by all effects combined equals $\hat{\eta}^2_{A, B, AB} = 450.00/2{,}700.00$, or .167. Using Smithson's SSPS script for noncentral F-distributions according to the instructions in Smithson (2001, p. 14)[13], I estimated the noncentral 95% confidence interval for $\eta^2_{A, B, AB}$ as 0–.280. Thus, the observed result $\hat{\eta}^2_{A, B, AB} = .167$ is just as consistent with a population proportion of total explained variance as low as $\eta^2_{A, B, AB} = 0$ as it is with population proportion of total explained variance as high as $\eta^2_{A, B, AB} = .280$, with 95%

---

[13]*psychology.anu.edu.au/people/smithson/details/CIstuff/Noncoht2.pdf*

confidence level. The values of partial $\hat{\eta}^2$ for the individual effects and their corresponding noncentral 95% confidence intervals for partial η^2, also calculated using Smithson's script, are reported next. As an exercise, show how the values of partial $\hat{\eta}^2$ were calculated for each individual effect and interpret all results:

Effect	Partial $\hat{\eta}^2$	Interval
A	.032	0–.164
B	.011	0–.087
AB	.135	0–.280

CHAPTER 7

Measurement

Measurement is the Achilles' heel of
sociobehavioral research.

—ELAZAR PEDHAZUR AND LIORA SCHMELKIN (1991, p. 2)

It is important that researchers know about measurement. This is because the product of measurement, or scores, is what you analyze. However, if the scores do not have certain essential characteristics, such as reliability and validity, then your results may be meaningless. Likewise, it is critical to wisely select among alternative measures of the same attribute, when such a choice exists. This chapter emphasizes the crucial role of measurement in behavioral science research. I define the concepts of score reliability and validity and outline ways to evaluate these characteristics. Attention is drawn to widespread but false beliefs about score reliability in particular that lead to bad measurement-related practices. Finally, two recent advances in measurement theory are briefly described, including item response theory and generalizability theory. This chapter is not a substitute for a full course in measurement, but I hope that it will at least help you to make better choices about measurement in your own study.

Chapter Scope

Because measurement is such a broad topic, I need to delineate the bounds of this discussion. Emphasized here is the measurement of attributes of research participants, either people or animals. This kind of measurement for people is called **individual-differences assessment**. There is a branch of measurement in psychophysics devoted to analyzing the relation between the physical characteristics of stimuli, such as sounds, and their corresponding psychological experiences (perceptions), such as loudness. Psychophysical measurement is not covered here, but see the comprehensive work by Gescheider (1998) for more information.

Also emphasized in this chapter is **classical test (measurement) theory**, which dates roughly to 1900 with the development of the theory of measurement error by the British psychologist Charles Edward Spearman and the 1905 publication of the original Binet–Simon scales of mental ability. Briefly, classical test theory is concerned with the:

1. Decomposition of observed scores (X) into systematic or "true" (T) and error (E) components.

2. Evaluation of the population relations between X, T, and E.

3. Estimation of the reliability of the observed scores.

Analysis of score reliability then leads to the analysis of score validity. Classical test theory has been influential in the behavioral sciences and is still the predominant model. More modern approaches to measurement, including reliability generalization and item response theory, are briefly described at the end of the chapter.

Finally, measurement is dealt with here more from a research perspective rather than from an applied perspective. Researchers are usually interested in comparing groups or conditions, such as treatment versus control. Measures that can be administered to whole groups at a time are often fine in research. In applied measurement, the focus is on the correct derivation and interpretation of scores for individual people. Accordingly, many measures in applied testing are intended for individual administration only. An example is cognitive ability tests administered by school psychologists to children referred by their teachers. There are published standards for test publishers and users that spell out requisite characteristics of tests for applied measurement. For instance, the *Standards for Educational and Psychological Testing* was developed jointly by the American Educational Research Association, the American Psychological Association, and the National Council on Measurement in Education (1999), and it addresses technical issues of test use in education, psychology, and employment settings. Along similar lines, the Joint Committee on Testing Practices (2004) of the American Psychological Association developed the *Code of Fair Testing Practices in Education* as a guide for both professionals and nonprofessionals (e.g., parents) concerning good testing practices.[1]

The Critical Yet Underappreciated Role of Measurement

Measurement, design, and analysis make up the research trinity (Chapter 3). Referring to the close connection between measurement and analysis, the British physicist and philosopher Norman Robert Campbell (1920) wrote that "the object of measurement is to enable the powerful weapon of mathematical analysis to be applied to the subject matter of science" (pp. 267–268); that is, the output of measurement is the input for analysis. Consequently, researchers in all sciences need both strong conceptual knowledge of and practical skills about measurement.

Unfortunately, there has been a substantial decline in the quality of instruction about measurement over the last 30 years or so. For example, about one-third of psychology PhD programs in North America offer no formal training in measurement, and the directors of only about one-quarter of these programs judged that their students were competent in methods of score reliability or validity assessment (Aiken et al., 1990). The situation is just as bad at the undergraduate level. For example, measurement courses are not even offered in the majority of "elite" undergraduate psychology programs (Frederich et al., 2000). This poor state of affairs puts students in a difficult spot: They may be expected to select measures for their research, but many lack the skills needed in order to critically evaluate those measures. Thompson and Vacha-Haase (2000) made the wry observation that many psychology and education graduate students, who were admitted in part based on Graduate Record Examination scores, may be unable to intelligently explain those scores. There is also widespread poor reporting about measurement in our research literature. Just how these reports are flawed is considered later. As noted in the quote at the beginning of this chapter, measurement is indeed a real weakness in the behavioral sciences.

Fortunately, there are some bright spots in this otherwise bleak picture. If you have already taken a measurement course, then you may be at some advantage in a research seminar course. Otherwise, you are strongly encouraged to seek out and take a measurement course at some point in

[1] *www.apa.org/science/fairtestcode.html*

your educational career. Some undergraduate programs offer a measurement course even though it is not required (i.e., it is an elective). If no measurement course is available in your academic program, then look to others at the same university. For instance, students in psychology programs where a measurement course is not offered may be allowed to take this course in an education program. Aiken et al. (1990) reminded us that formal coursework is not the only way to learn about measurement. Some more informal ways include participation in seminars or workshops and self-study. The list of recommended readings at the end of this chapter should be helpful for the latter. A great way to learn about measurement is to work with a research supervisor who works in the area of assessment or test development. These supervisors may specifically study the score reliability and validity of various kinds of measures. Finally, be aware that there are graduate programs in measurement. Graduates of such programs are highly skilled in measurement, and nowadays they are also in high demand.

Measurement Process Overview

There are three essential steps in the measurement process. They are actually cyclical because refinements or problems at a later step may require a return to an earlier step. These steps are basically the same in studies where the participants are people or animals. There may be some additional complications when people are studied, but the basic concepts are the same. In other words, it is a myth that measurement is not an issue in animal studies. The three steps of measurement as described by Thorndike (2005) are listed next and discussed afterward:

1. Identify (define) the attribute(s) that is (are) to be measured.

2. Determine the set of operations by which the attribute(s) may be isolated or displayed for observation.

3. Select a scale through which numbers are assigned to cases that indicate the degree of the attribute(s).

Hypothetical Constructs

The first step in the measurement process reminds us that we do not measure a whole thing (person or animal), but instead just its attributes. If an attribute of interest is a physical characteristic, such as height, then the rest of the measurement process is pretty easy. About all that is required in this case is to select an apparatus for obtaining the scores and a scale for reporting those scores, such as a portable height measure with gradations in millimeters. However, a higher level of abstraction is often required in behavioral science research. This is because we are often interested in measuring aspects of **hypothetical constructs**, which are explanatory variables that are not directly observable. As defined by Nunnally and Bernstein (1994), a construct

> reflects a hypothesis (often incompletely formed) that a variety of behaviors will correlate with one another in studies of individual differences and/or will be similarly affected by experimental manipulations. (p. 85)

Suppose that a researcher wishes to study whether a drug affects discrimination learning in animals. Discrimination learning is actually a construct because it is manifested only indirectly through behavior (i.e., differential responses to select sensory characteristics of stimuli). The researcher must decide exactly how discrimination learning will be measured. For example, what type of stimuli is to be discriminated (color, sound, etc.)? What kind of behavioral response will be recorded (bar press, maze running, etc.)? There are similar definitional issues for other constructs, such as that of intelligence, for which there is no single, definitive observed measure that covers all aspects of this construct. Indeed, this construct is particularly complex because the domain of related observable variables that could indicate intelligence is large and rather loosely defined. Constructs in animal studies may typically be more narrowly defined, but animal researchers must also deal with construct definition.

Operational Definitions

The second step concerns **operational definition**, which involves the specification of a set of operations to render an attribute amenable for measurement. These procedures should be standardized such that the same result is obtained for each case by different investigators. An operational definition can include both a method and a particular instrument. For example, a tape measure is an appropriate instrument for measuring the length of a long jump in track and field, and laying the tape from the end of the starting board to the first mark made in the sand is an accepted way to display length to the eye (Thorndike, 2005). At higher levels of abstraction, an attribute's definition may affect its operational definition. For instance, just what type of ability will be measured in a study of intelligence? Verbal, visual–spatial, memory, artistic, or social, among other possibilities? The measurement of different attributes of intelligence may require operational definitions that are specific to each particular domain.

Scaling and Multi-Item Measurement

In the third step, the results of the procedures implied by the operational definition are expressed in quantitative terms, that is, as numbers (scores), which indicate the degree of the attribute present. A critical issue here is the selection of a **measurement scale** or a **metric** for the scores. A scale provides an internally consistent plan for generating scores and also describes their numerical properties. One such property is the level of measurement of the scores (i.e., nominal, ordinal, interval, or ratio). A related property is whether the score units are considered equal or not (true for interval or ratio scales only).

Measurement scales are usually established by convention. That is, there is almost never an absolute, God-given scale for any variable (Nunnally & Bernstein, 1994), and this is just as true in the natural sciences as in the behavioral sciences. For example, there is more than one scale for measuring temperature (Celsius, Fahrenheit, Kelvin). Only one of these scales generates scores at the ratio level of measurement because its zero point is absolute (Kelvin), but all three scales have equal intervals based on a particular definition (i.e., a convention). For example, one degree Celsius is defined as $1/100$ of the difference between the freezing and boiling points of water (respectively, $0°$ C and $100°$ C). Selection of which temperature scale to use is a matter of both convenience and tradition, but all three scales describe temperature in a consistent way.

Selecting a measurement scale in animal studies is usually more straightforward than in studies with people. Scores in animal studies tend to be closely linked to the operational definition, and their scales may have numerical properties similar to those for physical measurements. For example, a frequency count for a discrete behavior can be viewed as a ratio scale with equal intervals. These properties are maintained if raw counts are converted through a linear transformation to a different metric, such as to proportions (e.g., .10 of all responses are of a particular type). Scales for reaction time (e.g., seconds) or response speed (e.g., the inverse of reaction time in seconds multiplied by 100) have similar numerical proper-

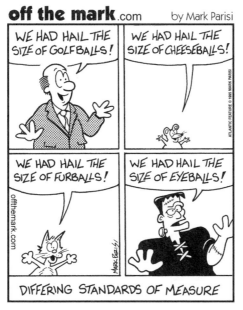

Sometimes the choice of measurement scale depends on your perspective. Copyright 1995 by Mark Parisi. Reprinted with permission.

ties. The scales just mentioned are also natural ones that almost present themselves in studies where the researcher wishes to analyze how quickly an animal performs some behavior.

The problem of how to scale numbers that quantify more abstract attributes is more difficult. For example, there is typically no obvious scale for scores that estimate the degree of hypothetical constructs for people, such as leadership ability. It can also be difficult to specify the numerical properties of scales for hypothetical constructs. Again, these challenges are usually dealt with by turning to convention. In classical test theory, the convention followed most often involves the use of **multi-item measures** (Nunnally & Bernstein, 1994). An item is the basic unit of a psychological measure. It is a question or statement expressed in clear terms about a characteristic of interest. An item is also a "mini" measure that yields a molecular score that can categorize people into only a very limited number of categories. Consider the following item from a hypothetical life satisfaction questionnaire:

I am happy with my life. (0 = *disagree,* 1 = *uncertain,* 2 = *agree*)

The response format for the item just presented is a **Likert scale**, along which respondents indicate their level of agreement with a statement. The numeric scale for this item (0–2) can distinguish among only three levels of agreement. It would be hard to argue that the numbers assigned to the three response alternatives of this item make up a scale with equal intervals.

A variation is to specify an item scale where only the endpoints are labeled but the gradations in between are not. An example for the item "I am happy with my life" is a 7-point rating scale where the lowest endpoint is labeled "strongly disagree" and the highest endpoint "strongly agree." In general, scales with about 5–9 points (i.e., 7 ± 2) may be optimal in terms of reliability and people's ability to discriminate between the scale values. You should know that selection of a numerical scale can affect how people respond to an item. For example, Schwarz, Knäuper, Hippler, No-elle-Neumann, and Clark (1991) asked people to rate their success in life along an 11-point scale. When the numeric values ranged from 0 ("not all successful") to 10 ("extremely successful"), about one-third of the respondents endorsed the values 0–5. However, when the numeric values ranged from –5 ("not at all successful") to +5 ("extremely successful") for the same question, less than 15% endorsed the corresponding values –5 to 0. Perhaps respondents interpreted the scale 0–10 as representing the absence (0) or presence (1–10) of life success. This is consistent with a unipolar (unidimensional) view of this construct. In contrast, the scale –5 to +5 may suggest that absence of life success corresponds to zero, but the negative values refer to the opposite of success, or *failure* in life. That is, this numeric scale with negative and positive values, including zero at the midpoint, may suggest a bipolar (bidimensional) view of life success. Accordingly, Schwarz et al. recommended that researchers match the numeric values for items with the intended conceptualization of the construct as unipolar or bipolar.

However an item is scaled, people's responses to individual items can be inconsistent over time, depending on their mood on a particular day or whether they misread the item and inadvertently give the wrong response. Besides, the degree of satisfaction with one's life or perceived life success are probably complex constructs that cannot be adequately captured by responses to a single, global question. These limitations of **single-item measures** are partially ameliorated by constructing multi-item measures where responses across a set of items are summed to form a total score. The total scores are then analyzed, either directly as raw scores or after converting them to a different scale, such as to standard score metric where the mean equals 100.0 and the standard deviation equals 15.0, among many other possibilities for standard score metrics. Total scores tend to have superior psychometric properties compared with responses to individual items. For instance, total scores tend to have a greater range than item scores and thus potentially allow for making finer discriminations among people. The tendency for responses to individual items to be affected by random factors tends to cancel out when item scores are summed. If a person makes a mistake on one item, the impact on the total score summed over, say, 50 items may be slight. A set of items may better capture various facets of a construct than a single item. Finally, total scores tend to be more reliable than item scores, which means less measurement error when total scores are analyzed compared with item scores. Given all these advantages, we almost never assess constructs using single-item measures.

We usually assume that total scores form at least an interval scale, or that the units of the total score are equal in terms of the relative amounts of the construct they indicate. For example, we usually take for granted that the difference between 25 items correct and 35 (i.e., 10 points) on a 100-item multiple-choice test reflects that same amount of change in knowledge as the 10-point difference between the total scores of 75 and 85. The assumption of equal intervals justifies the application to total scores of parametric statistical methods that require interval scales, such as the ANOVA. In reality, this assumption is often difficult to justify, and is thus suspect (Thorndike, 2005). However, Nunnally and Bernstein (1994) noted that many measurement scales that are assumed in the natural sciences to be interval are probably only ordinal at best, so the behavioral sciences are not unique in this regard.

In practice, though, the likelihood that total scores from psychological tests do not really form interval scales is not generally a problem, especially when means or correlations are analyzed. This is because just about any kind of transformation of the scores from one measurement scale to another that preserves the rank order of the scores has relatively little effect on statistical results associated with means or correlations. This includes effect size statistics and statistical tests (e.g., t and F) calculated for sample means or correlations. A score transformation that preserves rank order is a **monotonic transformation**, and such transformations are permissible for ordinal scales. For example, taking the square root of a set of scores ($X^{1/2}$) generates new scores where the rank order for the corresponding original and transformed scores is unchanged. Any linear transformation of the scores also preserves rank order, including the conversion of raw scores to standard scores. The Pearson correlation r_{XY} is not affected by linear transformations of the scale of X or Y, and its value may change relatively little given a monotonic transformation. Means on X and Y could change after a transformation, but they will do so by expected amounts. This is all to say that it often makes little difference whether measurement scales for total scores are ordinal or interval in many standard kinds of analyses.[2]

Resources for Finding Measures

The problem of how to find a suitable psychological measure for use with human research participants is perennial. There are two basic choices: Construct your own or find an existing measure. The former is not a realistic option for students or researchers who conduct substantive research that is not specifically measurement oriented. This is because it is difficult to construct a measure with (1) clear and unambiguous items that (2) measure a common underlying domain where (3) the scores are both reliable and valid. It is certainly *not* a matter of writing a set of items that, based on their wording, *appears* to measure a particular construct, specifying item response alternatives where each is assigned a unique numerical value and then calculating total scores across all items. This is how so-called tests are constructed for articles in popular magazines, such as *Cosmopolitan*, that promise to reveal some inner truth about yourself. Just whipping up a set of items is fine for entertainment's sake, but not for research. I hope that it will be clear after reading this chapter that whether a test actually measures what it should can be determined only through a series of empirical studies.[3]

The other, more realistic alternative—especially for students—is to find an existing measure. There are again two choices: Use a commercial (published) measure or a noncommercial one. Commercial tests are marketed and sold by test publishers. These tests are usually covered by copyright protection, which means that it is illegal to make photocopies of a paper

---

[2]Nunnally and Bernstein (1994) pointed out that level of measurement may be critical in some more sophisticated types of analyses. One example is trend analysis, where the researcher tries to estimate whether the functional relation between two variables has linear, quadratic, or other, higher-order trend components.

[3]There is generally no problem with making your own questionnaire that collects background information about participants, such as their age, gender, level of education, academic program, and so on. These questions should be asked in a clear way, and the layout of the questions in a paper-and-pencil questionnaire or in a virtual dialog box (for computer administration) should be easy to follow.

questionnaire or to copy a computer disk (CD) or DVD with commercial test administration software. For paper-and-pencil measures, test publishers may charge separately for the questionnaire booklet, the answer sheet, and scoring templates (if any). In other cases there may be separate charges for the computer scoring of a set of completed questionnaires. The cost of using a commercial test can be substantial even in relatively small samples. The fact that a measure is published, however, is no guarantee that it is actually worthwhile to use. That is, a commercial measure should be subjected to the same careful scrutiny as any other measure.

Another issue about commercial tests is the matter of **test user qualifications**, which refer to a level of knowledge, experience, or professional credentials considered necessary for optimal test use. Various professional associations, such as the American Psychological Association, the American Association for Counseling and Development, and the Canadian Psychological Association, have recommended that test publishers limit access to certain kinds of tests to qualified individuals as a kind of safeguard for responsible test use. This is especially true for standardized tests of cognitive ability, scholastic achievement, personality, or mental health status intended for individual assessment in applied settings. Test publishers will not generally sell these kinds of tests to individuals without the expected educational or professional credentials. The former often includes at least a master's degree in psychology, education, or a related field where tests are used, and the latter includes professional licensure in these fields.

Noncommercial measures are not published by a test publisher, and copyright protection may not apply to them. They may be described in journal articles where the contents of the whole measure (i.e., the items with response alternatives and scoring instructions) are listed in an appendix. Noncommercial measures are often constructed for research use in particular populations. If the author(s) also report(s) in the article information about the psychometric characteristics of the measure—namely, evidence for score reliability and validity—then that noncommercial measure could be considered for use in your own study.

Listed in Table 7.1 are printed and Internet resources for finding information about psychological tests. All of these resources *describe* tests, which means that they inform readers about test authorship, the intended purpose of the test, the population for which the test was devised and their language, test length and format (e.g., paper-and-pencil vs. computer-administered), scoring methods, and costs (if any). However, only two of these resources (indicated in the table) also explicitly *evaluate* tests, which

TABLE 7.1. General and Content-Specific Resources for Finding Information about Tests

Commercial tests

Spies, R. A., & Plake, B. S. (Eds.). (2005). *The sixteenth mental measurements yearbook.* Lincoln: Buros Institute of Mental Measurements, University of Nebraska.[a]

Buros Institute of Mental Measurements. (n.d.). *Test reviews online!* Retrieved April 13, 2007, from *buros.unl.edu/buros/jsp/search.jsp*[a]

Murphy, L. L., Spies, R. A., & Plake, B. S. (Eds). (2006). *Tests in print VII.* Lincoln: Buros Institute of Mental Measurements, University of Nebraska–Lincoln.[b]

Maddox, T. (2003). *Tests: A comprehensive reference for assessments in psychology, education, and business* (5th ed.). Austin, TX: PRO-ED.[b]

Noncommercial tests

Goldman, B. A., & Mitchell, D. F. (2002). *Directory of unpublished experimental mental measures* (Vol. 8). Washington, DC: American Psychological Association.[b]

Both commercial and noncommercial tests

Educational Testing Service. (2007). *Test link overview.* Retrieved April 13, 2007, from *www.ets.org/testcoll/*[b]

[a]Describes and evaluates.
[b]Describes only.

means that readers are provided with at least one critique of the test by a professional reviewer. Authors of test reviews base their reports on inspection of all test materials and also on results of empirical studies with the test. These reviews can provide invaluable summaries of the strengths and weaknesses of a test.

The resources listed in the top part of Table 7.1 concern commercial tests. The *Mental Measurements Yearbook* (MMY), now in its 16th version (Spies & Plake, 2005), is the "bible" in printed form for descriptive and evaluative information about psychological tests published in English. New versions of the MMY are released now about every 2 years. The MMY is available as a reference work in many university libraries. Some libraries permit students to search an electronic version of the MMY (i.e., a database) for no charge, which is very convenient. Otherwise, individual test reviews can be purchased from the publisher of the MMY through the Internet (see Table 7.1). Measures are indexed in the MMY by test name, acronym (e.g., TTS for the hypothetical Test of Typing Skill), author name, publisher, type of administration (e.g., group vs. individual), and test category (achievement, personality, etc.). Searching by test category may be the best way to start when you know what type of test is sought, but you do not know the name of a particular test.

The entry in the MMY for each test includes descriptive information, one or two professional reviews, and reviewer references. A test is reviewed in a recent version of the MMY if it is new, revised, or widely used since it was reviewed in a previous version. The publisher of the MMY, the Buros Institute of Mental Measurements (n.d.), lists in a Web page the names of all the tests reviewed in the 9th (1985) through the 16th (2005) versions of the MMY.[4] It is important to understand that a reviewed test is not itself available in the MMY. To use a test reviewed in the MMY, it must be purchased from the publisher.

Two other printed general reference works listed in Table 7.1 describe commercial tests but do not evaluate them. One is *Tests in Print VII* (TIP; Murphy, Spies, & Plake, 2006), which is basically a companion work to the MMY. The TIP volume is a comprehensive bibliography of all commercially available tests published in English. Each test listed there is briefly described, and whether a test has been reviewed in the MMY is also indicated. The other printed reference listed in Table 7.1 that just describes commercial tests is the reference volume by Maddox (2003). This work offers brief descriptions of tests from education, psychology, and business and also for populations with physical or sensory impairments.

The resource listed in the middle part of Table 7.1 is a directory of noncommercial psychological measures by Goldman and Mitchell (2002). Included in this work (the eighth in a series) are descriptions of noncommercial measures constructed by researchers and described in articles published in psychology, sociology, or education journals. The Goldman and Mitchell volume lists tests from works published 1996–2000, and the original measure is presented in the text of many of these articles. Measures are not evaluated, but the information given in Goldman and Mitchell may at least indicate whether a particular noncommercial measure is potentially useful.

Listed in the bottom part of Table 7.1 is an electronic database of both commercial and noncommercial tests compiled by Educational Testing Service (ETS). This database, called Test Link (TL), is not freely accessible to the general public. Instead, libraries purchase a subscription to TL on behalf of their students and faculty, so check with your library about access. The TL database is a searchable electronic directory of more than

[4]*www.unl.edu/buros/bimm/html/catalog.html*

25,000 psychological tests. Some of these tests date to the early 1900s (i.e., they are more historical than usable), but one can in a search restrict the date range to a certain limit (i.e., no earlier than 1990). A total of about 1,100 tests listed in TL are noncommercial measures that are reproduced in *Tests in Microfiche* (TIM), which is updated annually by ETS. If your library has access to a specific noncommercial test reproduced in TIM, then you are permitted to reproduce and use the original version of the test in your own research. However, you are not generally permitted to modify a test without the explicit permission of the test's author.

There are additional resources about tests in specific content areas, including human sexuality (C. Davis, Yarber, Bauserman, Schreer, & Davis, 1998), sport and exercise sciences (Ostrow, 2002), and family assessment (Touliatos, Perlmutter, Straus, & Holden, 2001). The works just cited each contain reproductions of dozens of original measures.

Adapting or Translating Tests

It is *not* a simple matter to either adapt an existing test, such as for use in a special population, or to translate it into another language. Indeed, there are so many potential pitfalls here that I strongly recommend that you do not try to adapt or translate a test unless you have appropriate supervision (e.g., you are working on a measurement-related project). Reasons for this cautionary tone are now explained. Some ways to adapt or modify a test include changing test instructions, dropping items or adding others (e.g., the test is shortened), and changing test stimuli (e.g., pictorial objects are presented in gray scale instead of in color), among others. However, modifying test content or its administration changes the conditions of measurement, and such changes may reduce the precision of the scores (i.e., decrease reliability) or alter what they measure (validity). Such problems are critical for standardized tests of ability. Correct interpretation of scores from such tests depends on uniformity of the testing situation.

There are similar concerns about translating a test into a different language. For example, it is a myth that anyone who knows the two languages is capable of producing a suitable translation. There is much variability among the skills of even professional translators, and different translators working from the same source will not typically produce the same translation. Up to three different types of bias may be introduced when translating a test (Van de Vijver & Hambleton, 1996). There are special statistical methods that may detect these three forms of bias, but they may require large samples in both language groups:

1. **Construct bias** where a translation ignores cross-cultural differences in the conceptualization of the construct.

2. **Method bias** where the effect of the way in which a test is administered (e.g., by an adult authority figure) on scores is greater for one group than another.

3. **Item bias** or **differential item functioning** where individual items do not have the same psychometric properties in the translated version due to anomalies, including poor item wording for a particular group.

Evaluation of Score Reliability and Validity

Suppose that you find an available psychological measure that seems suitable for your purposes and population of research participants. It is now time to evaluate the evidence for the reliability and validity of its scores. Let us first define these terms, though.

Definitions

Score reliability concerns the degree to which the scores are free from random error. Examples of random error include inadvertent clerical errors in scoring and incidental factors specific to a testing session, such as illness or fatigue. If the scores have no reliability, they are basically random numbers, and random numbers measure nothing. In contrast, scores are reliable if they are precise, consistent, and repeatable. This means that (1) scores from the same case remain nearly the same on repeated measurements, and (2) scores within a group maintain their rank order from one measurement to another (Thorndike, 2005). **Score validity** concerns the soundness of inferences based on the scores; that is, whether they measure what they are supposed to measure, but also not measure what they are not supposed to measure (Thompson & Vacha-Haase, 2000). Score reliability is a necessary but insufficient requirement for score validity. This means that reliable scores may also be valid, but unreliable scores cannot be valid.

It is important to know that reliability and validity are attributes of scores in particular samples, not of tests. This is because a test is not reliable versus unreliable or valid versus not valid across all possible samples or uses of it (Thompson & Vacha-Haase, 2000). This means that (1) you should not rely solely on information about score reliability and validity published in other sources, such as test manuals. This is especially true if the characteristics of samples described in published sources are very different compared with those in your own sample. For example, a test that yields reliable scores for adults with no mental health problems may not do so within a sample of teenagers who are psychiatric inpatients. Accordingly, Thompson and Vacha-Haase stated that the minimal acceptable evidence of score quality would involve an explicit comparison of relevant sample characteristics (e.g., age and gender) in your sample with the same features reported in published sources. It is much better to also (2) summarize in written reports the evidence for score reliability and validity within your own sample(s).

Widespread Poor Practices

Too many researchers fail to report enough information about score reliability and validity. For example, Vacha-Haase, Ness, Nilsson, and Reetz (1999) found that there was no mention of reliability in about one-third of the articles published from 1990–1997 in three different counseling or psychology journals. Only about one-third reported reliability coefficients for the scores actually analyzed in the study, and the rest described score reliability information from previous studies only. The latter practice is known as **reliability induction**. However, too many authors who invoke reliability induction fail to explicitly compare characteristics of their sample with those from cited studies of score reliability (Vacha-Haase, Kogan, & Thompson, 2000).

Thompson and Vacha-Haase (2000) and others have speculated that a cause of these poor reporting practices is the apparently widespread but false belief that it is *tests* that are reliable or unreliable, not scores in a particular sample. That is, if researchers believe that reliability, once established, is an immutable property of the test, then they may put little effort into evaluating reliability in their own samples. They may also adopt a "black box" view of reliability that assumes that reliability can be established by others, such as a select few academics who conduct measurement research. This false belief also implies that it is wasteful to devote significant resources to teaching about measurement. Similar kinds of false beliefs that lead to other poor practices about research, especially about statistical tests, were described in earlier chapters.

Reliability Coefficients

A reliability coefficient, designated here as r_{XX}, is interpreted as one minus the proportion of observed score variance that is due to random error. Thus, the theoretical range of r_{XX} is 0–1.00. If r_{XX} = .70, for example, then it is estimated that $1 - .70 = .30$, or 30% of observed variance is due to error. As r_{XX} approaches zero, the scores become more and more like random numbers. It can happen in actual samples that observed reliability coefficients are less than zero ($r_{XX} < 0$), or even less than –1.0 (e.g., r_{XX} = –6.25). A negative reliability coefficient is usually interpreted as though its value were zero, but such a result indicates a serious problem with the scores (e.g., Thompson, 2003, p. 13). As r_{XX} approaches 1.00, there is less and less random error; if r_{XX} = 1.00, the scores are perfectly concise, but reliability coefficients in actual samples are practically never this high.

There is no "gold standard" as to how high a reliability coefficient should be in order to consider score reliability as "good," but some guidelines are offered: Reliability coefficients around .90 are generally considered "excellent." For individually administered tests used in clinical or educational settings, however, .90 is about the minimum acceptable level of score reliability. Values of r_{XX} around .80 may be considered "very good," and values around .70 are "adequate." Scores from a test used to compare groups in a research study should have at least adequate reliability. If r_{XX} < .50, then most of the observed score variance is due to random error, and this is probably an unacceptably high level of imprecision in most situations. As implied by these guidelines, reliability coefficients are interpreted in an absolute sense. Although it is possible to test a reliability coefficient for statistical significance (e.g., divide r_{XX} by its standard error and interpret the resulting ratio as a z statistic), this information is typically of no value. This is because it is possible in a large sample that a very low reliability coefficient could be statistically significant. However, as noted by Abelson (1997b):

> And when a reliability coefficient is declared to be nonzero [based on statistical tests], that is the ultimate in stupefyingly vacuous information. What we really wish to know is whether an estimated reliability is .50'ish or .80'ish. (p. 121)

Considered next are different types of score reliability and how to estimate them.

Types of Score Reliability

Because there is more than one kind of random error, there is more than one type of score reliability. Some, but perhaps not all, of these kinds of score reliability may be relevant for a particular test. Various classical methods to assess score reliability rely on a general strategy: The test is subdivided into two or more equivalent fractions from either a single administration or multiple administrations, and score consistency across the fractions is estimated by r_{XX}. For example, **test–retest reliability** involves the readministration of a test to the same group on a second occasion. The fraction of the test in this case is 1.0 because the same test is given twice. If the two sets of scores are highly correlated, then error due to temporal factors may be minimal.

Other classical methods to assess reliability require just a single test administration. **Interrater reliability** is relevant for subjectively scored measures: If two independent raters do not consistently agree in their scoring of the same test given to the same participants, then examiner-specific factors are a source of random error. **Alternate-forms reliability** involves the evaluation of score stability across different versions of the same test. This method estimates the effect of **content sampling error** on scores; that is, whether variation in items drawn from the same domain leads to changes in rank order across the two forms. A drawback to this method is that it requires two equivalent forms of the test, which takes twice the effort of developing a single form.

Another kind of score reliability that estimates content sampling error but requires a single administration of just one form of the test is **internal consistency reliability**. In this method, each item in a test is treated as a one-item test. If responses across the items are consistent—that is, the items are positively correlated with one another—then the internal consistency reliability may be high. If so, the items may reflect a relatively homogeneous domain. Otherwise, item content may be so heterogeneous that the total score is not the best unit of analysis because it does not measure a single attribute. The most widely reported estimate of internal consistency reliability is **coefficient alpha**, also called **Cronbach's alpha**. The lowercase Greek letter alpha (α) is often used to designate this coefficient. Because the same symbol was used in earlier chapters to represent the a priori level of statistical significance, the symbol α_C is used here to refer to Cronbach's alpha. A conceptual equation is

$$\alpha_C = \frac{n\,\bar{r}_{ij}}{1 + (n-1)\,\bar{r}_{ij}} \qquad (7.1)$$

where n is the number of items (*not* group size) and $\bar{r}_{ij}$ is the average Pearson correlation between all item pairs. For example, given $n = 20$ items with a mean interitem correlation of .30, then

$$\alpha_C = 20\,(.30)/[1 + (20-1)\,.30] = .90$$

Internal consistency reliability is greater as there are more items or as the mean interitem correlation is increasingly positive. Another way to describe the requirement for positive mean interitem correlations in order for the value of α_C to be relatively high is to say that the correlations between items scores and the total score, or **item–total correlations**, should generally be positive. A calculational formula for α_C is presented next:

$$\alpha_C = \frac{n}{n-1}\left(1 - \frac{\sum s_i^2}{s_{\text{Total}}^2}\right) \qquad (7.2)$$

where $\sum s_i^2$ is the sum of the variances for the n individual items and s_{Total}^2 is the variance of the total score across all the items. For items that are dichotomously scored, such as 0 for wrong and 1 for correct, item variance is calculated simply as $s^2 = pq$ where p is the proportion of people who got the item correct (score = 1) and q is the proportion who got it wrong (score = 0); also $p + q = 1.0$. When all of the items are dichotomously scored, there is a special equation for calculating internal consistency reliability known as **KR-20**, which stands for the 20th formula in a seminal article by Kuder and Richardson (1937). The formula for KR-20 is presented next:

$$\text{KR-20} = \frac{n}{n-1}\left(1 - \frac{\sum p_i\,q_i}{s_{\text{Total}}^2}\right) \qquad (7.3)$$

where $p_i\,q_i$ is the variance of the ith item. Remember that KR-20 is good only for tests where all items are dichotomously scored.

Because Cronbach's alpha is affected by the mean interitem correlation, it is sometimes necessary to use **reverse scoring** or **reverse coding**, in which scores for items in a scale that are negatively worded are reversed in a positive direction, in order to match the scores for other positively worded items, or vice versa. This outcome of reverse scoring is that negative correlations between positively worded items and negatively worded items in their original scores are converted to positive correlations. Consider this set of three items about health status all with the same 3-point response format (0 = *disagree*, 1 = *uncertain*, 2 = *agree*):

1. My general health is good.
2. Often I do not feel healthy.
3. I worry little about my health.

People who agree with the first and third items (score = 2) just presented will tend to disagree with the second item (score = 0), which is negatively worded. Likewise, those who agree with the second item (score = 2) will tend to disagree with the first and third items (score = 0). These response patterns may lead to a negative correlation between the scores for the first and second items and also between the scores for the second and third items. These negative interitem correlations will lower the value of Cronbach's alpha, perhaps even to $\alpha_C < 0$. To avoid this problem, a researcher could use a computer to recode the scores on the item 2, specifically, to transform a score of 0 to a score of 2 and transform a score of 2 to a score of 0. (The score of 1 for "uncertain" is not changed.) This basically changes the item 2 to a positively worded item in terms of its reversed scores. Now the correlations between the scores for all three pairs of items should be positive.

A related kind of score reliability is **split-half reliability**. In this method, a single test is partitioned into two equivalent halves that are comparable in terms of item content and difficulty. A common way to split a test where the items become increasingly difficult is to assign the odd-numbered items to one half-test and the even-numbered items to the other half-test. The two halves of the test formed this way should be roughly equivalent in terms of difficulty. After the whole test is administered, the two halves are separated for scoring. Given an odd–even split, two scores are calculated for each case, one for the total across the odd-numbered items and another for the total across the even-numbered items. The correlation between these two sets of scores adjusted for the total number of items on the full-length test is the split-half reliability coefficient. If the two halves reflect the same content, then the split-half reliability coefficient should be high. A drawback to this method is that it is sensitive to how the test is split. That is, there are typically many different ways to split a test (odd–even, first half–second half, etc.), and each one may yield a different estimate of the split-half reliability coefficient. One way around this problem is just to report the value of coefficient alpha. This is because the value given by α is the average of all possible split-half reliability coefficients for a particular test.[5]

A brief example will illustrate the potential advantages of estimating more than one type of measurement error for a hypothetical test of impulsivity. The format of the test is a structured interview where the responses are recorded but scored later by the examiner. The scoring is not objective. Values of different types of score reliability coefficients are reported next: interrater reliability $r_{XX} = .85$; $\alpha_C = .90$; 3-month test–retest $r_{XX} = .80$; 1-year test–retest $r_{XX} = .30$. Based on these results, we can say that (1) there is a reasonable level of agreement about scoring between independent raters; (2) the items of the test seem to reflect a homogeneous content domain; and (3) scores maintain their rank order quite well after a shorter period of time, but not over a longer period.

Statistical Software and Reliability

In order to evaluate the internal consistency reliability of the scores of a multi-item measure, you must save the item responses in the raw data file. Suppose that a symptom checklist has 20 items. The checklist yields a total score that indicates overall level of illness. This total score is also a dependent variable in the analysis. To estimate the internal consistent reliability of checklist scores, each of the 20 items must be represented as a variable in the data file, and the variable for each item contains the responses of the participants for that item. If only the total score is saved, however, then internal consistency reliability cannot be estimated.

Some statistical computer programs have special modules for reliability analyses. For example, the Reliability procedure in SPSS calculates internal consistent reliability coefficients. It also generates item descriptive statistics, such as correlations between each pair of items and item–total correlations. The Reliability/Item Analysis module in STATISTICA has similar capabilities. It also provides a set of interactive what-if procedures that estimate reliability given particular changes to an existing test (e.g., it estimates reliability after adding or deleting items).

---

[5]The total number of possible splits for a test with n items equals $[.5(n!)]/[(n/2)!]^2$. If there are $n = 20$ items, for example, the total number of possible splits equals $[.5(20!)]/[(20/2)!]^2 = 92{,}378$! Fortunately, α_C for a 20-item test is the average across all these possible split-half reliability coefficients.

Factors That Influence Score Reliability

Score reliability is affected by characteristics of the sample, the test itself, and the testing situation. In practice, all three sets of factors may jointly affect score reliability (i.e., there are interaction effects). This is why reliability is not an immutable, unchanging characteristic of tests. Score reliability may vary with sample demographic characteristics, including age, gender, ethnicity, or level of education. The variability of the sample on the measured attribute is also a factor. Specifically, reliability coefficients tend to be lower in samples with narrower ranges of individual differences but higher in more diverse samples, assuming a linear relation between the observed scores and the underlying dimension (construct). The reason is straightforward: range restriction tends to reduce absolute values of correlations, and some kinds of reliability coefficients are correlations.

Properties of tests that affect score reliability include item content: Score reliability tends to be higher when the items reflect a single content domain than when they do not. This is the type of reliability—internal consistency—estimated by Cronbach's alpha. Another is scoring: Objectively scored tests are less susceptible to scoring error than subjectively scored tests. A third factor is length: Score reliability generally increases as more items are added (i.e., the test is longer), and it tends to decrease as tests are made shorter.

There is an equation in classical test theory called the **Spearman–Brown prophesy formula**, and it estimates the effect on score reliability by changing test length. Suppose that r_{XX} is the reliability coefficient for scores of the original test and k is the factor by which the length of the test is theoretically changed. If $k = 2.0$, for example, then the modified test will have twice as many items as the original; if $k = .5$, then the modified test will have half as many items. The Spearman–Brown equation is

$$\hat{r}_{kk} = \frac{k\, r_{XX}}{1 + (k-1)\, r_{XX}} \qquad (7.4)$$

where $\hat{r}_{kk}$ is the estimated score reliability of the modified test. Suppose that $r_{XX} = .75$ for a test with 50 items. A researcher wants to shorten the test to only 10 items (i.e., $k = 10/50$, or .20). How much less precise are the scores expected to be on the shorter test? Applying Equation 7.4, the estimate is

$$\hat{r}_{kk} = .2\,(.75)/[1 + (.2-1)\,.75] = .38$$

In other words, the estimated score reliability of a 10-item test, given $r_{XX} = .75$ for the original 50-item test, is only .38, which is awful (i.e., < .50). Note that Equation 7.4 generates an *estimated* reliability. The *actual* (observed) score reliability of a test where items are either added or deleted must be calculated in a particular sample. The Spearman–Brown prophesy formula also assumes that any items added to a test have the same psychometric characteristics as the original items. However, if the new items are worse in quality than the original items, then the actual score reliability may be lower than that indicated by the prophesy formula. If the new items are better, then the actual reliability of the expanded test could be even higher than the estimated value.

Characteristics of the testing situation also affect score reliability. One is guessing on a knowledge test, or the effects of passing or failing items due to blind luck, such as on a multiple-choice test. Guessing is a source of measurement error because it affects correlations between items. Temporary factors, such as fatigue or stress, can affect test scores on one occasion but not another (i.e., temporal instability). Systematic differences in the content of alternative forms can also reduce score precision. An example is a makeup examination in a university class that does not cover the same content as the original examination. The particular method used to obtain the scores is another factor. For example, the precision of reports about past illegal behavior may depend on the source (e.g., self-report vs. police records).

Consequences of Low Score Reliability

There are several detrimental effects of low score reliability. Poor reliability reduces the effective power of statistical tests, which means that it lowers the chance of getting statistically significant results, given a real effect in the population. It attenuates effect sizes, including standardized mean differences and correlation effect sizes, below their true absolute values, and it increases the amount of sampling error associated with a particular effect size statistic.

Unreliability in the scores of two different variables, X or Y, attenuates their correlation. This formula from classical test theory shows the exact relation:

$$\max \hat{r}_{XY} = \sqrt{r_{XX}\, r_{YY}} \qquad (7.5)$$

where max $\hat{r}_{XY}$ is theoretical (estimated) maximum absolute value of the correlation. That is, the absolute correlation between X and Y can equal

+1.00 only if the scores on both variables are perfectly reliable. Suppose that r_{XX} = .10 and r_{YY} = .90. Given this information, the theoretical maximum absolute value of r_{XY} can be no higher than $(.10 \times .90)^{1/2}$, or .30. Assuming that X is the predictor and Y is the criterion, then predictive power is reduced by poor score reliability on X. The correlation r_{XY} is a validity coefficient, and it is a datum in the evaluation of one aspect of the validity of scores on X, their criterion-related validity. Other forms of score validity are described next.

Types of Score Validity[6]

Most forms of score validity are subsumed under the concept of construct validity, which concerns whether the scores measure the hypothetical construct the researcher believes they do. Thus, construct validity concerns the *meaning* of scores vis-à-vis the underlying dimension the scores are presumed to reflect. Because hypothetical constructs are not directly observable, they can be measured only indirectly through the observed scores. Because a set of scores from one measure is unlikely to capture all aspects of a construct, there is no single, definitive test of construct validity, nor is it typically established in a single study. Construct validation studies are not limited to purely observational (nonexperimental) studies. Experimental manipulation of certain variables to evaluate whether scores changed in predicted ways on other variables can also be used to study construct validity. Major types of threats to construct validity were described in Chapter 3 (e.g., see Table 3.2). Many of these involve problems with how the construct is defined (e.g., overly narrow or broad) or operationalized (i.e., the selection of measurement methods). Another is poor score reliability.

One facet of construct validity is **content validity**, which concerns whether test items are representative of some domain. Expert opinion is the basis for establishing content validity. For example, whether a set of math problems adequately reflects the expected skill domain for grade 2 students is best judged by grade 2 teachers or other qualified experts in education. Another facet of construct validity is **criterion-related validity**, which concerns whether a measure (X) relates to an external standard (criterion, Y) against which the measure can be evaluated. These relations are estimated with validity coefficients, often represented with the symbol r_{XY}.

---

[6]Part of this presentation is based on Kline (2005, pp. 60–61).

Concurrent validity is when scores on the predictor X and the criterion Y are collected at the same time; **predictive validity**, when the criterion is measured later; and **postdictive validity**, when the criterion is measured before the predictor. Suppose that scores on X are from an IQ test given at age 10 years and scores on Y reflect level of occupational attainment at age 30 years. If $r_{XY} = .15$, for example, then childhood IQ scores have little predictive validity concerning occupational attainment in adulthood.

Convergent validity and discriminant validity involve the evaluation of measures against each other instead of against an external criterion. A set of variables presumed to measure the *same* construct shows **convergent validity** if their intercorrelations are at least moderate in magnitude. Suppose that the intercorrelations among three different types of reading tests, such as letter recognition, word recognition, nonsense word reading, are all > .70. These high intercorrelations support the claim that these three tasks all measure a common ability; that is, there is evidence for convergent validity. In contrast, a set of variables presumed to measure different constructs show **discriminant validity** if their intercorrelations are not too high. Suppose that we develop X as a measure of the effort expended to complete a task and Y as a measure of the outcome of that effort. If $r_{XY} = .90$, then we can hardly say that we are measuring two distinct constructs, effort versus results. Instead, we must conclude from the data that X and Y measure the same basic thing, that is, there is a lack of discriminant validity.

Messick (1995) described construct validity from a somewhat different perspective that emphasizes both score meaning and social values in test interpretation and use. The latter concerns whether a particular interpretation of test scores produces desired social consequences, such as the accurate and fair assessment of scholastic skills among minority children. In his integrated model, Messick emphasized the six aspects of validity summarized next:

1. **Content aspect**, which corresponds to content validity (i.e., item representativeness).

2. **Substantive aspect**, which refers to theoretical rationales or models for observed consistencies in scores (i.e., explanations for score reliability and patterns of intercorrelations).

3. **Structural aspect**, or the match of the item scoring system to the presumed structure of the construct (e.g., whether the underlying

dimension is presumed to be unipolar or bipolar and whether the item response scaling is consistent with this view).

4. **Generalizability aspect**, or whether score properties and interpretations generalize across variations in persons, settings, or tasks (i.e., external validity).

5. **External aspect**, which integrates the concepts of convergent and discriminant validity, the use of multiple measurement methods, and criterion-related validity.

6. The **consequential aspect**, or the value implications of score interpretations as related to issues of bias, fairness, and distributive justice.

Messick's unified concept of validity has been especially influential in education, where consequences of test use are of great concern.

Checklist for Evaluating Measures

Presented in Table 7.2 is a checklist of descriptive, practical, and technical information that should be considered before selecting a measure for use in your study. Not all of these points may be relevant in a particular project, and some types of research have special measurement needs that may not be represented in Table 7.2. If so, then just modify the checklist in the table to better reflect your particular situation. Carefully review the stated purpose of the test, what it is intended to measure, and the characteristics of the samples in which the measure was developed. Calculate costs taking account of both fixed expenses (e.g., for test manuals) and ongoing expenses (e.g., answer sheets and scoring services), if any. Potential limitations of the measure should be directly acknowledged by the test author(s). The author(s) should have academic or professional affiliations consistent with having expertise in test construction. Note the publisher (if any) and date of publication, too. A measure that is quite old (e.g., published in 1964 and not updated since) may be obsolete. Consider administration details, such as the time needed to give the test and skill requirements for those who will do so, special materials or equipment needed, and whether individual administration is required. Review test documentation for information about how to correctly derive and interpret scores, evidence for score reliability and validity, and results of independent reviews of the measure.

TABLE 7.2. Checklist for Evaluating Potential Measures

General

- Stated purpose of the measure
- Attribute(s) claimed to be measured
- Characteristics of samples in which measure was developed (e.g., normative sample)
- Language of test materials
- Costs (manuals, forms, software, etc.)
- Limitations of the measure
- Academic or professional affiliation(s) of author(s) consistent with test development
- Publication date and publisher

Administration

- Test length and testing time
- Measurement method (e.g., self-report, interview, unobtrusive)
- Response format (e.g., multiple choice and free response)
- Availability of alternative forms (versions)
- Individual or group administration
- Paper-and-pencil or computer administration
- Scoring method, requirements, and options
- Materials or testing facilities needed (e.g., computer and quiet testing room)
- Training requirements for test administrators or scorers (e.g., test user qualifications)
- Accommodations for test takers with physical or sensory disabilities

Test documentation

- Test manual available
- Manual describes how to correctly derive and interpret scores
- Evidence for score reliability and characteristics of samples (e.g., reliability induction)
- Evidence for score validity and characteristics of samples
- Evidence for test fairness (e.g., lack of gender, race, or age bias)
- Results of independent reviews of the measure

Recent Developments in Test Theory

Two more modern theories of measurement are briefly described next. They are not typically covered in much detail in undergraduate-level courses in measurement, but each theory has been so influential that you should at least know about them.

Item Response Theory

Item response theory (IRT), also known as **latent-trait theory**, is a modern alternative to classical test theory. It consists of a group of mathematical models for relating an individual's performance across individual items to the underlying construct, such as the true (latent) level of ability. Referring to ability, represented in a basic **two-parameter IRT model,** are two factors that predict the probability of a correct response to each individual item as a function of ability. One is item difficulty; the other is item discrimination. Highly discriminating items are useful for more exactly pinpointing a test taker's ability, if the items are not too easy or too difficult for that person. In a **three-parameter IRT model**, an additional factor that represents the effects of guessing on the probability of a correct response is also included in the model. This parameter is known as a **lower asymptote**, and it indicates the probability that a test taker with low ability would guess the correct answer. There is also an **upper asymptote**, which is the estimated probability of getting the item correct by a test taker of high ability. The graphical expression of an IRT model for an individual item is known as an **item-characteristic curve** (ICC). In general, an ICC represents a nonlinear or S-shaped functional relation between ability and the probability of a correct response. An example of an ICC for a hypothetical item is presented in Figure 7.1. Ability is represented on the X-axis on a scale where the mean is zero and the standard deviation is 1.0. The probability of a correct response as a function of ability is represented by the curve in the figure. Where the curve intersects the Y-axis corresponds to a guessing parameter. Specifically, the ICC in Figure 7.1 assumes that test takers of low ability (3 standard deviations below the mean) have about a 20% chance of guessing the correct answer. The discrimination of the item is represented in the portion of the curve with the steepest slope. In the figure, the steepest part of the ICC falls at an ability level about one-half a standard deviation above the mean. That is, this item may be too difficult at lower ability levels, and also too easy at higher levels. Instead, this item better discriminates within more average levels of ability.

The mathematical bases of IRT allow for some sophisticated kinds of applications that are not so feasible in classical test theory. One is **tailored testing**, in which the computer selects a subset of items from a much larger set that may optimally assess a particular person, and their order of presentation depends on the test taker's pattern of responses. For example, if the examinee fails initial items, then easier ones are presented. Testing stops when more difficult items are consistently failed. In tailored testing, reliability coefficients can be calculated for each individual person. In classical test theory, reliability coefficients are estimated for whole groups only. The same IRT framework can also be applied to the evaluation of potential item bias, that is, whether an item behaves differently for children who are members of ethnic minorities or not, for example. A related application concerns whether a test item means the same thing in two different

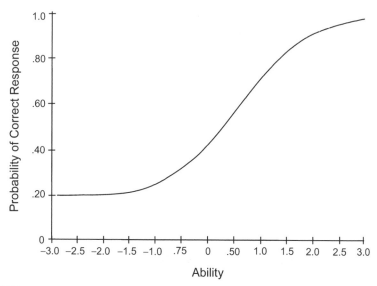

FIGURE 7.1. An item-characteristic curve for a hypothetical test item.

languages. See Embretson and Reise (2000) for a clear introduction to IRT suitable for students with at least a year of graduate statistics.

Generalizability Theory

Another modern measurement theory is that of **generalizability theory**, or **G-theory**. Like classical test theory, G-theory is concerned with the estimation of measurement error. In classical test theory, each type of measurement error (content, interrater, etc.) is usually estimated in separate studies. In the typical study of test–retest reliability, for example, time sampling error is estimated over just two occasions, and no other source of measurement error is estimated. In contrast, in a generalizability study, or **G-study**, different sources of measurement error, known as **facets**, can be simultaneously studied. Facets in a G-study can include raters, time, forms (item sets), and settings, among other possibilities. Also, each facet can include more than two levels. For example, the consistency of test scores over four different occasions and across five different raters can be estimated without difficulty in a G-study. That is, multiple facets can be studied together in the same investigation. The various facets included in a G-study represent ways in which it may be possible to generalize any specific result, such as from one setting to a larger number of settings. It is also possible to estimate **measurement error interaction effects**, which are joint effects among two or more facets that create yet more measurement error than either alone. For example, interrater reliability could be lower or higher depending on the particular form scored by them. In contrast, classical test theory offers no direct way to estimate measurement error interactions.

The mathematical model for computing results in a G-study is the same general linear model that underlies ANOVA and multiple regression. Accordingly, it may be possible to analyze data from a G-study using a conventional ANOVA procedure in a computer program for general statistical analyses. Just as in a standard ANOVA, it is usually possible in a G-study to partition observed score variance into different components, in this case main and interaction effects of facets concerning measurement error. The variance components are then represented in a **generalizability coefficient**, or **G-coefficient**, which estimates how various facets combine to affect score consistency and is analogous to a reliability coefficient (r_{XX}) in classical test theory. The results of a G-study can also inform a decision study, or a **D-study**, in which effects of alternative measurement plans are estimated. For example, effects on score consistency of using different numbers of raters (e.g., 2 vs. 10) or tests of different lengths (e.g., 10 items vs. 100 items)—or any combination of these two facets—can be estimated in a D-study. In general, G-theory is so flexible in its potential application that the possibilities mentioned here just scratch the surface of this multifactor model of score consistency. See Thompson (2003, Chs. 3, 13–16) for a clear introduction to G-theory in the context of reliability generalization.

Summary

Unfortunately, the curricula in too many educational programs at both the undergraduate and graduate levels about measurement is poor or nonexistent. Students need strong knowledge in this area if they are to select good measures for use in their research, and increasingly this knowledge must come from self-study instead of from professors in formal classes. In studies of people, it is scores from multi-item measures that are analyzed most often. These scores should be evaluated for their reliability or degree of precision. In classical test theory, the susceptibility of scores to various types of measurement error, such as time sampling error and content error, is estimated with reliability coefficients. Never forget that reliability is a property of scores in a particular sample, not of tests in an absolute way. Also report information about score reliability. It is best to report this information based on results in your own sample. If you instead report this information from another source such as a test manual—that is, you rely on reliability induction—then assure your readers that the characteristics of your sample are similar to those of samples described in that other source. Although score reliability is a prerequisite for score validity, the former does not guarantee the latter, so it is necessary to evaluate score validity, too. The most general form of score validity is construct validity, which concerns the correct interpretation of the scores. Construct validity is established over a series of empirical studies, not in any single investigation.

RECOMMENDED READINGS

Thorndike (2005) is an excellent undergraduate-level book about measurement theory. It is oriented for education students, but is general enough for other areas, too. Nunnally and Bernstein (1994) is a graduate-level book about measurement theory that covers both classical test theory and more modern approaches. Thompson (2003) gives a clear introduction to score reliability, including reliability generalization.

Nunnally, J. C., & Bernstein, I. H. (1994). *Psychometric theory* (3rd ed.). New York: McGraw-Hill. (Graduate level)
Thompson, B. (Ed.). (2003). *Score reliability*. Thousand Oaks, CA: Sage.
Thorndike, R. M. (2005). *Measurement and evaluation in psychology and education* (7th ed.). Upper Saddle River, NJ: Prentice Hall. (Undergraduate level)

EXERCISES

1. Comment: $\alpha_C = .80$; thus a total of 80% of the observed variability is systematic (not measurement error).

2. The score reliability for a questionnaire with 10 items is $r_{xx} = .35$. Estimate the reliability if 10 items were added to the questionnaire.

3. For the same 10-item questionnaire where $r_{xx} = .35$, estimate how many items would need to be added in order for score reliability to be at least .90.

4. For an achievement test where the items are presented in order of increasing difficulty, the split-half reliability coefficient based on an odd–even item

split is .90, but the internal consistency reliability is .70. Explain this pattern of results. Which one is correct?

5. Give two specific examples of how low score reliability can reduce observed effect sizes. (Hint: Think of measures of association and standardized mean differences.)

6. Presented next are scores on five dichotomously scored items (0 = wrong, 1 = correct) for eight cases (A–H). Calculate internal consistency reliability for these scores using the formula for KR-20 and also using the more general equation for α_C (respectively, Equation 7.3, Equation 7.1). For the latter, you should use a computer program for statistical analysis. If your program has a reliability procedure, use it to verify your calculations:

```
A: 1, 1, 0, 1, 1          B: 0, 0, 0, 0, 0
C: 1, 1, 1, 1, 0          D: 1, 1, 1, 0, 1
E: 1, 0, 1, 1, 1          F: 0, 1, 1, 1, 1
G: 1, 1, 1, 1, 1          H: 1, 1, 0, 1, 1
```

7. Presented next are scores on five dichotomously scored items (0 = wrong, 1 = correct) for eight cases (A–H). Calculate the internal consistency reliability for these scores. Interpret the results:

```
A: 1, 1, 1, 1, 0          B: 0, 0, 1, 0, 1
C: 1, 1, 0, 1, 1          D: 1, 1, 0, 0, 0
E: 1, 0, 0, 1, 0          F: 0, 1, 0, 1, 0
G: 1, 1, 0, 1, 0          H: 1, 1, 1, 1, 0
```

8. You are developing a group-administered test of math skills for grade 4 students. There is good evidence for score reliability. Identify relevant types of score validity and give examples of how to assess each.

PART III

SKILLS

CHAPTER 8

Practical Data Analysis

Begin with an idea. Then pick a method.

—LELAND WILKINSON AND THE TASK FORCE ON STATISTICAL
INFERENCE (1999, p. 598)

Sometimes students—and, truth be told, full-fledged researchers, too—look forward to statistical analyses with as much enthusiasm as a trip to the dentist for a root canal. In this chapter I try to ease the figurative pain by giving practical suggestions for conducting your analyses. These suggestions (1) are often not part of standard statistics courses, in which conceptual knowledge is usually emphasized; and (2) concern both general strategies and specific tips for getting the analyses done in a straightforward and efficient way. First, the need for a simple, clear plan for conducting the analyses is emphasized. How to efficiently use a statistical computer program when conducting a complex analysis is considered next. Finally, this chapter also addresses how to make sure that your data are actually ready to be analyzed through data screening.

Vision First, Then Simplicity

A successful analysis requires two things: (1) a vision of what is to be estimated (i.e., the goal), and (2) a plan to use the simplest technique to do so (i.e., the means). Without a clear goal, an analysis may be aimless, and much time can be wasted generating computer output of no real value. A paraphrase of a well-known verse from the book of Proverbs is that without vision, people fail to flourish (or worse). The same is generally true about your analyses: Without a good sense of direction to guide you, the process can be ineffective and frustrating.

The vision part concerns the fundamental question of the research, or the problem that motivated your study in the first place. Just as when you select a design, think first about your research hypotheses before making a choice about how to analyze the data. This choice can be guided by some of the same principles, too. For example, you should consider what you are capable of doing concerning the analysis and what resources are available, such as help from your supervisor or other, more senior students working in the same laboratory. The process just mentioned should help you to identify what is ideal versus what is possible. Next, ask yourself, what do you wish to learn in the analysis; that is, what is the goal? In nonexperimental studies, this goal is often to estimate the direction and magnitude of the relation between variables of interest, controlling for other variables. In experimental studies, the goal is often to estimate the direction and magnitude of the effect of an independent variable (factor) on a dependent (outcome) variable, again controlling for other variables. But if one variable affects another, then the two will generally be related, so the goal in experimental studies can often be rephrased as a matter of estimating the relation between variables of interest, just as in nonexperimental studies. Know the questions you are asking before you begin the analysis, but at the same time be open to unanticipated findings within the data. That is, you are trying to discern the story the data help tell, and sometimes this story has a surprise ending.

Thinking about effect size is a good starting point for planning your analysis. First, formulate a basic set of questions about effect size magnitude between variables of interest that should be estimated. Next, consider the design of your study and how the outcome variables are measured. The former concerns how other variables in the analysis are controlled (e.g., specification as covariates vs. factors), and the latter determines the level of measurement of scores (e.g., categorical or continuous). Finally, match the simplest statistical technique that will estimate the effect sizes, given the design and measurement. As noted by Wilkinson and the Task Force on Statistical Inference (1999), this is not a trivial task considering the large variety of statistical methods now available.

Wilkinson and the Task Force on Statistical Inference (1999) wisely recommended that you conduct a **minimally sufficient analysis**; that is, use the simplest technique that will get the job done instead of a more complicated technique. They also warned against choosing a complicated technique as a way to impress readers or deflect criticism. The latter refers to the maladaptive hope that readers will be so intimidated by the statistics that they will not ask tough questions. *Also, it is critical that you really understand what your results mean,* and this is harder to do when you use unnecessarily complicated statistical techniques. This also means that unless you have some basic idea about how the computer calculates the results for a particular technique and can also interpret the output, you should question whether that technique is appropriate (Wilkinson and the Task Force on Statistical Inference, 1999). Another rule of thumb about comprehension is that *you should be able to write a correct, one-sentence definition of every number listed in a table where statistical results are reported.* For instance, if you conduct an ANOVA, you should be able to explain every number in an ANOVA source table, including the sums of squares, mean squares, p values, and effect sizes. Otherwise, you are not ready to use ANOVA in an informed way.

For undergraduate-level research projects, the classical technique of multiple regression (MR)—which includes ANOVA as a special case—is usually sufficient when the criterion (dependent variable) is continuous and there are multiple predictors. That both continuous and categorical predictors can be analyzed together gives MR much flexibility. That standard regression methods can also be extended to analyze dichotomous outcome variables, such as survived or not, gives you even more options. The analytical method just described is logistic regression (Chapter 4), and it is easier to understand logistic regression when you begin with a good working knowledge of MR.

If there are at least two continuous outcome variables, then multivariate methods, such as MANOVA, can theoretically be used. These techniques have the advantage that they control for correlations among multiple outcome variables (and among multiple predictors, too). In my experience, though, they are not good options for use in undergraduate research projects, at least not without much help from the supervisor. This is because multivariate techniques are complicated and ordinarily taught at the graduate level. Accordingly, supervisors should resist the temptation to encourage their undergraduate students to use these techniques, except if they are willing to do a good deal of coaching. As mentioned, there is little point in using a state-of-the-art technique if you do not understand it, especially when a simpler technique can provide a sufficient answer (Wilkinson, and the Task Force on Statistical Inference, 1999). Besides, a multivariate analysis often winds up as a series of univariate analyses conducted for individual dependent variables. These univariate effects are typically analyzed with MR or ANOVA, so good skills with univariate techniques are often sufficient when analyzing multiple outcome variables. The same concerns about potential excessive complexity applies to structural equation modeling (SEM) (Chapter 4). The techniques that make up SEM are also multivariate methods that are not ordinarily taught at the undergraduate level.

There are now several different commercial computer tools for conducting statistical analyses on personal computers, including SPSS, SAS/ STAT, STATISTICA, Systat, and Minitab, among others.[1] All work much the same way and offer similar capabilities for standard statistical analyses. They differ in their capabilities to conduct some more advanced kinds of analyses, but all of the computer packages just mentioned are good general choices for students or new researchers. There are even student versions of all these packages available at a reduced cost. However, student versions may be restricted regarding the availability of more advanced methods or feature lower limits on the number of cases or variables that can be analyzed. Wilkinson and the Task Force on Statistical Inference (1999) noted that even more important than choosing a specific computer tool is understanding what the results mean and being able to verify them. The latter means in part that values in the output match your intelligent "guesstimates" about what is plausible for certain statistical results. Suppose that the correlation between two variables reported in the output is .95. A value so high may be implausible, given what the researcher knows about the variables. Implausible results can be caused by errors in the dataset, such as incorrectly entered scores. It has also happened that incorrect statistical results have been printed by popular computer programs due to software errors (bugs).[2] When in doubt, the output of one computer program can be compared with that of another. If the two do not agree, then a problem is indicated. As noted by Wilkinson and the Task Force on Statistical Inference, using a highly regarded computer tool does not relieve you of the responsibility to verify the plausibility of your results.

Statistical computer tools also typically generate much more output

[1]There are also some free statistical utility programs or calculating Web pages available over the Internet (e.g., *freestatistics.altervista.org/en/index.php* and *statpages.org/javasta2. html*).

[2]Before Microsoft issued a patch to eliminate this bug, the spreadsheet program Excel 2007 may have displayed the value "100,000" for calculations that actually yielded the result "65,535" (Johnston, 2007).

than would ever be reported. Specific suggestions about the kinds of statistical information that should be reported are offered in the next chapter, but part of becoming a researcher is knowing how to selectively read output in order to find the essential information, and to ignore the rest.

Managing Complex Analyses (Batch to the Future)

About all modern programs for statistical analyses available on personal computers have a graphical user interface (GUI), in which the user controls the analysis by manipulating virtual icons, windows, and menus that represent information or actions available. A well-designed GUI can make a computer program easier to use because it frees you from learning a specific command language. However, there are two potential drawbacks to a GUI in programs for data analysis. First, the availability of "push-button analyses" through no- or low-effort programming could encourage use of the computer in uninformed or careless ways. For example, it is possible through a GUI to specify a very complex kind of statistical analysis without knowing anything about the technique. Steiger (2001) made the point that the emphasis on ease of use in advertisements for statistical computer tools (e.g., "statistics made easy!") can give the false impression that all you need to do is to click on a few virtual buttons and the computer takes care of the rest. Nothing could be further from the truth. As mentioned, you must understand both the conceptual bases of your analyses and how to interpret the output, and no computer program can do this for you. Treat the computer as a tool of your knowledge, not its master.

Second, controlling a statistical program through a GUI works best in simpler analyses, but doing so can actually be an obstacle in more complex analyses. A complex analysis does not necessarily mean a large number of cases or variables. For this discussion, a complex analysis is one in which many new variables are calculated by the computer from existing variables, or when it is necessary to select several different subsets of cases based on their patterns of scores. Suppose that variables V1 to V6 are already in the data file but there is a need to create a new variable, VN, as follows:

$$VN = .25 \times V1 + 1.50 \times V2 + .75 \times V3 + 9.60 \times V4 + .35 \times V5 + .80 \times V6$$

In the GUI for a statistics program, you would select from a menu the option to calculate a new variable. A graphical dialog box for the compute variable command would appear, and in that box you would type the numeric expression for VN just presented. Then after clicking with the mouse cursor on the "OK" button, the dialog box closes and the computer calculates scores on VN for all cases, given its equation. So far, no problem, except that some statistical computer programs may not "remember" the original equation for VN. That is, the scores on VN are added to the data file, but the equation you originally entered for VN is not recorded or retained. If you forget to record the equation and fail to recall it later (very likely), then there may be no record anywhere about the definition of VN. A different kind of problem can arise if you make a typing mistake when entering the equation for a new variable in a GUI dialog box. For example, you may have inadvertently typed "25 × V1" as part of the equation for VN instead of ".25 × V1." After clicking on the "OK" button, the equation you just entered disappears, and you may have missed the error.

A similar problem can arise when you need to select subsets of cases for analysis. Suppose that the variables AGE (in years), GENDER (1 = woman, 2 = man), SES (socioeconomic status; 1 = low, 2 = middle, 3 = high), BMI (body mass index), and CT (cholesterol test score) are in a dataset. You wish to conduct a statistical analysis with data from men at least 45 years old from low SES households with CT scores of least 240 or BMI scores greater than 30 only. This pattern can be described by the following logical expression:

$$\text{Select if } [(\text{GENDER} = 2 \text{ and AGE} \geq 45 \text{ and SES} = 1)$$
$$\text{and } (\text{CT} \geq 240 \text{ or BMI} > 30)]$$

If the pattern for a case satisfies this expression, then that case is selected for further analysis; otherwise, it is omitted. Suppose that in the GUI for a statistical program, you pick the option to select cases. In the dialog box for the select cases command, you type a logical expression similar to the one just presented. After clicking on the "OK" button, the dialog box closes and the computer selects the appropriate subset of cases. However, the original logical expression you typed in the GUI may not have been recorded by the computer. The failure to notice a typing mistake in the select cases dialog box presents a similar problem.

A solution to the difficulties just discussed is to control a statistics program in batch mode instead of through a GUI. In **batch mode**, lines of commands (code, syntax) that describe the data and analyses are entered directly into an editor window that may be saved later as a text file. The syntax is later executed through some form of a "run" command, and the output appears in a new window or is saved in a separate file. Batch mode is an older way of controlling computer programs that has been histori- cally associated with mainframe computers. About 30 years ago, computer software for statistics was available on mainframe computers only, and back then about all students and researchers worked in batch mode.

You might think that batch mode is obsolete nowadays. However, it is actually not, and here is why: Many modern statistics programs for per- sonal computers, such as SPSS and SAS, offer batch mode processing as an alternative to a GUI. It is true that batch mode is not as easy as working in a GUI. This is because you must first learn the command language for a par- ticular statistics program in order to use its batch mode. Each command must be entered perfectly or else the analysis may fail, so batch mode can be rather tedious. Nevertheless, there are significant advantages of batch mode that can outweigh these drawbacks.

In batch mode, the command file in which program syntax was en- tered also serves as the archive for your analysis. This means that all com- mands—including those that specify the calculation of new variables or case selection—are stored in this file. The command file is also your record of all statistical analyses conducted and specifications of your data file. If you later forget something important about the analysis, then just review the command file. A typing mistake that does not result in an error mes- sage (e.g., "25 × V1" instead of ".25 × V1") is easily fixed by editing the com- mand file and then rerunning the analysis. Also, the command file along with your data file can be electronically transmitted to someone else, who could then reproduce all your analyses.

In some statistics programs, certain types of analyses or output may be available only in batch mode. For example, depending on the particular version of SPSS for personal computers, there is a procedure known as MANOVA that is available in batch mode only; that is, there is no option for this procedure in any menu of the GUI. However, a different proce- dure, General Linear Model (GLM), can be selected through the GUI. Both the MANOVA and GLM procedures analyze repeated-measures data and multivariate data, but the formats of their outputs are somewhat dif- ferent. Some researchers (like me) find that certain types of statistical in- formation is better reported in MANOVA output than in GLM output for the same data. These people may prefer to use MANOVA in batch mode than use GLM through the GUI.

Another advantage of batch mode is that it often supports the conduct of secondary analyses with summary data. Most researchers (and students, too) work with raw data files when conducting their analyses. You may be surprised to learn, however, that the raw data themselves are not necessary for many kinds of statistical analyses. For example, it is possible for a computer to conduct a one-way ANOVA using only group means, standard deviations, and sizes (i.e., n). A repeated-measures ANOVA can be calculated using only these summary statistics and the correlations between the levels of the within-subject factor, and the computer requires only the correlation matrix, standard deviations, and means in order to conduct a standard MR analysis. Thus, a secondary analysis can be conducted by someone who does not have access to the raw data but to whom sufficient summary statistics are available. For example, readers of a journal article can, with the right summary information, either replicate the original analyses or conduct alternative analyses not considered in the original work. Most meta-analyses are secondary analyses conducted with summary statistics taken from primary studies.

Presented in Table 8.1 are two examples of syntax for batch mode processing in SPSS. The syntax for the first example in the table concerns the calculation of a new variable, VN, and case selection. The second line of code in this example specifies that the data are stored in the external SPSS raw data file named "datafile.sav." The third line, the compute com-

TABLE 8.1. Examples of SPSS Syntax for Batch Analyses

Example 1

```
comment compute and select.
get file 'datafile.sav'.
compute VN=.25*V1+1.50*V2+.75*V3+9.60*V4+.35*V5+.80*V6.
descriptives variables=VN/statistics=all.
temporary.
select if (GENDER=2 & AGE>=45 & SES=1 & (CT>=240 or BMI>30)).
descriptives variables=VN/statistics=all.
```

Example 2

```
comment oneway anova with summary statistics.
matrix data variables=GROUP rowtype_ DV/factors=GROUP.
begin data
1 n 50
2 n 55
3 n 65
1 mean 66.25
2 mean 60.25
3 mean 69.30
1 sd 23.50
2 sd 23.25
3 sd 22.95
end data.
oneway DV by GROUP/statistics=descriptives/matrix=in(*).
```

mand, instructs the computer to calculate VN as a weighted combination of variables V1 through V6, which are already in the data file. The fourth line requests descriptive statistics for the whole sample on VN. The next two lines temporarily select a subset of cases—low-income men who are at least 45 years old with high scores on either a CT or a BMI—for one analysis. This analysis generates descriptive statistics on VN for this subgroup only (last line in Example 1 in the table). The second example in Table 8.1 concerns a statistical analysis conducted with summary statistics, not raw scores. In this example, the second line of syntax specifies the "Matrix Data" command, which in SPSS is used to read in summary statistics. In this case, the sizes, means, and standard deviations for three groups are read (lines 3–9), and then a one-way ANOVA conducted with these group descriptive statistics is requested (last line).

For relatively simple statistical analyses with few case selections or computations of new variables, it may be more bother than it is worth to use batch mode. For more complex analyses, however, batch mode offers some distinct advantages. Once mastered, you may also find that using batch mode for complex analyses is actually more efficient and faster—and thus easier—than using a GUI in computer programs for statistics.

Data Screening[3]

It is understandable that you might be eager to begin the analyses right after entering all your scores in a computer data file. However, there are many data-related problems that can so adversely affect the analysis that the results may be nonsense. The aphorism "garbage in, garbage out" is relevant here as it reminds us that the quality of computer output depends on the accuracy of the input. *Thus, it is critical to check the data for problems before conducting any substantive analyses.* Failure to do so can mean frustration after the discovery of data-related errors that rendered a set of analyses useless. This frustration may turn to embarrassment if problems are found only after reporting the results at a conference or, even worse, in print.

The discussion that follows emphasizes basic data screening for univariate analyses, especially for the classical techniques of MR and ANOVA. There are also methods for screening data at the multivariate level, but this

---

[3]Part of the presentation in this section is based on Kline (2005, pp. 48–58).

topic is not covered here (see Tabachnick & Fidell, 2007; Ch. 4, for more information). Fortunately, many instances of data-related problems at the multivariate level are detectable through data screening at the univariate level. You should understand that it is not possible to cover all aspects of data screening in a single section. Indeed, entire books are devoted to some topics in this area, such as that of missing data. Instead, this presentation is intended as a brief introduction that points out major options for screening data that should be useful in student research projects.

The basic steps of univariate data screening are summarized in Table 8.2. They are presented in the table in the same general order in which they are usually carried out. The basic tasks of each step are summarized in the table, too. You can use this table as a checklist for screening your own data. The data screening steps listed in Table 8.2 are elaborated next.

Proofread for Data Entry Errors

The very first thing to do in data screening is simple—*look at the data* (Wilkinson and the Task Force on Statistical Inference, 1999). This means

TABLE 8.2. Basic Steps of Univariate Data Screening

1. Proofread for data entry errors.
    a. Scan data file for incorrect values.
    b. Compare data file entries for each case against original records.

2. Assess univariate descriptive statistics.
    a. Check for out-of-range values.
    b. Identify extreme scores (outliers).
    c. Plausible mean, range, and standard deviation?

3. Check distribution shape.
    a. Calculate indexes of skew and kurtosis.
    b. If necessary, transform variables.
    c. Check results of transformations.

4. Evaluate amount and nature of missing data.
    a. Do incomplete cases differ from complete cases on other variables?
    b. Select an option to deal with missing data (delete cases; impute values).
    c. Check results with and without missing data.

5. Inspect bivariate relations.
    a. Check correlations for pairwise multicollinearity.
    b. Inspect scatter plots for curvilinearity, heteroscedasticity.
    c. Analyze the distribution of residuals.

to visually scan the data file for entries that are obviously incorrect, such as a score of 300 when the highest possible score is 30. This is not too difficult a task for datasets with even a few hundred cases but not a large number of variables (e.g., < 20). Next, proofread the data file against the original data records, such as paper-and-pencil questionnaires completed by research participants. It is so easy to make a typing mistake during manual data entry that errors are almost guaranteed even in small datasets. Proofing the data file works best when carried out by someone other than the person who originally entered the scores. Another kind of check is when two different people independently enter the same set of scores in two different data files. Any discrepancies would indicate a problem, but this tactic would not identify when the same data entry mistake was made by both people. Even careful proofing may not detect all data entry errors, so more formal methods are needed.

Sometimes students analyze archival or existing datasets (i.e., someone else collected the data), so it may not be possible to proof the data file against original records. *Do not assume that a data file given to you has been carefully screened.* That is, always carry out steps 2–5 in Table 8.2 for any raw data file before analyzing it.

Assess Univariate Descriptive Statistics

Use the computer in the second step of data screening (Table 8.2) to calculate descriptive statistics (e.g., the mean, standard deviation, and lowest and highest values) for each variable. Carefully inspect these values—especially the lowest and highest ones—for **out-of-range scores** with impossible values for a particular variable. Such scores may be the result of a data entry error or the failure to specify a missing data code. Suppose that the range of valid scores for some variable is 10–80. A researcher decides to enter a value of "99" in the data file for cases with missing values on that variable but forgets to specify the meaning of this value in a data editor. Without this specification, the computer will treat the value "99" as a valid score. Also, some computer tools for statistics assume by default that an empty field, or a "blank," indicates a missing value, but others may treat a "blank" as a score of zero, or a valid score. Check the documentation for your computer tool.

This is also the time to check for **outliers**, or extreme scores in a distribution. There is no universal definition of "extreme," but a common heuristic is that scores more than 3 standard deviations beyond the mean may be outliers. Univariate outliers are easy to find by inspecting frequency distributions of z scores (i.e., $|z| > 3.00$ indicates an outlier). In a small dataset, even a few outliers can greatly affect the results. Let us assume that an outlier is not due to a data entry error or the failure to specify a missing data code; that is, it is a valid score. One possibility is that the case with the outlier does not belong to the population from which you intended to sample. Suppose that a senior graduate student audits a lower-level undergraduate class in which a questionnaire is distributed. The auditing student is from a different population, and his or her questionnaire responses may be extreme compared with those of the other students.

If it is determined that a case with outlier scores is not from the same population as the rest, then it may be best to remove that case from the sample. Otherwise, there are ways to reduce the influence of extreme scores if cases with them are retained. One option is to convert extreme scores to a value that equals the next most extreme score that is within 3 standard deviations of the mean. Another is to transform the variable with outliers. Transformations are also a way to deal with severe nonnormality and are discussed later. After correcting out-of-range scores and dealing with outliers, recalculate the descriptive statistics for these variables to verify that your corrections resulted in plausible values for the scores. However, do not assume that outliers are always just nuisances to be eliminated from the dataset or converted to a less extreme value. Sometimes they present an opportunity to learn something new. This is because an outlier can be seen as an unexpected event, one that goes against expectations or a general rule. There are times in the natural sciences when an outlier indicates a knowledge gap for which there is no apparent explanation. The search for such an explanation could lead to a new discovery. In the behavioral sciences, the presence of cases from an apparently different population when such is not expected could present a similar prospect. This saying, attributed to the science fiction author and biochemist Isaac Asimov, is apropos for outliers if they prompt a reaction of puzzlement from a researcher: "The most exciting phrase to hear in science, the one that heralds new discoveries, is not 'Eureka!' but 'That's funny . . .'."

Check Distribution Shape

This is the third step in data screening (Table 8.2). Traditional test statistics for continuous variables, such as t and F, assume normally distributed population distributions. This assumption is indirectly evaluated by examining whether sample distributions are approximately normal. Recall that it is a mistake to assume that t and F are so robust against violation of the normality assumption that distribution shape does not matter, especially when the sample size is not large (Chapter 5). Thus, you should assess the degree of departure from normality in sample distributions and take corrective action in clear cases of nonnormality.

Skew and kurtosis are two ways that a distribution can be nonnormal, and they can occur either separately or together in the same variable. Briefly, **skew** means that the shape of the distribution is not symmetrical about its mean, and **kurtosis** means that the distribution is peaked or flat relative to a normal distribution. For each of skew and kurtosis there are two types, positive and negative. **Positive skew** means that most of the scores are below the mean, and **negative skew** means that most of the scores are above the mean. Presented in the top part of Figure 8.1 are examples of distributions with either positive skew or negative skew compared with a normal curve. **Positive kurtosis** means that the distribution has heavier tails and a higher peak relative to a normal curve. A distribution with positive kurtosis is described as **leptokurtic**. A distribution with **negative kurtosis** has lighter tails and is flatter compared with a normal curve; such a distribution is described as **platykurtic**. Presented in the bottom part of Figure 8.1 are examples of distributions with either positive kurtosis or negative kurtosis compared with a normal curve.

Skew is generally easy to detect by looking at graphical frequency distributions or histograms of the original scores. However, a drawback to these types of displays created by some statistical computer programs is that the user may be unable to specify the number of intervals (classes, bins) or bars in the graph. This is because the computer may automatically pick the number of intervals based on the total number of scores (N). The width of each interval is then determined by dividing the overall range by the number of intervals. For instance, the computer may "decide" that there will be 10 intervals in the frequency distribution for a set of 200 scores. The range of the distribution is 50, so the width of each interval will equal $50/10$, or 5. If the user wants fewer or more intervals, then he or she may be out of luck. Another drawback is that one cannot reconstruct the individual scores from a frequency distribution or histogram when the number of intervals is less than the range for the whole distribution.

Two other types of visual displays helpful for detecting skew are stem-and-leaf plots and box plots. A **stem-and-leaf plot** summarizes distribution shape and shows extra detail regarding individual scores. Each score in a stem-and-leaf plot is split into a "stem" part and a "leaf" part. The "leaf" is usually the last digit, and the "stem" is all the other digits to the left of the "leaf." Presented in the left side of Figure 8.2 is a stem-and-leaf plot for

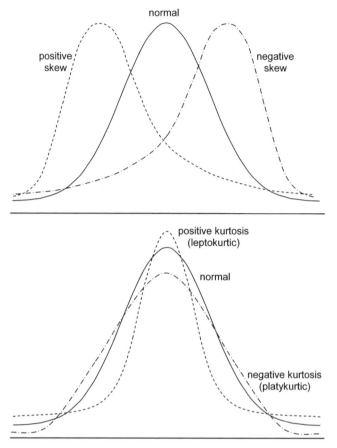

FIGURE 8.1. Distributions with positive skew or negative skew (top) and with positive kurtosis or negative kurtosis (bottom) relative to a normal curve.

a set of scores, $N = 64$. The lowest score in the distribution is 10 and the highest is 27. The latter score is an outlier that is more than 5 standard deviations above the mean ($M = 12.73$, $SD = 2.51$, $z = 5.69$). In the stem-and-leaf plot of Figure 8.2, the numbers to the left side of the vertical line ("stems") represent the "tens" digit of each score, and each number to the right ("leaf") represents the "ones" digit. The number of "leaves" for each "stem" indicates the frequency of that score. The shape of the stem-and-leaf plot in the figure indicates positive skew.

Presented in the right side of Figure 8.2 is a **box plot**—also called a **box-and-whisker plot**—for the same set of scores. The bottom and top borders of the rectangle in a box plot correspond to, respectively, the 25th

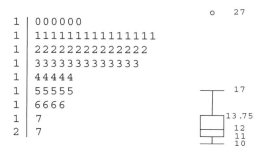

```
1 | 000000
1 | 111111111111111
1 | 222222222222222
1 | 333333333333333
1 | 44444
1 | 55555
1 | 6666
1 | 7
2 | 7
```

FIGURE 8.2. A stem-and-leaf plot (left) and a box plot (right) for the same distribution ($N = 64$).

percentile (or first quartile) and the 75th percentile (or third quartile). The bottom border of the rectangle in a box plot is referred to as the **lower hinge** and the upper border as the **upper hinge**. The total region in the rectangle of a box plot represents 50% of the scores. The line inside the rectangle of a box plot represents the median (or second quartile). The "whiskers" of a box plot are vertical lines that connect the lower and upper hinges with the lowest and highest scores that are not extreme, or outliers. The length of the whiskers show how far the nonextreme scores spread away from the middle of the distribution. Skew is indicated in a box plot if the median line does not fall at the center of the rectangle or by "whiskers" with unequal lengths. In the box plot of Figure 8.2, the lower and upper hinges are, respectively, 11 and 13.75; the median is 12; and the lowest and highest scores that are not extreme are, respectively, 10 and 17. The highest score of 27 is extreme and thus is represented in the box plot as a single open dot beyond the upper "whisker." The box plot in the figure indicates positive skew because there is a greater spread of the scores above the median (and mean, too). Also, a box plot is better at showing outliers than stem-and-leaf plots (Figure 8.2).

Kurtosis is harder to spot by eye, especially in distributions that are more or less symmetrical. Thus, there is a need for more precise measures of skew and kurtosis. The most common measures of skew and kurtosis that allow the comparison of different distributions to the normal curve are calculated as follows:

$$\text{skew index} = \frac{S^3}{\left(S^2\right)^{3/2}} \qquad \text{kurtosis index} = \frac{S^4}{\left(S^2\right)^2} - 3.0 \quad (8.1)$$

where the terms S^2, S^3, and S^4 are known as, respectively, the second through fourth **moments about the mean:**

$$S^2 = \Sigma\,(X - M)^2/N, \; S^3 = \Sigma\,(X - M)^3/N, \text{ and } S^4 = \Sigma\,(X - M)^4/N \quad (8.2)$$

The sign of the skew index indicates the direction of the skew, positive or negative, and a value of zero indicates a symmetrical distribution. The value of the kurtosis index in a normal distribution also equals zero; otherwise, its signs indicate the type of kurtosis, positive or negative.[4] There are no absolute standards for saying when there is so much skew or kurtosis that corrective measures should be taken, but some suggestions can be offered. Variables with absolute values of the skew index greater than 3.0 are described as "extremely" skewed by some researchers. There is less agreement about the kurtosis index. A conservative rule of thumb is that absolute values of the kurtosis index greater than 10.0 may suggest a problem, and values greater than 20.0 may indicate a bigger one. For the data in Figure 8.2, the value of the skew index is 3.10, and the value of the kurtosis index is 15.73. In computer output, values of the skew and kurtosis indexes may be reported along with their standard errors. The ratio of the value of either the skew index or the kurtosis index over its standard error is interpreted in large samples as a z-test of the null hypothesis that there is no population skew or kurtosis, respectively. However, these statistical tests may not be very useful in large samples because even slight departures from normality may be statistically significant. And in small samples, great departures from normality may not be statistically significant. In other words, the statistical test associated with a skew or kurtosis index is generally not very useful.

One way to deal with extreme skew or kurtosis is with **transformations**, which means that the original scores are converted with a mathematical operation to new ones that may be more normally distributed. For example, transformations that may normalize positively skewed distributions include square root, logarithmic, and inverse functions (respectively, $X^{1/2}$, $\log_{10} X$, and $1/X$). All the transformations just mentioned but applied to the original scores subtracted from the highest score plus 1 may remedy negative skew. Odd-root (e.g., $X^{1/3}$) and sine functions tend to bring outliers from both tails of the distribution in closer to the mean, and odd-power transformations (e.g., X^3) may help for negative kurtosis. All the transformations just mentioned are monotonic in that they do not change the rank order of the scores.

---

[4]Some computer programs calculate the skew index as $S^4/(S^2)^2$ (compare with Equation 8.1). In this case, a value of 3.0 indicates a normal distribution, a value greater than 3.0 indicates positive skew, and a value less than 3.0 indicates negative skew.

There are many other kinds of transformations, and this is one of their potential problems: It can be difficult to find a transformation that works for a particular set of scores (i.e., there may be much trial and error). Also, some distributions can be so severely nonnormal that basically no transformation will work. Another potential drawback of transformations is that the scale of the original variable is lost. If that scale is meaningful, such as the level of education in years, then its loss could be a sacrifice. Also, interpretations of the results of statistical analyses of transformed scores do not apply to the original scores. For example, the level of statistical significance (i.e., p) found for a transformed variable may not apply to the original variable. See Hartwig and Dearing (1979) for more information about transformations.

Evaluate Amount and Nature of Missing Data

This is the fourth step in data screening (Table 8.2). The topic of how to analyze incomplete datasets is complicated. Entire books are devoted to it (e.g., P. E. McKnight, McKnight, Sidani, & Figueredo, 2007), and state-of-the-art techniques require graduate-level quantitative skills. Even these modern techniques may only reduce bias due to missing data but do not eliminate it. Emphasized next are classical techniques for dealing with missing data that are of greater use to students. Some suggestions for mitigating limitations of these techniques are also considered.

Ideally, researchers would always work with complete datasets, ones with no missing values. Otherwise, prevention is the best approach for avoiding missing data. For example, questionnaire items that are clear and unambiguous may prevent missing responses, and completed forms should be reviewed for missing responses before research participants leave the laboratory. In the real world, missing values occur in many (if not most) datasets, despite the best efforts at prevention. Missing data occur for many reasons, including hardware failure, software bugs, data entry errors, missed appointments by participants, and attrition of cases (e.g., they withdraw from the study), to name a few. A few missing values (e.g., less than 5% missing on a single variable) in a large dataset may be of little concern, especially if the reason for data loss is accidental, such as when hardware sporadically fails. Accidental data loss is random, which means that whether scores are missing or not is unrelated to participants' true status on that variable or on other variables. Selection among methods to deal with the missing observations in this case is pretty much arbitrary in that the method used tends not to make much difference.

It is a more serious problem when data loss exceeds, say, 10–15% of the scores on a variable *and* the reason for data loss is systematic, not accidental. A systematic data loss pattern means whether scores are missing or not predicts participants' true status on that variable or on other variables. If so, then results based on cases with no missing data may not generalize. For example, patients who dropped out of a drug treatment study may have experienced worse side effects than patients who remained, and results based only on the latter will not reflect this situation.

Two sets of classical techniques for handling missing observations are described next. One is based on **available-case methods**, which involve the exclusion of incomplete cases from the analysis. In **listwise deletion**, cases with missing scores on *any* variable are excluded from the analysis, that is, the analysis is conducted with complete cases only. This method can greatly reduce the effective sample size if missing observations are scattered across many records, but it has the advantage that all analyses are based on the same subset of cases. Not so with **pairwise deletion**, in which cases are excluded only if they have missing observations on the variables involved in a particular analysis. Consequently, the effective sample size can vary from analysis to analysis, and each could be based on a different subset of cases. Suppose that $N = 150$ for a sample with missing values on some variables. If 135 cases have no missing values on either X or Y, then the effective sample size for computing r_{XY} is 135. If fewer or more cases have valid scores on X and W, however, then the effective sample size for r_{XW} will not be 135. This feature of pairwise deletion can cause regression analyses to fail due to the calculation of a pattern of correlations that would be mathematically impossible to observe in a sample with no missing data. Of the two, listwise deletion is generally preferred.

A second set of classical methods is **score imputation**, in which each missing score is replaced (imputed) by an estimated score. The most basic method is **mean substitution**, in which a missing score is replaced by the overall sample average on that variable. A variation for grouped data is **group-mean substitution**, in which a missing score in a particular group is replaced by the group mean. Group-mean substitution may be preferred when group membership is a factor in the analysis and there are missing observations on the outcome variables. Both methods are simple, but they can distort the distribution of the data by reducing variability. Suppose in a dataset where $N = 75$ that five cases have missing values on the first variable. Substituting the mean of the 70 valid cases will result in the mean for $N = 75$ cases and the mean for $N = 70$ cases after substitution both being equal. However, the variance for the $N = 70$

scores before substitution will be greater than the variance for the $N = 75$ scores after substitution.

A more sophisticated method is **regression-based imputation**, in which each missing score is replaced by a predicted score using MR based on nonmissing scores on other variables. Suppose that there are five trials in a learning task, and each trial yields a continuous score. Due to equipment failure, the score for Trial 4 for some cases is not recorded. In this method, specify Trials 1–3 and 5 as predictors of Trial 4 (the criterion) in an MR analysis based on scores from all complete cases (i.e., ones with valid scores on Trial 4). From this analysis, record the values of the four unstandardized regression coefficients $(B_1–B_3, B_5)$ and the intercept (A) (i.e., the constant). An imputed score for Trial 4 is the predicted score $(\hat{Y}_4)$, given scores on the other four trials (designated with X below), the regression coefficients, and the intercept, as follows:

$$\hat{Y}_4 = B_1 X_1 + B_2 X_2 + B_3 X_3 + B_5 X_5 + A$$

Because it uses more information, regression-based substitution takes better advantage of the structure in the data than mean substitution. However, it is best to generate predicted scores based on data from the whole sample, not from just one particular group (e.g., the treatment group only). This is because regression techniques can be adversely affected by range restriction, which can happen when scores from a particular group are less variable compared with scores for the whole sample. Because it uses more information, regression-based imputation may be the preferred classical method overall.

When there are few observations missing randomly, it often does not matter which of these classical techniques is used. However, *none* of the classical techniques is really adequate for dealing with higher levels of data loss (e.g., > 10–15% missing on any variable), especially if the data loss pattern is systematic instead of accidental. Specifically, none of the classical techniques can be expected to somehow correct the results for bias due to a data loss pattern that is systematic. Some more state-of-the-art methods may do a better job in this regard, but even these more complex methods are not a miraculous cure for bias. So what, then, is a student to do when faced with a serious missing data problem? Three suggestions are offered, one rational and the other two statistical:

1. Try to understand the nature of the underlying data loss mechanism, and then accordingly qualify your interpretation of the re-

sults. Suppose that a much higher proportion of patients in a treatment group drop out of a study than patients in a control group. At the least, inform your readers of this fact and caution them that results about the treatment may generalize only to patients who stick it out, not to all patients who could theoretically be treated.

2. A statistical comparison of cases who dropped out of the study with those who did not on other variables, such as pretests, may help to identify the nature of the data loss mechanism. Suppose it is discovered that treated cases who dropped out have more of a severe or chronic form of an illness than treated cases who remained in the study. These results would suggest that the treatment may work best for patients with an acute or less severe form of the illness.

3. If the selection of one option for dealing with missing data instead of another (e.g., mean substitution vs. listwise deletion) makes a real difference in the results, then it is best to report both sets of findings. This makes it clear to all that your results depend on how missing observations were handled.

Some state-of-the-art techniques for dealing with missing data are briefly mentioned now. These methods may require specialized software and, as mentioned, are not really suitable for undergraduate-level student research projects. However, if you go on to graduate school, then you may have occasion to use these techniques, given that missing data is such a common problem. Some contemporary techniques are extensions of imputation methods that take into account even more information than regression-based substitution. In **pattern matching**, the computer replaces a missing observation with a score from another case with a similar pattern of scores across other variables. In **random hot-deck imputation**, the computer separates complete from incomplete records, sorts both sets so that cases with similar patterns on background variables are grouped together, randomly interleaves (shuffles) the incomplete records among the complete records, and then replaces missing scores with those from the same variable from the nearest complete record. There is also a family of **model-based imputation methods** that replace a missing score with an estimated value from theoretical distributions that model both the complete data and the incomplete data. Some of these techniques, such as the **expectation–maximization method**, use a series of regressions to first derive predicted scores for each individual missing observation, and these estimates are further refined through additional analyses with the whole dataset. See Allison (2002) for more information about these advanced methods for dealing with missing data.

Inspect Bivariate Relations

This is the final step in data screening (Table 8.2). Described next are a total of four different potential problems that can affect regression analyses. The first is **multicollinearity**, which occurs when correlations between some variables are so high (e.g., > .85) that estimation with the computer results in an error message. This can happen because certain mathematical operations are impossible or unstable due to denominators in some ratios that are close to zero. Sometimes multicollinearity occurs when what appears to be two separate variables actually measure the same thing. Suppose that X is the number of items correct and Y is the speed with which the problems were solved. If $r_{XY} = .95$, then two variables measure basically the same thing and thus are redundant. One or the other could be analyzed, but not both. It is easy to spot pairwise multicollinearity simply by scanning a correlation matrix. A special kind of multicollinearity is harder to detect this way, but it is easy to avoid. This special case occurs when both total scores and their constituent variables are analyzed together. Suppose that a questionnaire has five items, and a total score is summed across all five items. Because the total score is determined by the five items, it is actually collinear with the items. Either the five items or the total score could be analyzed, but not both together in the same analysis.

A second problem concerns linearity. Recall that the Pearson correlation r estimates only the degree of linear association between two variables. For this reason, it can happen that the value of r is about zero even though there is a strong curvilinear association. Consequently, inspecting a correlation matrix is not sufficient to spot curvilinear relations; a much better way is to visually inspect scatterplots. Presented in Figure 8.3 is a scatterplot in which a curvilinear association—specifically, a quadratic one—between X and Y is apparent. However, the value of the Pearson correlation for these data is only $r_{XY} = -.047$. The linear regression line for these data, which is also shown in the figure, clearly does not reflect the quadratic association between X and Y. If one looked just at the near-zero Pearson correlation for these data, one might falsely conclude that these two variables are unrelated. One of the exercises at the end of this chapter concerns how to estimate a curvilinear association with **MR**.

The third and fourth regression-related problems are considered next.

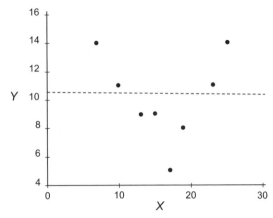

FIGURE 8.3. Scatterplot with a curvilinear (quadratic) association and the linear regression line.

Statistical tests of correlations assume that the **residuals,** the differences between observed and predicted scores (i.e., $Y - \hat{Y}$ calculated for each case), are normally distributed and have uniform variances across all levels of X. The latter characteristic is known as **homoscedasticity**. Its opposite, **heteroscedasticity**, can be caused by outliers, severe nonnormality in either X or Y, or more random error at some levels of X or Y than others. A transformation may correct heteroscedasticity due to nonnormality.

Two types of graphical displays are helpful to evaluate the assumption of normally distributed residuals. The first is a **normal probability plot**, which shows the relation of actual (observed) scores in a distribution to ones expected in a normal curve. When a computer creates a normal probability plot, the scores are arranged from lowest to highest. The percentile equivalent of each score is found, and these percentiles are converted to z scores assuming a normal distribution. The expected z scores are then plotted against the actual values. An alternative is to plot the expected cumulative probabilities against the observed ones. The plotted points will lie close to a straight line if the distribution is reasonably normal. The second type of graphical display is a simple frequency distribution or histogram of the residuals, not of the original scores. The shape of the distribution of residuals should approximate a normal curve.

Presented in Figure 8.4 is a scatterplot with scores from a small sample ($N = 18$). One of the cases has an extreme score (40) on Y, which is more than 3 standard deviations above the mean ($M_Y = 13.78$, $SD_Y = 8.09$, $z = 3.24$). For these data, $r_{XY} = -.074$, and the linear regression line is nearly horizontal. However, these results are affected by the outlier. When the outlier case is removed (i.e., $N = 17$), then $r_{XY} = -.772$, and the new regression line clearly better fits the remaining data (see Figure 8.4). Presented in the top part of Figure 8.5 is the normal probability plot for the standardized residuals (i.e., the residuals converted to z scores) for the data in Figure 8.4 with the outlier included ($N = 18$). The plotted points of the expected versus observed cumulative probabilities for the residuals do not fall along a straight line. Presented in the middle part of Figure 8.5 is the histogram of the standardized residuals for the same data with a superimposed normal curve. Both kinds of displays just described indicate that the residuals for the data in Figure 8.4 are not normally distributed when the outlier is included.

Inspection of the scatterplot of the standardized residuals and the standardized predicted scores ($\hat{z}_Y$) can be helpful for evaluating the assumption of homoscedasticity. If the residuals are distributed evenly around zero throughout the entire length of this scatterplot, then homoscedasticity is indicated. Presented in the bottom of Figure 8.5 is this type of scatterplot for the data in Figure 8.4 with the outlier included. The distribution of the residuals is clearly not uniform around zero across the predicted scores, which suggests heteroscedasticity. Many regression modules in statistical computer programs can optionally plot all the kinds of displays presented in Figure 8.5, and some statistical packages, such as SPSS, have separate regression diagnostics modules. See Fox (1991) for

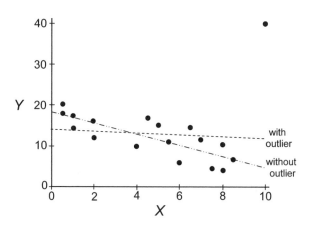

FIGURE 8.4. Scatterplot with outlier ($N = 18$) and the linear regression lines with and without ($N = 17$) the outlier.

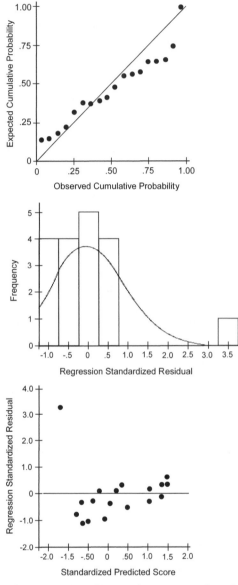

FIGURE 8.5. Plots for regression diagnostics: a normal probability plot of the standardized residuals (top), a histogram of the standardized residuals (middle), and a scatterplot of the standardized residuals and predicted scores (bottom) for the data in Figure 8.4 with the outlier included (N = 18).

more information about graphical and statistical ways to evaluate assumptions about the residuals in regression analyses.

Summary

Begin your statistical analyses only after you have carefully prepared and screened your data for potential problems. Visually scan your data file in order to spot obvious problems, and then use the computer to calculate descriptive statistics for every variable. It is also helpful for continuous variables to inspect graphical displays of distributional characteristics, such as stem-and-leaf plots, box plots, or frequency distributions. Look for scores that are out of range or are outliers. If you plan to use a statistical method that assumes normal distributions, then use corrective measures, such as transformations, to remedy severe skew or kurtosis. Before conducting regression analyses, inspect bivariate scatterplots for the presence of nonlinearity, the presence of outliers with respect to the regression line, or heteroscedasticity. Some basic ways to deal with missing observations include case deletion, mean substitution, or regression-based substitution, but none of these methods can remove bias due to a systematic data loss pattern. After screening the data, conduct a minimally sufficient analysis using a technique that you understand. When in doubt, ask others for help instead of reporting statistical results that you could not explain in person. Keep in mind the goal of your analyses by referring often to the basic questions you want to address. Be ready to be surprised by your data, but avoid excessive analyses, or fishing expeditions, that are not directly connected with your hypotheses.

RECOMMENDED READINGS

Hartwig and Dearing (1979) described various kinds of graphical display techniques for understanding datasets. Stem-and-leaf plots and box plots are just two of these methods. The work by Pallant (2007) is a comprehensive guide to using SPSS from the stages of data coding and entry to the statistical analyses. Roth (1994) provides an accessible review of classical options for handling missing data.

Hartwig, F., & Dearing, B. E. (1979). *Exploratory data analysis*. Newberry Park, CA: Sage.

Pallant, J. (2007). *SPSS survival manual: A step-by-step guide to data analysis* (3rd ed.). Maidenhead, Berkshire, UK: Open University Press.

Roth, P. L. (1994). Missing data: A conceptual review for applied psychologists. *Personnel Psychology, 47,* 537–560.

EXERCISES

1. Enter the 64 scores represented in the stem-and-leaf plot in Figure 8.2 into a data file. Use a computer tool for statistics and calculate for these scores basic descriptive statistics (e.g., $M = 12.73, SD = 2.51$, etc.) and values of the skew and kurtosis indexes (respectively, 3.10, 15.73). Also create a box plot for these data like the one in Figure 8.2.

2. Presented next are the scores that correspond to the scatterplot in Figure 8.3. They are reported as (X, Y) for a total of eight cases:

    $$(7,14), \quad (10,11), \quad (13,9), \quad (15,9),$$
    $$(17,5), \quad (19,8), \quad (23,11), \quad (25,14)$$

    Use a computer program for statistics to reproduce the scatterplot in Figure 8.3. Calculate for these data the correlation $r_{XY} = -.047$. Now create a new variable, X^2. In a regression analysis, specify that both X and X^2 are the predictors of Y. Report the multiple correlation from this analysis. Create the scatterplot with the regression "line" from this analysis. Explain the results.

3. Presented next are the scores that correspond to the scatterplot in Figure 8.4. They are reported as (X, Y) for a total of 18 cases:

    $$(4,10), \quad (2,12), \quad (1,14), \quad (.5,18), \quad (4.5,17), \quad (5,15),$$
    $$(5.5,11), \quad (6,6), \quad (6.5,14.5), \quad (7,11.5), \quad (8,4),$$
    $$(7.5,4.5), \quad (8.5,6.5), \quad (8,10.5), \quad (10,40), \quad (.5,20),$$
    $$(1,17.5), \quad (2,16)$$

    Use a statistics computer tool to create figures for regression diagnostics similar to those presented in Figure 8.5 for these same scores.

4. Presented next is a small dataset where scores for each case are reported as (Y, X_1, X_2, X_3):

    $$(12,11,10,10.5), \quad (14,10,9,9.5), \quad (15,13,6,9.5),$$
    $$(12,10,7,8.5), \quad (8,6,8,7), \quad (10,8,15,11.5),$$
    $$(5,8,4,6), \quad (12,9,14,11.5), \quad (9,2,8,5)$$

    Using a computer tool for statistics, specify X_1, X_2, and X_3 as the predictors of Y in a regression analysis. However, this particular analysis will fail. Figure out why.

5. Presented next are scores for 10 cases reported as (X, Y, W) and where a missing observation is coded as −9. Enter these scores into a data file with the appropriate missing data specification. Calculate the bivariate correlations using listwise deletion, pairwise deletion, and mean substitution. Describe the results:

    (−9,15,−9), (12,23,48), (13,25,38), (−9,18,38),
    (15,20,39), (13,15,35), (17,−9,36), (18,24,47),
    (19,21,42), (17,−9,−9)

CHAPTER 9

Writing

Few people write well; many people revise well.

—MARTHA DAVIS (2005, p. 103)

Strong writing skills are important for students. Students in advanced educational tracks, such as specialization or honors programs, are usually required to write more than other students. The ability to write well is also critical for researchers. Writing is the main way that researchers communicate about their work, so it is a core professional activity. It is also critical for writing applications for funding agencies in order to receive financial support for your work. Scientific writing involves communicating not only with words but also with numbers and graphics, so it is a complex task. Considered in this chapter are general principles of good scientific writing and practical suggestions for writing manuscripts based on empirical studies, such as for student thesis projects or journal articles. Writing a master's thesis or doctoral dissertation is even more demanding. However, learning how to write good, focused, manuscript-length works will contribute to writing a graduate-level thesis and also applications to funding agencies.

Plagiarism and Academic Integrity

Students should know about **plagiarism**, which is a form of academic misconduct where someone takes claim for the work or efforts of others without proper citation or authorization. Plagiarism can be seen as a form of theft, not of property but ideas, which is the currency of research in particular and academia in general. To make the matter more personal, imagine how you would feel after writing the results of your research project if another student submitted your manuscript and received credit for it, but not you. As a student writer, you should know how not to get in trouble regarding plagiarism. Not only is plagiarism a violation of your personal honor code, it compromises basic principles of scientific integrity, too. Many universities have Web pages about plagiarism and also offer free counseling about how to avoid it. Suggestions for avoiding plagiarism include keeping detailed notes about sources, learning how to appropriately paraphrase what is said in published sources, and correctly citing and referencing these works. Because it is hard to differentiate accidental plagiarism from intentional plagiarism, universities may censure students who commit plagiarism regardless of the excuse. Some penalties include failing the course in which plagiarism was committed, the placing of a permanent letter about the incident in the student's academic record, or requiring the student to take an additional course about library research that does not count toward his or her degree. It is easy to find resources about plagiarism—use them, especially when in doubt.

Writing as Learning

It helps to view writing as a learning activity. This means that writing is not just for conveying what you already know; it also helps authors to better understand the subject matter. This is because writing forces one to synthesize his or her knowledge in order to express it in ways that others can understand. It is said that one does not really know something until it can be explained to others. It is one thing to do so orally, but quite another to do it in writing. This is because writing is a more formal means of communication than speaking and thus requires a higher degree of organization. Also, the struggle to put thoughts into written words often requires authors to reexamine their initial understanding. An implication of the view of writing as learning is that it is not necessary to have all of one's thoughts clearly organized before starting to write. The exercise of writing will itself help to bring order to those thoughts.

Getting Started

The hardest part about writing for many authors is getting started. For many, staring at a blank page (virtual or physical) at the beginning of a writing project is unnerving. Writing is also an individual task in that there are different ways to begin, so you may need to experiment with different methods. Some authors first write an outline and then later add sentences in paragraph form. An outline can have a formal structure with headings and subheadings labeled in the standard way or consist of a simple list of points. Others use **freewriting**, which is a kind of brainstorming where one just writes sentences as they come to mind without trying to evaluate them yet. These sentences can take any form, such as series of questions to be answered in each section of the document. The goal is to commit ideas to written words in order to get started. It helps some authors to explain their ideas to another person before beginning to write. This is a type of speaking-as-learning activity that can help to organize one's thoughts. Another tactic is to write the abstract first; this forces you to reflect on the overall message of the study. M. Davis (2005, pp. 21–26) described additional types of prewriting activities.

However you get started, try not to spend too much time on prewriting activities. One reason is that a prewriting activity can become a form of procrastination. Another is that writing is a circular or iterative process where the beginning and end are really the same thing. That is, one starts to write by writing, and one concludes by writing. This adage attributed to the American author Gertrude Stein (1874–1946) expresses this idea more lyrically:

To write is to write is to write is to write is to write is to write is to write.

What an author needs most of all in the early stages of writing is a rough draft, which is then extensively revised, usually many times, but it is a critical milestone.

The Role of Style Guides

There are two kinds of style guides for authors of scientific articles. The first is a **technical style guide** about acceptable organization, layout, format, wording, punctuation, and so on for manuscripts submitted to journals. Recommendations about the use of language that is not sexist or derogatory and about statistical results that should be reported may also appear in such guides. In the behavioral sciences, the *Publication Manual* of the American Psychological Association (APA; 2005) is the technical standard for many journals. There are also now many websites devoted to the basics of APA style. Students who submit theses may be required to follow a particular technical style guide. The second type is a **writing style guide**, which is a resource that details grammar rules and principles of composition and word usage. One of the best-known general style guides is *The Elements of Style* by Strunk and White (2000). There are also specific writing style guides for students and researchers in the social sciences (e.g., Northey & Tepperman, 2007; Richards & Miller, 2005).

Students often find both kinds of style guides to be intimidating. A technical style guide is basically a list of rules that can stretch over hundreds of pages. A writing style guide is packed with grammar rules, but many university students have had relatively little exposure to formal grammar. For two reasons, though, there is no need to fear style guides. First, a technical style guide can be mastered only after repeated usage over many writing projects. This experience gives a context for the technical requirements, which may not be obvious after writing a single paper. Second, many people can write well without being to able to articulate specific grammar rules (i.e., they "write by ear"). However, consulting a writing style guide many times gradually increases one's knowledge of grammar. So relax and consult a writing guide whenever needed—which is probably every time you write.

General Principles of Good Writing

Some general principles of good writing of any kind are considered next.

Maladaptive Beliefs

There are several myths about writing that are a factor in serious procrastination, even among experienced writers such as university professors (Boice, 1990). Some of the more common false beliefs are listed next and discussed afterward: Good writers

1. Are born, not made.

2. Do not begin writing until they have a large block of uninterrupted time and are inspired.

3. Work best in a binge style or under pressure and finish a draft in a single long session.

4. Do not believe in rewriting because they are afraid to lose the spontaneity of the first draft.

5. Do not share their writing with others until it is polished and perfect.

There are some people who seem to take naturally to writing, but the reality is that most of us need lots of practice before we become better writers. Accordingly, it is more adaptive to recognize that most good writers are edited, not born. Another reality of writing is that most of us do not have large, uninterrupted blocks of time that can be devoted to writing. Instead, writing is something that must usually be fitted into busy personal or professional schedules. Indeed, if you wait for a large chunk of free time for writing, then you might never start. It can help to schedule specific times for writing, even if that time is relatively short, such as an hour or so. Sometimes just a bit of focused effort in a short time can help you to identify how to start writing (or rewriting) in the next session. It is also a mistake to wait until you are "in the mood" to start writing or feel inspired about what is to be written. This myth ignores the role of writing as learning. It is better to get in the mood by actually starting to write than waiting around for the mood to somehow strike out of the blue.

A romanticized view of a writer is of someone who, facing an impending deadline, sits down in a single long session and, binge style, produces a complete draft. A related myth is that the first draft of real writers is basically the final version that needs only proofing. These beliefs are also quite maladaptive. Writing produced under these conditions is likely to be poor. As with other complex tasks, writing may require several work sessions over a sufficient time period well before any deadline. This is true because the biggest part of writing is often revising. First drafts are only the beginning because good writers extensively revise them, perhaps so much so that the final version bears little resemblance to the first. A great way to improve a draft is to let others read it and offer comments. Remember not to take negative comments as a personal slight; instead, view them as grist for the improvement mill. It can also help to put your manuscript aside, and then come back to it after a few days. In coming back fresh, you may find ways to improve the text that you would otherwise miss because you were too close to the work. Finally, learn your own personal foibles, such as ways you may avoid beginning to write or rationalizations about such avoidance. This is not an easy thing to do, and can even be painful, but we can best overcome personal bad habits when we are aware of them.

Simple, Clear, Active

Good writing is efficient and concise. This means that, in general, a shorter text is better than a longer one, if the two convey the same basic information. Use words that are familiar and organized in sentences that are short and direct instead of long and complicated. Use unfamiliar words only if necessary, such as when defining technical terms. Otherwise, the use of unfamiliar words may exclude some readers. Also avoid **inflated diction**, which results from choosing pretentious words instead of simpler ones, such as "utilize," "facilitate," or "subsequent to" instead of, respectively, "use," "help," or "after." There is no need to spice up scientific writing by adding a foreign-language phrase, so avoid it. As they say, *nie wszystko się godzi, co wolno.*[1] Long, convoluted sentences are more difficult to follow than shorter ones, and it is easier to make a grammatical mistake in a longer sentence, too. This does not mean you should use short sentences only. This type of presentation quickly becomes monotonous, and it comes across as a literary form of machine gun bursts. It is better to vary sentence length in order to hold readers' interest, and to vary sentence openings, too. Text can grow tedious for readers if too many sentences start with the same word, such as "the," "I," or "this."

Another characteristic of good writing is use of the active voice instead of the passive voice. In the **passive voice**, the subject receives the action, as in "The data were analyzed by the researcher with the SuperStat computer tool." In the **active voice**, the subject of the sentence performs the action, as in "The researcher analyzed the data using the SuperStat computer tool." The active voice is generally preferred because it is more direct and not as wordy as the passive voice. Also, overuse of the passive voice can make the text seem bland and monotonous. In the past, the passive voice was preferred in scientific writing in part because it comes across as more impersonal and objective (e.g., "it was decided to" [passive] vs. "I decided to" [active]). However, this is changing, and more scientific writers use the active voice nowadays. This means that scholarly writing is increasingly becoming more like good writing in other, nonacademic venues. This change also acknowledges that even scientific authors have their own direct and personal voice.

---

[1]Few readers probably understood this Polish expression—which roughly means, not everything allowed is good—and that is the point.

The first passage of text that follows breaks practically every suggestion about writing just offered. Compare this passage with the second one,
which is written in a much clearer style:

✘ It was determined by the committee that a new process will be
   implemented subsequent to a manager becoming cognizant of a
   sales decline of 10% in his or her division that will facilitate the goal
   of corrective action, resulting in a review of the ongoing decision-
   making process that led up to the original problem, the making of
   recommendations to impact on the problem in a positive way, and
   utilizing all available personnel and resources.

✓ The committee decided to begin a new review process. If a division
   manager reports a sales decline of 10%, then that manager will
   conduct a review with all relevant personnel. The goals of the
   review are to identify contributing factors and suggest corrective
   actions.

Good writers also use words correctly. For example, there are certain
pairs of words that are often confused in writing. Listed in Table 9.1 are
some of these word pairs especially relevant for scientific writing. Reported
in the table for each pair is the correct definition of the words and examples
of their correct and incorrect usage. For example, the words "affect" and
"effect" are sometimes incorrectly substituted for one another when used
as nouns or verbs. Another pair is the words "relationship" and "relation."
Reserve use of the former for animate objects only. For example, it is poor
style to say, "Weight has a *relationship* with blood pressure," because weight
and blood pressure are inanimate, specifically, they are variables. Variables
may be related (i.e., they covary), but they do not have relationships with
one another. See the writing style guides cited earlier for more extensive
lists of commonly misused words.

Finally, avoid **anthropomorphism**, the attribution of uniquely human characteristics to abstract entities or inanimate objects. For example,
the phrase "This research found …" is an anthropomorphism because
"research" is an abstract entity that cannot "find" anything—only people
(i.e., researchers) can do so. For the same reason, the phrase "The theory
says …" is also an anthropomorphism. It is better to say something like
"Smith (2007) claimed …" or "An implication of the theory is … ," neither
of which are anthropomorphisms.

TABLE 9.1. Commonly Misused Words in Scientific Writing and Examples of Correct Usage

Words	Correct usage
accept, except	*accept* (v), take something offered; *except* (v), exclude something; *except* (p), used before naming excluded things The student will <u>accept</u> ~~except~~ the job offer. The teacher ~~accepted~~ <u>excepted</u> the student from the field trip.
affect, effect	*affect* (n), emotion, feeling; *effect* (n), result, consequence; *affect* (v), product a change; *effect* (v), make something happen This will not <u>affect</u> ~~effect~~ your health. The ~~affect~~ <u>effect</u> of your work was a good grade.
allusion, illusion	*allusion*, applied or indirect reference; *illusion*, misleading image The speaker made an <u>allusion</u> ~~illusion~~ to Dante. The mirror gave the ~~allusion~~ <u>illusion</u> of depth.
although, while	*although*, not temporal, in spite of; *while*, temporal, at the same time <u>Although</u> ~~While~~ it is a known fault, it was not detected. ~~Although~~ <u>While</u> it rained, the roof leaked.
because, since	*because*, not temporal, for that reason; *since*, temporal, after that time He left home <u>because</u> ~~since~~ he wanted to find a job. <u>Since</u> leaving home he has found no job.
elicit, illicit	*elicit* (v), bring out, evoke; *illicit* (adj), unlawful The reporter tried to <u>elicit</u> ~~illicit~~ information. The report concerned ~~elicit~~ <u>illicit</u> commercial activity.
fewer, less	*fewer*, plural, countable items; *less*, singular, noncountable items The are <u>fewer</u> ~~less~~ mechanical failures now. Repairs cause ~~fewer~~ <u>less</u> delay now.
principle, principal	*principle*, basic truth or law; *principal*, head of school, sum of money The basic <u>principle</u> ~~principal~~ of the theory is unproven. A new ~~principle~~ <u>principal</u> was hired.
relationship, relation	*relationship*, a type of kinship between animate objects; *relation*, for inanimate objects, or refers to a relative Do you have a personal <u>relationship</u> ~~relation~~ with her? Is there a ~~relationship~~ <u>relation</u> between weight and blood pressure?
that, which	*that*, for restricted clauses, provides essential meaning; *which*, for unrestricted clauses, provides incidental detail The car <u>that</u> ~~which~~ was parked here was stolen. The car, ~~that~~ <u>which</u> was parked here, was stolen.
then, than	*then*, time transition, in that case; *than*, used to make a comparison First we walk <u>then</u> ~~than~~ we run. She is taller ~~then~~ <u>than</u> he.

Note. v, verb; p, preposition; n, noun.

Read and Listen

One way to become a better writer is to read good writing. This helps you to develop a sense of the organization, tenor, and flow of effective writing. Readers can view just about any kind of good writing, fiction or nonfiction, as a model for effective communication with words. In the sciences, the writing quality of articles in the best journals tends to be good, and a well-written article in the same area as your own research can be a helpful example. It also helps to read aloud a draft of your own writing, or listen as someone else reads it to you. Sometimes the experience of hearing one's own writing gives a new perspective. For example, if a sentence sounds awkward or drags on for too long when you hear it, it needs revision. Reading text aloud is also a good way to catch punctuation or other kinds of writing mistakes that affect meaning or logic. Remember that good scientific writing is *not* conversational in tone, which means that one does not write in the same style as one speaks. Spoken speech is often so loosely structured that it violates basic requirements for clearness and conciseness. A more formal style with a high degree of organization is needed for scientific writing.

Principles of Good Scientific Writing

The single most important requirement for good scientific writing is good content. This means that the (1) hypotheses tested are meaningful and based on solid ideas, and (2) the design, methods, and analyses are all technically correct and appropriate for the problem. If the basic research question is not relevant or the methods or analyses are seriously flawed, then why would anyone bother to read such a paper, even if well written?

Elefteriades (2002) offered these general tips for writing scientific papers. Some of these points are elaborated in the next section about how to write specific parts of a manuscript:

1. Keep it brief and concise.

2. The title must be descriptive, and the abstract should convey all cardinal findings.

3. Avoid excessive literature review and excessive use of tables and figures.

4. Make clear the weaknesses of the study, and avoid superlatives in describing your own work.

Brevity and conciseness in scientific writing are critical, especially for journal articles. Not only is journal space limited, but the typical scientific reader is pressed for time. Consequently, it is necessary to write using a minimum of words, tables, figures, and references. Elefteriades (2002) noted that it is often possible to cut a great deal out of an initial draft of a scientific paper without detracting in a significant way from substance. My own rule of thumb is that the first draft of a manuscript can usually be shortened by 50% through elimination of unnecessary material. This degree of reduction may sound drastic, but a better paper is the usual result. As suggested by Trujillo (2007), "Every sentence must be written for a reason and the shorter, the better" (Transition to Academia section, para. 4).

You should write for a general reader, that is, your manuscript should be understandable by someone who is intelligent but not really familiar with your specific research area. Accordingly, avoid the use of pretentious jargon, and when technical language is needed, use only words or terms for which there are no everyday-language equivalents. The use of unnecessary jargon to "dress-up" common sense or the obvious is a shortcoming of some writing in the behavioral sciences. Reporting too many statistics can also make the text unnecessarily complicated. Perhaps some behavioral science authors emphasize jargon or statistics in order to make the work seem more credible or comparable with studies in the natural sciences. However, the best writing in the natural sciences is also clear, free of hollow jargon, and written for a general science reader.

Take care not to exaggerate when writing about mental or physical health problems. Specifically, do not overstate the base rate of a particular disorder, and do not claim without citing proper evidence that the base rate of that disorder has recently increased. Unfortunately, in both the professional and general media there is a tendency to commit both kinds of errors just mentioned. A warning signal to the critical reader is use of the word "epidemic" in the title or text. For example, it has been reported in the mass media and in some journal articles that there is an "epidemic" of depression among children and adolescents, and specifically that this problem has increased in the last decade. However, there is no evidence for an actual increase in the rate of childhood depression over the last 40 years (Costello, Erkanli, & Angold, 2006). Likewise, the oft-repeated claim that obesity kills upwards of 300,000 people annually in the United States is a gross exaggeration (Gibbs, 2005). Finally, claims that there has been a rapid, recent increase in the general rate of mental disorders—perhaps in response to the stresses of our times—are without basis (Kessler et al., 2005). Serious health or mental problems should not be minimized, but no one benefits from the use of alarmist language.

Writing Sections of Empirical Studies

This mantra relayed to me by Bruce Thompson (personal communication, September 7, 2007) gives a good perspective on the topic of this section: In rank order, the six most important things in writing manuscripts are (1) title, (2) title, (3) title, (4) abstract, (5) first paragraph, (6) last paragraph; begin strong, end strong! These ideas are elaborated next.

Title and Abstract

The title and abstract are the most visible parts of your work. Many people decide whether to read a whole article based on its title or abstract, and many electronic bibliographical services depend on titles to select, index, and classify articles. Your title must be descriptive and complete yet also concise. A title should generally be about 12 words in length, or at most about 20 words. Use simple word order and combinations in the title, and do not use abbreviations or acronyms. Listed next are three example titles, the first too skeletal, the second too verbose, but the third is just about right:

- ✘ EFA Results for Asthma Symptom Ratings

- ✘ A Preliminary Attempt at Using Exploratory Factor Analysis as a Means toward Understanding the Factor Structure of Symptom Ratings from Patients with Asthma at Varying Degrees of Severity

- ✓ Exploratory Factor Structure of Asthma Symptoms as a Function of Illness Severity

The abstract should clearly and briefly convey to a general reader both the rationale *and* the results of your study. An abstract that mentions the results only in passing at the end with the empty phrase, "The findings and implications of this study are discussed," and gives no further detail,

TABLE 9.2. Examples of Poor and Better 120-Word Abstracts

Poor

A within-subject, auditory LI paradigm was used to assess whether patients with a diagnosis of schizophrenia are slower to learn a CS–UCS association given repeated unpaired exposure to the CS. Results of previous studies indicated little evidence of LI deficits in a between-subject, visual and auditory paradigm that verifiably detects LI in normal control participants and that was also found to be disrupted by acute treatment with dopamine agonists. Instead, a general learning deficit was found among the schizophrenia patients in these studies. In this study, a within-subject, visual LI paradigm was used to assess LI deficits in acute and chronic schizophrenia patients. The results and their implications for the possibility that LI deficits are characteristic of schizophrenia are discussed.

Better

Latent inhibition (LI) refers to expected slower learning of a paired association between a conditioned stimulus (CS) and an unconditioned stimulus (UCS) when the CS is first experienced alone. Results of some earlier studies indicated that schizophrenia patients exhibit LI deficits, but later attempts to replicate these findings have been mixed. Results from our previous studies indicated general learning deficits but not LI deficits in schizophrenia patients, using a between-subject design with auditory and visual stimuli. In this study, we used a within-subject visual paradigm that detects LI in normal subjects and is disrupted by drugs that activate dopamine receptors. There was no evidence for LI deficits in schizophrenia patients. The robustness of LI deficits in schizophrenia patients is questioned.

Note. Both abstracts are based on Swerdlow et al. (2005).

is incomplete. An example of a poor abstract and a better abstract both based on the same study of latent inhibition in schizophrenia by Swerdlow et al. (2005) are presented in Table 9.2. The abstracts in the table are each 120 words long, the recommended maximum length in APA style. The poor abstract in Table 9.2 gives no indication of the results and is written in a less accessible way. The better abstract in the table gives the reader a much clearer sense of the research problem and the basic findings. (The longer, 200-word abstract in the original article is clear and informative.)

Introduction (Literature Review)

Beginning scientific writers tend to write literature reviews that are much too long for manuscripts. This happens because they try to write a comprehensive review of previous theory and results. This is fine for a dissertation (and often required, too) but not for a journal article, in which the literature review is typically quite short, about four to six paragraphs. Such brevity means that it is impossible to tell the story of a whole research area. Instead, just the story of the rationale of your particular study should be told in the introduction. This story has basically three parts, including (1) a statement of the basic research problem, (2) explanation of why the problem is important, and (3) an outline of what solution or step toward a solution is proposed. How to approach the writing of each part is considered next.

The basic research problem should be identified in the very first paragraph of your literature review (i.e., begin strong!). The details of the problem can be fleshed out in later paragraphs, but it is important in scientific writing to indicate *right away* the overall purpose of your study. In this sense, what the author of a scientific article does is just the opposite of what a good fictional storyteller does. The latter often lays out a series of events or background elements that lead up to the overall point, morale, or objective of the story (the climax). In scientific writing, the reader should be told up front the point of the story, which is the basic problem that motivated your study (anticlimactic). An example of a strong first paragraph from a recent article by McEwan and Anicich (2007) in a chemistry journal is presented in the top part of Table 9.3. This paragraph is written for a general scientific audience, and it makes clear the basic research problem.

The next few paragraphs (e.g., two to four) in the literature review should describe the context for the core research problem, or why it is important. This includes the definition of key terms, concepts, or issues so that the reader can better understand the problem. It also includes a *selective* (not exhaustive) review of results from key previous studies in the area and related unanswered questions. Also indicate in the text how your study will challenge or extend ideas and findings from previous work. These previous studies are not usually described in a serial, one-at-a-time manner. Instead, they are usually described in groups formed according to common characteristics, such as kinds or methods used or types of participants studied, among other possibilities. In-text citations of these works typically group several sources together. If A, B, and C are authors, then an example of a sentence with parenthetical multiple citation would be, "However, results in this area when researchers use an observational method are quite different (A, 2001; B, 2003; C, 2005)." If an individual previous study is exceptional or groundbreaking, then it could be described in its own paragraph. Otherwise, describing sets of studies is more efficient, and doing so identifies relevant patterns for readers.

In the last paragraph (or two) of the introduction, the specific hypotheses and general experimental design or methods should be *briefly* described. Details about the design will be elaborated in the methods sec-

TABLE 9.3. Exemplary First and Last Paragraphs of Literature Reviews

First paragraph[a]

The ion chemistry of Titan has been one of our main research topics since the announcement of the NASA/ESA Cassini/Huygens project. Our aim was to provide the support necessary for interpreting the data received from the INMS and NGMS experiments. This objective would be accomplished by providing laboratory data enabling the unique ion chemistry taking place in Titan's atmosphere to be described. At the time of the announcement of the phase A mission study in 1987, there were some theoretical models of Titan's atmosphere arising from the Voyager earlier fly-by missions and also from some ground-based observations. After an examination of the available information relevant to Titan in the literature, we realized many reactions were unknown. We then embarked on a laboratory measurement program targeting specific ion-molecule reactions to give us a better understanding of Titan's ion chemistry. We have included many of these new reactions in this review for the first time. We believe that we now have a very good database for modeling the ion chemistry of Titan, at least in its initial reaction sequences, at any altitude (McEwan & Anicich, 2007, p. 381).

Last paragraph

In sum, the present research is designed to examine a set of hypotheses regarding the influence of the color red on performance. Our foremost interest was in testing the hypothesis that red undermines performance on achievement tasks (Experiments 1–4); most of these experiments used an IQ test as the focal achievement task. We also sought to examine the degree to which individuals were conscious of the processes involved in the proposed inimical influence of red (Experiments 2–4). We anticipated that individuals' self-reported avoidance motivation, as well as their self-reported appraisals, perceptions, and moods, would be unrelated to the perception of red and, furthermore, that individuals would not be aware that perceiving red undermined their performance. Finally, we sought to move beyond self-report measures to examine the link between red and avoidance motivation with measures that do not require conscious access to activated motivational processes (Experiments 5–6). We hypothesized that the perception of red would evoke motivation to avoid failure, as indicated by both behavioral and psychophysiological markers of avoidance motivation (Elliot et al., 2007, p. 156).

[a]NASA, National Aeronautics and Space Administration; ESA, European Space Agency; INMS, ion neutral mass spectrometry; NGMS, noble gas mass spectrometry.

tion, but it is important to give the reader a sense of the "bigger picture" for your study at the conclusion of the literature review. Nothing about any of the results should be mentioned yet, however. Presented in the bottom part of Table 9.3 is an example of an excellent last paragraph in the literature review from Elliot, Maier, Moller, Friedman, and Meinhardt (2007).

Methods

This section can be challenging to write. It is basically a set of plans for replicating the original study. Just enough detail must be provided so that replication is possible, but not too much. That is, you must balance the goals of communication brevity versus completeness in the methods section. It can happen that this section for studies with complex designs is the longest in the manuscript. When results of multiple studies are reported in the same article, a separate methods section may be needed for each individual study. It can be difficult for others to really understand what the results mean if the methods section is not clearly written, so the need for good writing is great here. Use a narrative format (write in the past tense) throughout.

The typical methods section is divided into up to five or so labeled subsections. These include Participants (Subjects), Apparatus (or Materials), Measures, Procedures, and Data (Statistical) Analyses. A participants or subjects subsection is included in virtually all studies with, respectively, human or animal cases, but not all of the other subsections may be needed for a particular study. Sometimes authors combine the text for two subsections under a single label, such as "Apparatus and Procedure" or "Materials and Measures." When needed, different subsection labels can be used, such as "Design" for a study with a complex experimental design. Use the minimum number of labeled subsections for the methods section of a particular study. Considered next are suggestions for what to include in the text of major subsections.

The number and characteristics of the research participants are described in the participants subsection. If there is a single, undifferentiated group of participants, it is usually possible to describe the group with just text and no tables. For example, descriptive statistics for the average age (and standard deviation), proportions of participants who are men or women, or a breakdown of diagnostic categories could be given in a few sentences. However, if there are multiple groups that differ on several key demographic or other variables, then it may be better to report group descriptive statistics in a table and summarize those results in the text. Also clearly explain how the participants were selected, which helps readers to understand possible limits to the generalizability of the results. Likewise, interpretation of your results later in the manuscript should not go beyond what the sample warrants (Wilkinson & the Task Force on Statistical Inference, 1999). Also needed is a statement about how the participants or subjects (i.e., human or animal) were treated in accordance with ethical standards. In studies conducted with animals, provide as much information as necessary (e.g., the rat species) so that your study could be replicated with the same animal subjects.

An apparatus or materials subsection is needed for studies in which special equipment is used to control experimental conditions or record data, among other possibilities essential for carrying out the study. Give enough information about a physical apparatus, such as the brand and model number for a device purchased from a commercial supplier, to permit replication. If an apparatus is bespoke (custom-made), then consider including an illustration, drawing, photograph, or whatever is necessary to allow replication. If a questionnaire is used to collect data, then a measures subsection is needed in which the psychometrics characteristics of the scores are described plus any specific methods used for collecting the scores. Psychometric characteristics include information about score reliability and score validity in your sample (Chapter 7). In animal studies, outcome variables are usually based on operational definitions that associate observable behaviors with particular hypotheses or constructs. Complete definitions should be presented either in other subsections, such as "Procedures" or "Design," or in a separate subsection for this topic.

Give details about how each step of the investigation was carried out in the Procedures subsection. This includes instructions given to participants and information about specific experimental manipulations, such as randomization or counterbalancing, or about any other critical feature of the design. Describe any sources of anticipated attrition of cases due to factors such as dropout or noncompliance, and indicate how such attrition could affect the generalizability of the results. Also describe ways used to deal with experimenter bias, especially if the data were collected by a sole author.

A subsection about the statistical analyses is generally needed only if a special technique is used that is not standard or widely known in a particular area. For instance, there is no need to describe general characteristics of MR or the ANOVA because these are standard techniques in the behavioral sciences. If there is something special about the application of these techniques to your data that readers must know in order to replicate your analyses, however, then provide those details. If you are unsure about whether a particular statistical technique should be described in the methods section, consult related published works or seek the advice of your supervisor. If you wind up including a data analysis subsection, then you need to explicitly justify those analyses. You can do this in part by citing relevant works that provide a rationale for your use of a particular statistical technique. That is, the methods section may need citations, too.

Results

In brief articles, the results and discussion sections may be combined; otherwise, these are distinct sections with different goals. Specifically, the basic findings are described in the results section with little interpretation beyond that associated with explaining the outcomes of the analyses. Broader interpretation, including whether specific hypotheses were supported or not and possible implications of the results, are dealt with in the discussion section.

It helps to begin the results section with a brief reminder about the basic hypotheses associated with a particular analysis, especially if a different kind of analysis is required for each hypothesis. Next, describe complications, protocol violations, or other unexpected problems in data collection (Wilkinson & the Task Force on Statistical Inference, 1999), if any. A frequent complication is missing data due to participant dropout, failure of some participants to complete questionnaire items, or equipment failure, among other possibilities. Reasons for concern about missing observations and options for dealing with this problem were considered in the previous chapter. Clearly inform readers about how missing data were handled in your study. Unfortunately, too many authors ignore this advice. For example, Roth (1994) found that 65% of the analyses reported in 75 articles published in two different psychology journals were conducted with incomplete datasets, but in about 40% of these cases the authors did not indicate how they dealt with missing data. Also mention early in the results section about whether assumptions for your statistical analyses, such as normality, were met and also about any corrective steps taken, such as transformations. This is critical information that too many researchers neglect to report (but not you).

To write the rest of the results section, use text, tables, and figures to each communicate unique content. The text of the results section is for words and just a few select numerical values. The latter should be mainly descriptive statistics, including effect sizes, not inferential statistics. Too many numbers in the text can make it difficult to read, and tables are a better place for readers to scan a set of related numbers. Also, modern readers of journal articles in the behavioral sciences will be disappointed to find mainly inferential statistics in the results section, and they will rightfully conclude that the report is flawed (American Psychological Association, 2005). An example of the kind of text to avoid in the results section is presented next:

> ✘ A 2 × 2 × 2 (Instructions × Incentive × Goals) ANOVA was conducted with the number of correct items as the dependent variable. The three-way interaction was significant (F (1, 72) = 5.20, $p < .05$) as were all two-way interactions (Instructions × Incentive, F (1, 72) = 11.95, $p < .001$; Instructions × Goals, F (1, 72) = 25.40, $p < .0001$;

Incentive × Goals, $F(1, 72) = 9.25$, $p < .01$) and two of three of the main effects (Instructions, $F(1, 72) = 11.60$, $p < .01$; Goals, $F(1, 72) = 6.25$, $p < .05$).

Not only is the foregoing text chock-a-block with inferential statistics, it confuses substantive significance with statistical significance and also fails to inform the reader about effect size. A proper emphasis on effect size helps to avoid this kind of confusion. See Appendix 9.1 for an example of a better, more contemporary text that describes results from an actual study where effect sizes are also reported.

If possible—and it usually is for student research projects—report in tables or in an appendix sufficient descriptive statistics to permit a secondary analysis. That is, give the reader enough summary information so that he or she could replicate your major analyses. For ANOVAs conducted in between-subject designs, report the means, standard deviations, and number of cases for each cell (group or condition). For within-subject designs, also report the correlations across levels of within-subject factors, such as repeated-measures variables. For MR analyses, report the complete correlation matrix (not just values that are statistically significant), the standard deviations, and the means (Wilkinson and the Task Force on Statistical Inference, 1999). Also report complete source tables for analyses of variance for critical outcome variables. These tables should include the sums of squares, degrees of freedom, mean squares, F values, and effect sizes, such as estimated eta-squared ($\hat{\eta}^2$). In tables in which results of MR analyses are summarized, report both standardized regression coefficients (beta weights) and unstandardized regression coefficients, too. The latter are more useful for comparing results across samples with different variances on variables of interest.

Apart from tables for ANOVA and regression results, which tend to have pretty standard formats, there are too many other possible variations in table organization for reporting the results from other kinds of statistical analyses to cover them all. Some examples are presented in the APA *Publication Manual* (2005), including ones for results of analyses in structural equation modeling (SEM). Of course, many examples are available in journal articles. In any event, use the smallest number of tables necessary to report statistical results, and format the tables so that the visual layout is simple and clear. This means that related numbers are grouped together and with clear and meaningful labels for that kind of data analysis. A total of two to three tables should be sufficient for a study with a single method section and a results section. A larger number may be fine for a multiple-study report, but nevertheless keep the overall number of tables to the absolute minimum necessary to convey key results.

Many times it is unnecessary to include a figure in a journal article, so there is no general requirement of any kind for a figure. That is, include a figure only if it is good. A good figure conveys essential information that cannot be more efficiently summarized in words or tables. Tufte (2001) outlined related properties: A good figure should

1. Make large datasets coherent.

2. Present many numbers in a small space.

3. Reveal the data at different levels without distorting what the data have to say.

4. Illustrate the relation between at least two different variables.

5. Devote a minimum of ink (actual or virtual) to nondata detail.

6. Be presented with a clear purpose.

7. Be closely integrated with accompanying text.

8. Induce the viewer to think about substance, not about graphical design.

Unfortunately, too many figures found in scientific and other kinds of works are poor because they do not accomplish these goals. Principles for constructing effective graphical summaries of results are outlined in the next section.

Discussion

Remind readers in the very first paragraph about the basic purpose(s) of your study. Some authors next begin to summarize the main findings, but I prefer next to outline possible limitations to the generalizability, credibility, or robustness of the results. It is just as true in the natural sciences as in the behavioral sciences that no empirical study is perfect. Common sources of imperfection include the nature of the sample (e.g., relatively small and unrepresentative), an unforeseen confound, and missing data, among other possibilities. The good scientific writer openly acknowledges possible shortcomings and tries to explain how they may have affected the results. Indeed, readers will rightly feel suspicious if an obvious study weakness is not mentioned by the author. This is why the second or third sentence in the discussion section in basically all of my own empirical studies looks something like this: "Before specific results are discussed, some possible limitations to their generalizability are considered." Some authors prefer to mention possible limitations later in the discussion section, but I think that doing so right away is better.

The next major goal of the discussion is to close the circle of the article that began in the introduction. Summarize the essential findings of the study in relation to both the specific hypotheses tested (i.e., which hypotheses were supported or not) and results of earlier studies, which were often cited in the introduction. Connecting the results of the present study to those reported by others also builds a context to help readers better understand the research problem. Try to explain inconsistencies among the results of your study and those of previous studies. For example, is there something about cross-study variation in methods, samples, or other characteristics that could explain contradictory findings? This is often one of the explicit goals of a meta-analysis, but the author of a primary study should address these issues, too. However, do not in the discussion mention any result or pattern from your study that was not already described in the results section. That is, the discussion is no place for surprises concerning your findings.

Just as in the results section, use cautious, careful language that sticks close to the data when interpreting the findings in the discussion. Do not give the impression that the results of a single study are important outside of findings reported elsewhere in the literature (Wilkinson and the Task Force on Statistical Inference, 1999). This is consistent with the aspect of meta-analytic thinking that assumes that the impact of a single primary study is limited. *Be equally cautious about inferring causality, especially if randomization was not part of your design.* Although as students we are told time and again that "correlation does not imply causation," too many behavioral science authors seem to forget this essential truth. For example, Robinson, Levin, Thomas, Pituch, and Vaughn (2007) reviewed about 275 articles published in five different journals in the area of teaching and learning. They found that (1) the proportion of studies based on experimental or quasi-experimental designs (i.e., with researcher-manipulated variables) declined from 45% in 1994 to 33% in 2004. Nevertheless, (2) the proportion of nonexperimental studies containing claims for causality increased from 34% in 1994 to 43% in 2004. Recall that nonexperimental studies have no design elements that support causal inference (Chapter 3). Despite this fact, researchers in the teaching-and-learning area—and, to be fair, in other areas, too—may have become less cautious than they should be concerning the inference of causation from correlation.

Please do *not* conclude the discussion section with a variation on the typically banal, hackneyed call for future research on the topic. The criticism that little is ever concluded in the "soft" social sciences except for the need for ever more research was mentioned in Chapter 2. Sometimes more research is *not* needed, especially when it is quite clear after many studies that some result is nil (i.e., it is time to move on). Otherwise, it is more helpful to offer specific suggestions about how to improve research in the area, or to articulate new hypotheses (questions for future studies). This is how you end strong, not with an empty, reflexive call for more research.

References

Sometimes written almost as an afterthought, the reference section is very important, so proper diligence is needed here. The reference list is a record of your sources, and therefore it is critical that each entry in the list be correct. Otherwise, a reader will have trouble finding a cited work. It is distressing how easy it is to find incorrect references in published articles, so it seems that too many authors are not careful enough in this regard. Also, the reference list is a kind of contract that says that the author has actually read each work in the list. Accordingly, do not include in the references works that you have not read. In the past, authors used **indirect citation** in text when referring to a work not read by the author. For example, the citation "B (2005) (as cited in A, 2006, p. 32)" signals that the writer read only "A (2006)," in which "B (2005)" was mentioned on p. 32. Accordingly, the work "B (2005)" would not appear in the reference list. However, secondary citations are less acceptable nowadays, given increasing availability of works in digital format. That is, use primary sources, not secondary ones.

Effective Graphical Displays

Some types of graphs are infrequently seen in scientific publications because they convey little essential information. For example, pie charts waste space because the numbers represented in them can typically be more efficiently reported in text or a table. The same is generally true for bar graphs or line graphs for a single variable with a small number of categories. Scatterplots in which just a regression line for the linear association between two variables is shown without data points are also uninformative. This is because seeing just the slope and intercept of the line adds little to our understanding of the relation between the variables. Display of the data points gives information about outliers and also about the degree of nonlinearity in the relation (e.g., see Figure 8.3).

One often sees line graphics in journal articles that display the results of analyses of variance. Means in these graphics are often represented with dots or similar graphical symbols. In line graphics for factorial analyses of variance, lines are used to connect the dots for cell means from the same row or column of the whole factorial table. Better line graphics feature error bars (i.e., confidence intervals) around the symbol for each mean. Error bars indicate visually the degree of statistical uncertainty associated with each mean. A line graphic for means can be combined with other graphical techniques that represent distribution shape or outliers. For example, presented in Figure 9.1 is a line graphic for a 2×2 factorial ANOVA with a box plot (box-and-whisker plot) presented for each cell. The means in the figure are represented with solid dots. The bottom and top borders of the rectangle in each box plot correspond to, respectively, the 25th percentile (1st quartile) and 75th percentile (3rd quartile); the line inside the rectangle represents the median (second quartile); the vertical lines ("whiskers") connect the first and third quartiles with the highest scores that are not outliers; and the open circles depict individual outlier scores. Inspection of Figure 9.1 indicates the presence of outlier scores in the upper part of the distribution for cell A_2–B_2. These outliers pull the cell mean up relative to the median, and thus may be responsible for the apparent $A \times B$ interaction effect depicted in the figure.

A few words are needed about line graphics for means. Do not think that the presence of lines that connect dots (means) in such graphics suggests a continuous scale between those points. This is true even if each of these two points connected by a line correspond to an interval or ratio scale. Suppose that the drug dosages 5, 15, and 25 mg · kg^{-1} make up the three levels of factor A. In a line graph, means from these three conditions will be connected by a line that is straight between each of the two pairs of adjacent dosages (i.e., 5 and 15, 15 and 25 mg · kg^{-1}). This graphical necessity does not imply that the trend is linear across all possible intermediate dosages, such as dosages within the range 5–15. Because dosages within this range were not tested, whether the trend is linear or curvilinear over these levels is unknown.

Most data graphics in scientific publications are printed in gray scale. Used effectively, color in a data graphic can add useful information, but

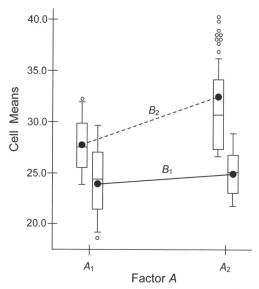

FIGURE 9.1. Example of a line graphic for a two-way interaction effect with box plots.

color is rarely necessary for the kinds of charts and figures used in the behavioral sciences. Indeed, the improper use of color can make a data graphic more difficult to understand. This is especially true if superfluous color is combined with other unnecessary features in a data graphic including a three-dimensional (3-D) perspective. The latter rarely adds anything to a data graphic and should generally be avoided. Tufte (2001) used the term **chartjunk** to refer to gratuitous visual elements of charts and figures that are not part of the minimum set required to communicate about a set of numbers. Presented in Table 9.4 is a set of 12 numbers about the relation between geographic region and quarterly sales. This dataset is so small that a figure is not really needed. Presented in Figure 9.2 is an example of chartjunk for the data in Table 9.4. It is displayed in an unnecessary 3-D perspective that makes it more difficult to see the basic numerical information. It also features the superfluous use of different geometric shapes to represent each series (regions).

Choose a scale for data graphics and use that scale consistently across all the graphs. However, do not select a scale that unnecessarily exaggerates small differences. Suppose over the course of a trading day in the stock market that the Dow Jones Industrial Average (DJIA) drops by 75 points, say, from a hypothetical value of 13,500 to one of 13,425. Plotted

TABLE 9.4. Tabular Display of a Small Dataset (Quarterly Sales by Region)

	Quarter			
Region	1st	2nd	3rd	4th
East	20	27	90	20
West	31	39	35	32
North	46	47	45	44

on a graph where the scale ranges from 13,400 to 13,500, a decline of 75 points could look dramatic because the trend will drop 75% of the height of the graph. However, a decline of this magnitude corresponds to only about one-half of 1% (.0056) of the value of the DJIA at the start of the trading day. The relative magnitude of this drop would be more apparent when plotted against a scale with a wider range, such as 8,000–15,000. Putting error bars around individual points in a data graph can also help the reader to understand the relative magnitude or degree of precision associated with each data point relative to the graph's scale. See Tufte (2001) for several examples of how selecting a scale with too narrow a range can exaggerate slight differences.

Ready for the Big Time

Later in your career, you may be in a position to write a graduate thesis, such as for a master's degree or a doctorate of philosophy, or a grant application for research funds. Writing on this level is more demanding than

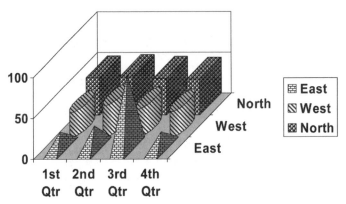

FIGURE 9.2. Example of chartjunk for the data in Table 9.4.

writing a manuscript-length scientific paper, but you need many of the same skills. These skills include the ability to clearly describe the rationale of your study, explain why the research question is worthwhile, and convey the results in such a way that everything makes sense to a general science reader. The latter is a key characteristic of both committees for graduate-level research projects and granting agencies in that committee members may have backgrounds in different areas than your own. This means that you need to write your document for what is basically a multidisciplinary audience. However, if you become practiced at writing smaller-scale research manuscripts for such audiences, then these skills will transfer to similar writing at higher levels.

The scope of a graduate thesis, especially a dissertation, is typically much broader than that of a 20- to 30-page research manuscript. For example, the length of just the literature review in a dissertation may exceed 30 pages, and some dissertation projects are made up of a series of smaller empirical studies. If so, then principles for writing a scientific paper can be broken down and applied to each individual study. It is more challenging when writing a larger document, such as a dissertation or book, to maintain a consistent voice, cadence, level of clarity, and perspective across all sections, especially if writing that document takes place over many months. It is often necessary to go back and revise work written earlier as later sections are written. This is due in part to the writing-as-learning phenomenon: Your understanding of the material may change as you write about it, and what you wrote earlier may not express your current level of comprehension. This is why writing on a larger scale often requires ongoing revision of both current and previously written sections. See Cone and Foster (2006) for advice about how to write a dissertation in psychology and related areas.

Writing a successful grant proposal is also a challenge. As the applicant, you must typically describe the rationale, approach, significance, and innovation of your project within a very limited space, perhaps just a few pages. Indeed, the length confines of a grant application are often even more restrictive than for a manuscript to be submitted to a journal. The description of the rationale and significance of your project must be compelling or else the proposed study will be seen as incremental, low-impact research. By "compelling," I am not referring to hyperbole or exaggeration; instead, I mean "beautiful" scientific ideas, ones that are based in a clear empirical foundation, address interesting problems, offer the promise of true advancement of knowledge by connecting what we know with what we should know, and are expressed in language that is clear and understandable to readers who are experts in their own areas, but perhaps not also in your particular research area. It is also important not to propose a project that appears too ambitious, given available resources. In the eyes of reviewers, such projects are at high risk for failure, so be realistic in what you propose.

It is also necessary in a grant application to clearly and accurately describe yourself as a credible researcher through the articulation of a clear plan for the proposed study. You are also required to report evidence of prior research productivity, including publications in high-impact, peer-reviewed journals, successful completion of previous funded research projects, and participation in collaborative research projects. It is also crucial to make clear to reviewers that you have the appropriate level of institutional support (e.g., you have a secure position) and minimum startup package or equipment needed for your proposed project. Otherwise, your project will be seen as a high-risk one. You also need a good sense of financial and budgetary matters concerning your project, often on a multiyear basis.

Writing successful grant applications is not easy, and this is true even for very experienced researchers. Another reality is that, in general, the minority of all grant applications are actually funded. So the standards are high, but so it should be whenever a researcher asks for the largesse of using someone else's money to conduct his or her particular research project. It helps that many funding agencies have special programs targeted toward new researchers. A book by Carlson (2002) deals with the writing of grant applications for nongovernmental agencies or nonprofit foundations. However, government funding agencies, such as the National Institutes of Health (NIH) in the United States or the Social Sciences and Humanities Research Council (SSHRC) of Canada, generally have strict requirements for grant applications. A recent book by Scheier and Dewey (2007) is a writing guide to NIH applications in the behavioral sciences, and it may be helpful to consult this or other related books for useful examples even if you never anticipate applying to NIH per se.

Summary

Very few of us are good writers by nature; instead, most good writers become so through practice, practice, and more practice. Try to identify your own maladaptive beliefs or ways of procrastinating concerning writing, and set aside specific times for writing in your schedule. In scientific writing, keep it clear and concise, and write for a general science reader. This means to avoid unnecessary jargon, especially when everyday words can be used instead. In the introduction, tell your readers right away about the basic research question addressed in your study, and then step back and describe its context and history. Because you usually have just a few paragraphs to "spend" on the introduction in manuscript-length documents, this description is typically not comprehensive. Instead, you should emphasize only the most relevant historical details, including results of previous studies, of the background for your study. Describe your procedures and methods in sufficient detail so that another researcher could replicate your study. Describe your findings using the clearest language possible, and do not report excessive statistics in the text. Use the minimum number of tables necessary to present sets of related numbers. Provide a figure to visually convey a finding only when that finding cannot be efficiently summarized in a table. Avoid chartjunk at all costs; in general, it is better to present no data graphics than bad data graphics. The discussion section should complete the story of your study by setting your findings in context and identifying unresolved questions in the area. The next chapter deals with another important medium for scientific communication, oral presentations.

RECOMMENDED READINGS

The books by Alley (1996) and M. Davis (2005) are excellent resources for general scientific writing. Both emphasize the need for clarity, conciseness, and simplicity. Tufte (2001) gives many examples of bad and better designs for data graphics. It also emphasizes the beauty and communication power of simplicity in the graphical display of numerical information.

Alley, M. (1996). *The craft of scientific writing* (3rd ed.). New York: Springer.

Davis, M. (2005). *Scientific papers and presentations* (2nd ed.). New York: Academic Press.

Tufte, E. R. (2001). *The visual display of quantitative information* (2nd ed.). Cheshire, CT: Graphics Press.

APPENDIX 9.1

Example Results Section

Wayne, Riordan, and Thomas (2001) studied whether outcomes of mock juror decisions about work-related sexual harassment (SH) cases varied as a function of gender. They randomly assigned a total of 408 women and men to one of four conditions in which the gender of the harasser or victim were manipulated. These conditions permitted study of less common forms of SH, including same-gender SH and cross-gender SH where the harasser is a woman and the victim a man. Along with mock juror gender, the overall design is a 2 × 2 × 2 factorial. The dependent variables included the verdict, amount of monetary damages, and degree of negative perception of the offense. The example results section presented next concerns the analysis of the negative perception variable only. A balanced design is assumed here ($n = 51$ in each cell), but the original design was unbalanced. However, the results assuming equal cell sizes are similar to those reported by Wayne et al. (2001).

Results

Negative Perception

It was hypothesized that mock jurors would in cross-gender SH perceive the behavior as more negative when the harasser is a man and when the jurors are female. It was also expected that same-gender SH would be rated more negatively than cross-gender SH, especially if both the harasser and victim are men. Reported in Table 9.5 are means and standard deviations on the negative perception variable for the whole design.

Reported in Table 9.6 are the results of the 2 × 2 × 2 factorial ANOVA conducted with the data from Table 9.5. All main and interaction effects together explain about 17% of the total observed variability in negative perception ratings ($\hat{\eta}^2 = .168$). Most of the overall explanatory power is due to the two-way interaction effect between harasser gender and victim gender (HG × VG), which by itself explains about 14% of the total variance ($\hat{\eta}^2 = .136$). Among the other effects, only the main effect of juror gender (JG) is statistically significant, and it explains an additional 2% of the total variance ($\hat{\eta}^2 = .017$). The remaining 1.5% of total explained variance is

TABLE 9.5. Cell Means and Standard Deviations for Negative Perception Ratings by Harasser, Victim, and Juror Gender

		Juror gender	
Harasser gender	Victim gender	Male	Female
Male	Female	12.62 (2.62)[a]	14.41 (2.93)
Female	Male	13.27 (3.28)	14.11 (3.03)
Male	Male	16.02 (1.97)	15.86 (3.07)
Female	Female	15.35 (2.67)	16.02 (2.22)

Note. From Wayne, Riordan, and Thomas (2001, p. 184). Copyright 2001 by the American Psychological Association. Adapted with permission of Julie Holliday Wayne (personal communication, November 15, 2007) and the American Psychological Association.

[a]M (SD); n = 51 for all cells.

due to all other effects besides the two just mentioned combined. Accordingly, only the HG × VG interaction and the JG main effect are analyzed further.

Presented in Figure 9.3 are the means for the HG × VG interaction effect with 95% confidence intervals. Contrary to expectations, cross-gender SH where the harasser is a woman was not rated as appreciably more serious (M = 13.69) than when the harasser is a man (M = 13.52). The value of Hedges's g for the contrast of these two means, calculated with the square root of the overall within-cells mean square (see Table 9.6) in the denominator, equals (13.69 − 13.52)/$7.59^{1/2}$, or .06, which is a relatively small effect size. As predicted, same-gender SH was generally rated as more serious than cross-gender SH. However, the mean for male–male SH (M = 15.94) was not appreciably higher than the mean for female–female SH (M = 15.69). For this particular contrast, g = .09. Another way to describe the two-way interaction is to say that for male harassers, the offense

TABLE 9.6. Analysis of Variance Results for Negative Perception Ratings

Source	SS	df	MS	F	$\hat{\eta}^2$
Victim gender (VG)	4.71	1	4.71	.62	.001
Harasser gender (HG)	.16	1	.16	.02	<.001
Juror gender (JG)	62.85	1	62.85	8.28[a]	.017
HG × VG	498.18	1	498.18	65.60[a]	.136
HG × PG	.09	1	.09	.01	<.001
VG × JG	20.20	1	20.20	2.66	.006
HG × VG × JG	28.65	1	28.65	3.77	.008
Total model	614.84	7	87.83	11.57[a]	.168
Within cells (error)	3,037.59	400	7.59		

[a]p < .05.

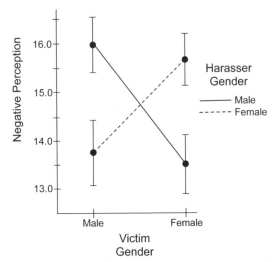

FIGURE 9.3. Mean negative perception ratings with 95% confidence intervals for the two-way interaction of victim gender and harasser gender.

is rated as more serious when the victim is a man than when a woman is a victim. Just the opposite is true for female harassers: The offense is seen as more serious if the victim is a woman than when the victim is a man (see Figure 9.3).

Analysis of the JG main effect, which explained about 2% of the total observed variance, is straightforward: The overall rated seriousness of SH across all combinations of harasser and victim gender was greater for female jurors ($M = 15.10$) than for male jurors ($M = 14.32$). The magnitude of the difference is about .30 standard deviations ($g = .28$).

CHAPTER 10

Presentations

There's the old axiom in design that said, "Less is more." They should have that printed on the outside of the PowerPoint box. It needs a warning label.

—LARRY NIGHSWANDER (quoted in Keller, 2003, p. 28)

Good presentation skills are essential for students and researchers alike. The former are often required to make presentations as part of a research seminar or thesis courses, and the latter often give presentations at scientific conferences. Two kinds of scientific presentations are considered in this chapter, oral presentations and poster presentations. Because oral presentations are usually more challenging, they are considered in greater detail. General principles for giving effective presentations are discussed and common mistakes to avoid are considered. Some of these mistakes happen when one misuses a computer tool for presentations, such as PowerPoint. Accordingly, the intelligent use of PowerPoint is a major theme of this chapter. It is hoped that the combination of principles, tips, and examples presented here will help you to give more effective presentations with greater confidence.

Challenges of Oral Presentations

Considered next are three potential obstacles to making effective oral presentations. Later sections address how to deal with these challenges.

Stage Fright

The very thought of making an oral presentation fills some people with dread. This is a kind of performance anxiety or stage fright that often involves the fear of coming across as inadequate, fumbling, or unprepared in front of an audience. There is a "fear of fear" aspect, too, in that some presenters worry about these things happening *because* they feel nervous. Listed next are some ways of looking at stage fright that I hope will reduce your concern about it:

1. *Stage fright is expected and completely normal.* Perhaps most presenters—even very experienced ones—feel some degree of anxiety before, less so during, their presentations. That is, do not conclude that you are somehow inadequate as a presenter just because you experience anxiety—conclude instead that your nervous system works properly!

2. *Stage fright can be positive.* During presentations, anxiety can actually lead to better outcomes. It can heighten the speaker's energy, posture, and attention to the audience so that performance is improved, not worsened. Fear can be your friend, if it drives you to achieve better results.

3. *Good presenters are made, not born.* There are some people who seem to be natural-born public speakers, but they are relatively rare. Most of us become better presenters through practice, which is also the best single way to deal with stage fright. This means that the experience of stage fright diminishes as one gives more presentations. See Alley (2003) for anecdotes about how some famous scientists renowned for their public speaking later in their career started out as a poor public speaker.

4. *Do not rely on PowerPoint to reduce anxiety; instead, rely on good content and preparation.* Some presenters seem to use PowerPoint as a sop for reducing their anxiety (e.g., they look more at the screen than at the audience). Instead, rely on preparing good content in the first place and then sufficiently rehearsing your presentation.

Finally, remember that courage is not doing something without fear; it means doing it even though you are afraid. But with enough practice, making presentations gets easier and easier.

Time Limits

Another challenge is that the lengths of oral presentations in academic settings are often restricted by rather tight time limitations, such as 20 minutes (or less). Limits on presentation time may be enforced by moderators or teachers, who are sometimes forced to stop speakers from continuing if the allotted time has expired. Although speakers often feel pressed by time constraints, 20 minutes is actually enough time to convey a fair amount of information, if the presentation is well planned. It also helps if your visual aids (i.e., slides) are not actually visual distracters.

PowerPoint as Tool or Hindrance

Students are often required to use PowerPoint in presentations. The justification is that experience will be gained with a computer tool that will be used again. Considering that about 30 million PowerPoint presentations are given each day and upwards of 10^{10}–10^{11} PowerPoint slides are created each year (Simons, 2004; Tufte, 2006), this rationale is plausible. There are other computer tools for presentations—Corel Presentations, Apple Keynote, and Lotus Freelance Graphics, among others—but all work generally the same way and create the same basic product. Consequently, the term "PowerPoint presentation" is used from this point on to refer to any computer-assisted presentation with electronic (digital) slides. Likewise, later discussion about problems with the use of PowerPoint is not specific to this particular tool but instead concerns the whole genre.

There is a certain art to giving an effective PowerPoint presentation, one that is practiced well by relatively few presenters. The truth to this observation becomes more apparent as one sees more and more PowerPoint presentations. For example, Paradi (2003, 2005) surveyed almost 900 people who regularly see PowerPoint presentations. A third of all respondents indicated that more than 50% of the presentations they see are poorly done. About 40% said that about the same proportion of presentations suffer from at least one annoying characteristic. These results are consistent with my own experiences, which is that few PowerPoint presentations are good, some are tolerable, but many are so flawed that the speaker's message is not effectively communicated. The fact that so many computer-assisted presentations are poor is ironic considering that PowerPoint is supposed to make it easier to give effective presentations. However, there are features of PowerPoint that, if used the wrong way, can actually make it

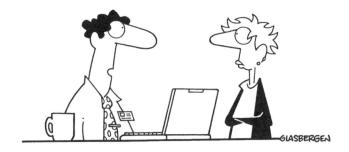

"What software would you recommend to give
my presentation so much flash and sizzle that
nobody notices that I have nothing to say?"

Copyright 2002 by Randy Glasbergen. Reprinted with permission.

more difficult to pull off a successful presentation. These ideas are elaborated next.

Problems with PowerPoint Presentations

There are some common problems with PowerPoint presentations. Once known, it may be easier for novice presenters to avoid making them in the first place. Listed in Table 10.1 are the top ten annoyances of PowerPoint presentations reported by respondents in surveys conducted by Paradi (2003, 2005). The percentages in the table do not sum to 100 because each respondent could have listed up to three annoyances. It is clear from the results listed in Table 10.1 that the most annoying feature mentioned by a majority of the respondents (61.7%) is the speaker who gives his or her talk by reading the text presented on the slides. This is a flagrant error and one of the best ways to ruin a presentation, and here is why: It insults the intelligence of an audience when the speaker seems to feel it is necessary to read text that is before all to see. It also frustrates people because they can read the same text much faster than it can be spoken aloud. Perhaps you have experienced the same frustration while watching an advertisement on television where a narrator reads every word that is also presented on the screen.

Near majorities (about 40%) of respondents in Paradi's surveys described three different characteristics of electronic slides as annoying (Table 10.1). Two of these concern text slides, including the selection of a font size that makes the text difficult or impossible to read (47.7%) and using full sentences instead of just a few words in bullet points (40.7%). A related annoyance is the use of too many different fonts in text slides (12.6%). These annoyances speak to an irony concerning PowerPoint: Computer presentation tools are ideal for presentations where it is essential to display images. Examples include presentations about works of art or architecture. In these cases, an image may be worth a thousand words. In scientific presentations, graphical representations of results or diagrams that illustrate essential concepts, such as the basic structure of a cell, can also convey much information at a glance and more efficiently than words. However, note that about one-quarter of survey respondents cited the use of overly complex diagrams or charts (22.0%) as a problem in PowerPoint presentations (Table 10.1). The capability to include video clips in PowerPoint presentations can also be invaluable. An example is when a video clip clearly illustrates a particular experimental procedure or result, such as how an animal solves a learning task, that is difficult to describe in words alone. However, perhaps most electronic slides shown during scientific presentations contain mainly text, and PowerPoint is just not as helpful for showing words.

The third general complaint mentioned by many survey respondents concerns the use of colors that make slides hard to see (41.2%). There

TABLE 10.1. Top 10 Annoying Features of PowerPoint Presentations

Annoyance	Percentage endorsing
Speaker reads slides	61.7
Text too small to read	47.7
Slides hard to see because of colors	41.2
Full sentences instead of bullet points	40.7
Moving/flying text or graphics	24.7
Annoying use of sounds	22.1[a]
Overly complex diagrams or charts	22.0
No flow of ideas; jumped around too much	18.9[a]
No clear purpose of the presentation	18.2[a]
Too many fonts used	12.6[a]

Note. These results are averaged across samples surveyed by Paradi (2003, 2005) with, respectively, 159 and 688 cases. The total sample size is 847 cases except where indicated. Reproduced with permission of Dave Paradi (personal communication, September 6, 2007).
[a] $N = 159$.

is a tendency among novice PowerPoint users to create slides with too many colors, or to use standard templates included with PowerPoint where colors, fonts, and graphical design elements are combined in preset formats. (Other terms for templates include master slides, master gallery, and themes.) Templates are supposed to allow the user to quickly create a presentation with a consistent graphical design by just adding their own content. Unfortunately, many templates for electronic slides are bad in that they combine colors and graphics in overly complex ways that make it difficult to see content. This point is elaborated later, but it is worth knowing now that some features of PowerPoint intended as conveniences can, if misused, result in a less successful presentation due to ugly, distracting, or annoying slides that make content less salient. As noted by M. Davis (2005), "it is better to have no visual aid than a bad visual aid" (p. 173).

Another set of annoyances listed in Table 10.1 concerns the use of irritating sounds (22.1%) or the display of text or graphics that move or fly around the screen (24.7%). Perhaps the most common form of the latter occurs within a single slide where first a title is shown which then is followed by a line-by-line display of additional bullet points added by the speaker. Some terms for this feature include the **slow reveal** or **build sequence**. Each new bullet point in a build sequence can be made to just simply appear or to swoop or rotate in from some starting point to its final position. These features plus others, such as transition effects where the image of one slide dissolves or fades into the next, are optional "bells-and-whistles" features that can be easily added to electronic slide shows. These features may be appealing to novice users of PowerPoint, who may see them as ways to add pizzazz to their presentations. However, just the opposite is true: These kinds of special effects can easily ruin the visual aids.

The remaining two presentation annoyances listed in Table 10.1 concern what the speaker says. About 18–19% of the respondents in Paradi's surveys mentioned the absence of a clear flow of ideas or purpose as significant flaws. These problems may have little to do with PowerPoint; instead, they concern how the speaker organized the presentation's content or conveyed it. However, a common mistake of novice presenters is to spend more time working in PowerPoint than thinking about the substance of the presentation. Another is to make too many PowerPoint slides, perhaps so many that what were once coherent ideas wind up being scattered across so many slides that the bigger picture is no longer apparent. Given all the annoyances just considered, it is clear that many speakers need help using PowerPoint.

Principles for Creating Effective PowerPoint Presentations

This discussion is organized around a general rule referred to here as the

$$IF / BP / 10, 20, 30, 3 \times 5 / NT / DDS / NC$$

rule for PowerPoint presentations. Each set of acronyms in this rule refers to a specific principle for giving effective PowerPoint presentations. Each is defined as follows: Ideas First (IF); Be Prepared (BP); 10 slides in 20 minutes, text font size is at least 30 points, and text slides should have no more than three bullets each with five words or less (10, 20, 30, 3 × 5); No Templates (NT); Drop-Dead Simple (DDS) design; and No Crap (NC) (sorry, strong talk is needed here). Presented in the appendix for this chapter is a set of slides and a handout for a hypothetical 20-minute presentation based on the classic study of bystander intervention by Darley and Latané (1968). These materials represent the application of the principles discussed next.

Ideas First

The principle of IF emphasizes the fact that the content of your presentation is more important than the visual aids (slides). This is especially true for scientific presentations, which in the end must be based on good ideas communicated in a clear, simple way. *Accordingly, you should spend more time working on presentation content than working in PowerPoint to create your slides.* Too many presenters get this critical part wrong by spending more time with PowerPoint than thinking about what they want to say. Students or researchers who start with PowerPoint first also run the risk that limitations of all presentation computer tools can potentially distort the communication of critical content.

Another implication of the IF principle leads to what may seem to be a radical suggestion nowadays: Leave the computer alone when first working out presentation content. Also put aside all other digital devices, including your cellular phone, BlackBerry, Bluetooth, or similar wireless device, and, yes, your Apple iPod or related kind of entertainment system. Rid yourself of potential distractions that can arise from digital gadgets in order to give yourself space and time to think. Use pencil and paper if you feel the need to record something, such as an outline or a key set of ideas.

This suggestion reflects the reality that a modern form of procrastination involves the use of computers in ways that waste time, such as checking e-mail or sending instant messages to friends (Steel, 2007). Faced with an impending deadline, a digital procrastinator is ultimately forced to productively use the computer, but with too little time to adequately prepare for a presentation. Bad ideas (because they are poorly thought out) communicated with bad visuals are the likely result.

Anholt (2006) gave some helpful advice for planning the content of a presentation, and it involves thinking in terms of threes. First, write three sentences that summarize the essential take-home message of your presentation. These are the critical points that, even if an audience member forgets everything else, communicate something of substance if he or she remembers them. Writing so little also forces you to concentrate on what's really important to convey in the presentation. These three sentences should say something about the core research problem, the methods used, and the results. An example of a three-sentence summary for the Darley and Latané (1968) study follows:

> Whether bystanders would intervene in an emergency was studied in an experimental setting where participants overheard an apparent epileptic seizure either alone, or that one or four unseen others were also present. The results are consistent with the hypothesis that the presence of other unseen bystanders predicts both a slower speed and lower likelihood of seeking help. The findings also support the idea that inaction in some emergencies may be related more to the bystander's response to other observers than to indifference to the victim.

Next, think about the three parts of a presentation: the introduction, body, and conclusion. In a scientific presentation, the introduction concerns the research question (problem, hypotheses—i.e., what motivated the study) and its context. The latter refers to the background information necessary to fully appreciate both why the study was conducted and the content of the rest of the presentation. The body is basically the methods and results sections of your talk, and it concerns how the study was conducted and what was found. The conclusion brings the presentation full circle in that the findings are related to the context and the implications of the results are mentioned, just as in the discussion section of a paper. In a 20-minute presentation, the introduction must be brief— say, no more than 5 minutes long—and the core rationale for your study should be stated right away, within the first few sentences you speak. That is, do not hold the audience in suspense by building up to the rationale; instead, say it first.

Next, write three lines of text for each of the three sections of the presentation (i.e., nine points altogether). A limit of three points per section again forces you to identify the most critical points that should be conveyed in each part of the talk. Each point in this outline can be elaborated during the presentation, so do not worry about listing all details yet. This is because the level of detail in each part of the presentation should be planned considering the audience. That is, target the presentation to the audience, which requires thinking about who will be in attendance and what kinds and amounts of detail would best serve their needs. Also, think carefully whether this outline sufficiently honors the essential take-home messages written earlier. If not, then accordingly alter the outline so that these points are emphasized.

Sometimes presentations are given to groups of insiders, those who are already expert in a particular field. Such audiences need little introduction to the research area, so presenters can start right away by describing hypotheses and methods. It happens more often that researchers present their findings to a mixed audience made up of some people who are quite familiar with the subject and others who are not. This is often true in research seminars where students make presentations to other students (and to the instructor, too) who may know relatively little about a particular research area. Audiences at presentations in general scientific conferences are also usually mixed. It is not easy to plan the depth of a presentation for a mixed audience, and just how to pick and choose which details to present is one of the hardest parts of making scientific presentations (Alley, 2003). Unfortunately, there are also no clear-cut rules or guidelines about how to specify the level of detail for a mixed audience, but some suggestions can be offered.

Perhaps the best thing to do is to prepare the presentation enough in advance so that you can try it out in front of a group of people who are intelligent but naïve concerning the research topic. These people could be classmates or members of a different research team (i.e., not your own). In preparing to speak to mixed audiences, presenters tend to error on the side of including too much detail. Besides possibly swamping the audience with facts not critical to understanding study objectives or results, packing too much detail in a presentation risks exceeding a time limit. Detail that is interesting but not critical can be dealt with in the question period, if an audience member wishes to ask about it. Thus, you can view the question period as a kind of a safety valve for reducing the pressure to cover everything in the presentation per se. Another kind of safety valve for including more advanced information is a handout, which is covered later.

Anholt (2006) described the method of **zooming in** for connecting the essential points of the introduction to the rest of the presentation. The goal of zooming in is to give the audience a context for what the presenter is about to say and show. One starts with a general perspective and then gradually the focus is turned to the presenter's particular study. For example, one can zoom in from an overarching principle, such as from a historical perspective about a particular research problem or from the perspective of a specific theoretical model. Doing so establishes a connection between your study and that of a larger body of work or general scientific principles. Zooming in also helps to set limits on the scope of a presentation by focusing the audience's attention on a set of relevant ideas or historical events.

Be Prepared

The motto of the Boys Scouts of America is "Be prepared!" For presenters, this motto means three things: First, be prepared for any technical problem, including the total inability to show electronic slides. Second, be prepared to deal with the fact that PowerPoint is a narrow-bandwidth tool for communicating results of scientific studies. This means that only quite limited amounts and quality of information can be conveyed through the sequential presentation of slides. (The presenter is also a low-bandwidth communication medium because he or she speaks more slowly than people can read.) The best way to deal with both problems just mentioned is to prepare a printed handout that accompanies the presentation. Third, be prepared by practicing the presentation beforehand. All these points are elaborated next.

Computer technology for presentations is wonderful when it works, but there are many technical glitches that can derail it (software bugs, hardware failures, damaged media, etc.). *A prepared speaker is never stopped by technical problems.* That is, always be prepared to give the presentation without computer support, and also without waiting those seemingly endless moments while others fuss with nonfunctioning computer or display hardware. One way is to bring along a set of acetates for an overhead projector with your slides printed on them. Many classrooms and smaller auditoriums have overhead projectors, and they can be used in an emergency when computer-assisted display is not available. If no overhead projector is available, then the prepared presenter can speak from the handout, and the audience can follow along. It also looks very impressive when a prepared speaker, who when faced with an apparent "catastrophe" (no computer support) that would derail most others, is nevertheless able to proceed right away with little delay and few ruffled feathers.

A handout for a scientific presentation should contain text, a few tables or figures (as needed), and a reference list. An annotated bibliography is often helpful for a mixed audience as is a list of acronyms or technical terms with definitions (i.e., a glossary). A reference list displayed on the screen is often illegible, and it disappears after a few moments. At minimum, include the same basic text and tables or figures that you intend to display in PowerPoint. This allows you to speak directly from the handout even without computer-assisted display. The handout can also be used to present more detail than could be shown in a PowerPoint slide. For example, a whole table of numerical results could be printed in the handout while only part of it is shown on screen. The on-screen portion could concern some basic pattern of results, but the rest of the details from the table are given in the handout. The same thing can be done with a figure: A basic version is presented on screen, and a more complete version is included in the handout. This way the audience members can shift their attention from the screen to the handout in order to get more information. The text in a handout can be in paragraph form which, unlike bullet points, is closer to "gold standards" of scientific communication: journal articles, book chapters, or technical reports. The use of outline form for text is fine in a handout, too, and it is less work to prepare.

A handout also involves the audience more directly in the presentation. Specifically, an audience member controls how he or she reads through a handout and selects from the available information. Otherwise, that person has a passive role when he or she just sits there and does nothing but watch and listen. It is also my experience that audiences value a handout because (1) it gives them something tangible to take away from the presentation, and (2) many speakers do not bother with preparing a handout. Accordingly, you can distinguish yourself as a conscientious speaker by distributing a handout. *However, the handout should not be printed in PowerPoint or similar computer tools.* Each page of a PowerPoint-generated handout contains the images of up to nine slides per page with additional room for handwritten notes. This type of handout is usually inadequate for scientific presentations. Small printed images of slides are often hard to see, such as when figures with multiple colors are rendered in gray scale in printed form. No value is added by a handout that shows just the slides. You should view the handout as a distinct product that is to be produced in a word processor, not a presentation computer tool. For a 20-minute presentation, a two-page handout is usually sufficient, and the layout can follow the basic form of a journal article or a newsletter. See Appendix 10.1 for an example of a handout.

You can use discretion about when to distribute a handout. When handouts are distributed just as you begin to speak, there is a tendency for audience members to start reading and perhaps not listen. It may be better to wait to distribute the handout until it is needed, such as when you ask the audience to divide their attention between the screen and handout. If the audience is large, however, then it is probably best to distribute the handout right away, because it can take several minutes to distribute a handout to all members in a large audience, which interrupts your presentation and wastes precious time, too. If the handout is not an essential part of the presentation (perhaps it serves mainly as a backup in the event of computer problems), then it could be distributed at the conclusion of your presentation.

A skilled speaker leaves enough time to practice the presentation before it is scheduled to be given. Practice sessions are invaluable for fine-tuning a presentation and building confidence. Practice should be done under conditions that closely resemble those of the actual presentation. This includes going through the whole presentation before a live audience and also timing these practice runs to make sure that the allotted time is respected. Remember that the actual presentation may take longer than practice presentations. This happens in part because good presenters pace themselves based on nonverbal audience feedback (e.g., slow down or elaborate more if people look confused).

As you become more familiar with your content, then also practice making eye contact with the audience. Too many speakers spend more time looking at notes or the screen than at the audience and thus miss out on making a "connection," an intangible but crucial part of oral presentations. Try to spread eye contact equally among the different audience members. This is in part to establish a connection with each audience member. Another reason to spread eye contact is to get nonverbal feedback from the audience and make adjustments accordingly. For instance, monitor whether people are engaged and whether they seem to understand your message. If necessary, adjust your presentation (e.g., slow down, speed up, speak louder, give additional concrete examples, and try a different wording) based on this feedback.

Always respect the time limit for your presentation. This is such a crucial point that it warrants special emphasis: *Good presenters never go beyond the time limit in the actual presentation.* Going over time not only violates the audience's expectations about the boundaries of your presentation but may also cheat speakers who follow out of some of their allotted time. It is much better to quickly wrap up and then give the audience its turn when the time limit for the formal presentation has expired. At the very end of your allotted time, you can also invite interested audience members to speak with you after the session is over, especially if not all questions were addressed within the time limit. See Alley (2003, Chs. 7–10) and Anholt (2006, Ch. 4) for more suggestions about how to prepare and deliver effective oral presentations.

10, 20, 30, 3 × 5

This rule concerns specific guidelines for the electronic slides. The 10, 20, 30 part of the rule is from Kawasaki (2005), and it means that a PowerPoint presentation should have 10 slides, last no more than 20 minutes, and have a minimum font size in text slides of at least 30 points. This rule has broad application. For example, 20 minutes is a typical time limit for classroom or conference presentations. Showing fewer rather than more slides helps to focus the audience's attention on what is really important, what you say. Novice presenters tend to show too many slides, which can water-down the basic take-home message. There may be no harm in showing a few more than 10 slides, especially if some key results can be clearly summarized with a diagram or smaller table. A slide with an outline of the talk is not usually necessary in a scientific presentation because everyone already knows the basic order (introduction, methods, etc.). However, once the number of slides reaches 20 or so, the speaker can wind up interacting more with the computer than the audience, due to the need to advance the slides so often. The rationale for using a large font size is clear: It limits the amount of text that can be put on a slide, and the text is easier to read, too.

The 3 × 5 part of the rule is for text slides, and it says that there should be no more than three bullet points per slide each expressed in about five words. As an alternative, all bullet points could be replaced by a single sentence that makes a crucial point, such as a bottom-line conclusion based on all results. A good text slide is simple and accomplishes two limited objectives: It gives audience members something to look at without annoying them, and it reminds the speaker about points to be covered in that part of the presentation. A slide with few words instead of whole sentences also prevents the speaker from reading the slide to the audience. If more text details are needed, then put them in the handout, not in your text slides.

No Templates

This rule says not to use the templates that are included with PowerPoint. Recall that templates are prepackaged combinations of colors, fonts, and graphics that make up a whole slide design. They are intended to make it easier to create a slide show because all the visual design work for the background is already done. However, there are two reasons why templates are a potential pitfall. First, some standard PowerPoint templates are used by so many people that it is easy to see two (or more) different presentations in the same session based on the same template. This gives these presentations a cookie-cutter appearance that can make content look less distinctive.

Second, many standard PowerPoint templates are pretty bad—if not downright awful—from a visual design perspective. This is because many are made up of so many different clashing colors or design elements that the background winds up competing with the foreground (i.e., your content) for attention. There are probably thousands of additional PowerPoint templates available over the Internet, some for free but others part of commercial packages. Many of these add-on templates are even *worse* than the ones that come with PowerPoint because they are designed to "wow" an audience. They may be so dazzling and garish that your content hardly stands a chance to be noticed. Remember that up to 10% of men have some degree of color blindness, and thus may have trouble discriminating red and green or blue and yellow, among other combinations. Use of the color pairs just mentioned in the same slide to make a visual distinction should thus be avoided.

Now, there is nothing wrong with tasteful use of color or graphics to enhance a slide's visual appeal. There is also truth to the expression that beauty is in the eye of the beholder concerning visual design. However, it is more important in scientific presentations to inform your audience than to entertain it. This includes the slide design, which as noted by M. Davis (2005) should "not detract from the science by calling attention to itself" (p. 156). How to design visually clean and simple slides is considered in the next section.

One should also avoid using the AutoContent wizard in PowerPoint. The AutoContent wizard is intended to help create a presentation of about 8–12 slides with ease, mainly for business contexts instead of scientific ones. The AutoContent wizard will create slides and suggest content relevant to a particular type of presentation, such as communicating bad news. A slide color scheme (template) is also automatically selected, but the user can usually specify later a different scheme. The AutoContent wizard thus automates much of the process of creating a slide show. However, it is easy for experienced viewers of PowerPoint presentations to spot an AutoContent-generated slide show because it has a cookie-cutter appearance.

Drop-Dead Simple

Readers who are warned against using templates or wizards to design their slides may feel anxious at the prospect of coming up with their own designs. Relax, there is really no need to worry. This is because the best designs for slides in scientific presentations are drop-dead simple, or DDS. For example, a white slide background with large text in a single font and color (black) and just one graphical element, such as thin color bar to separate titles from bullet points, is just fine. Indeed, such design simplicity with a lot of white space in text slides is consistent with the goal of emphasizing substance over style in scientific presentations. A simple slide design is also like a breath of fresh air for audiences too often annoyed by busy, buzzing, and booming PowerPoint slides (see Table 10.1). Simplicity is the new classy.

For text slides, a simple sans-serif font, such as Arial, is a good choice. Although fonts with serifs, such as Times Roman, are usually easier to read in print, computers may render sans-serif fonts clearer than fonts with serifs. In print, sans-serif fonts are often used for headlines, but bullet points in slides are basically headlines. An exception concerns equations, where a font with serifs may be best. This is because it can be hard to distinguish between certain Greek letters used in equations, such as a lower-case chi (χ), from uppercase letters in our Latin alphabet, such as X, in a sans-serif font. Use standard sentence case in your text slides. That is, capitalize as you would in print, but otherwise use lowercase letters. TEXT WHERE ALL LETTERS ARE UPPERCASE IS DIFFICULT TO QUICKLY READ AND PROJECTED ON A SCREEN LOOKS LIKE A VISUAL FORM OF SHOUTING. (See what I mean?) *Finally, check the spelling and grammar in each and every text slide.*

It is surprising how many text slides in scientific presentations
has speling or gramatical errors. (See how this looks?)

A few words are needed about slides in which results will be displayed. As mentioned, a table of numerical results that would be fine for a journal article may be too complicated to show in a slide. Only quite simple tables, such as ones with four or fewer rows and columns, are suitable for slides. Put larger tables in the handout, when it is necessary to convey more detailed information. Select the smallest number (including none) of simple, two-dimensional (2-D) graphical displays necessary to show the most critical findings. Do not use chartjunk-type displays with unnecessary features, such as 3-D format (Chapter 9). Text labels in figures or charts should be brief yet descriptive and displayed in a large font size. If the presenter needs a pointer to guide the audience through a graphic or illustration, then it may be too complicated for a slide.

It is easier to appreciate the elegance of DDS design by comparing bad PowerPoint slides with better ones. Presented in Figure 10.1 are two text slides (*see the color insert following p. 306 for Figures 10.1–10.4*). The bad text slide in the top part of this figure is based on a standard PowerPoint template (Capsules) that I have seen in dozens of presentations (i.e., the slide looks like a copycat). This slide is also jam-packed with text, most of which may be impossible to read from 20 feet away. The better text slide in the bottom part of Figure 10.1 features the use of a large font, only three simple bullet points, and lots of white space. Not only is the organization much cleaner in this better text slide, but it is also more readable.

Presented in Figure 10.2 are two title slides. The bad title slide in the top part of this figure features the use of bullet points with too many words displayed in too many different types and colors fonts and a garish background that makes the text hard to read. Many superfluous graphical images clutter the slide. A much simpler design for a title slide is presented in the bottom part of Figure 10.2. This better slide also has color, but it is used sparingly, as an accent only (i.e., it stays in the background). This slide also has a graphical image, but it is simple and does not compete for attention with the text, which is rendered in a uniform font.

Presented in Figure 10.3 are two slides that convey numerical results. The bad slide in the top part of this figure contains an example of chartjunk created using PowerPoint's chart editor. This 3-D frequency chart shows 12 numerical values rendered in too many colors and with nearly illegible legends. The same 12 numbers are presented in a simple 3×4 table in the better slide shown in the bottom part of Figure 10.3. The table in the better slide conveys exactly the same numerical information, but now it is easy to see the basic pattern. A simple 2-D line graphic rendered in black and white would also be a good way to display the same data points.

Presented in the top part of Figure 10.4 is a bad graphics slide with an overly complicated illustration. There is such a mish-mash of colors and images that the viewer hardly knows where to begin when looking at it.

The same basic informational elements are shown in a much simpler way in the better graphics slide presented in the bottom part of Figure 10.4. In this better slide, the flow of materials—in this case, images—from various sources or producers to consumers is much more obvious. See M. Davis (2005, pp. 315–322) for an example of a set of simple slides for a scientific presentation. Anholt (2006, Ch. 3) gives additional examples of both bad and good PowerPoint slides for scientific presentations.

No Crap

Here the term "crap" refers to any kind of optional special effect that can be added to a PowerPoint slide show. This includes superfluous sound or animation clips, special transition effects (wipes) between slides, and build sequences. *None* of these belong in a scientific presentation, and the inclusion of any one of them can annoy an audience. For example, I once saw a student presentation where a sound clip of a round of applause was played as each new slide appeared on screen. The audience thought it was cute the first time, but this initial good will turned to annoyance by the third slide and then to frank irritation by the end of the presentation (i.e., no one felt like clapping). A variation on an expression attributed to Confucius is relevant here: Slideshows should really be simple, but we insist on making them complicated.

Lessons from Multimedia Learning

Mayer (2001) described a set of empirically based principles for the effective use of multimedia presentations that are relevant to PowerPoint presentations. These principles and their implications are summarized next:

1. **Spatial contiguity principle, temporal contiguity principle**: Learning is better when corresponding words and pictures are presented near each other on the same page or screen (spatial). This presentation should also be simultaneous instead of sequential (temporal). *Implication:* Do not separate images from essential words that describe them across multiple slides, and do not gradually add text to images in a build sequence.

2. **Coherence principle**: Learning is better when extraneous words, images, video, and sound are excluded from the presentation. *Im-*

plication: The need to keep PowerPoint presentations free of these kinds of distractions was discussed earlier.

3. **Modality principle, redundancy principle**: People learn better from animation and narration than from animation and on-screen text (modality) and better than from animation, narration, and on-screen text (redundancy). *Implication:* Here animation means a substantive video clip (it is real content), not an unnecessary special effect (crap). The presenter should use spoken words only to describe the video while it is playing.

4. **Individual differences principle**: Multimedia design effects are stronger for low-knowledge than for high-knowledge learners. *Implication:* It is even more important to design presentations that respect the design principles discussed earlier when the audience is relatively unfamiliar with the content.

Other PowerPoint Issues

Some additional substantive issues about the use of PowerPoint are discussed next.

Why Use PowerPoint?

If substantive video or sound clips are to be included as part of a presentation, then PowerPoint or a similar computer tool is a good way to combine text, images, and media files into an integrated slide show. Otherwise, there may be little need to use PowerPoint. A good alternative is to use a word processor to create your slides, convert the word processor document to Adobe Portable Document Format (PDF), and then use Adobe Reader to display the PDF file.[1] The command "View | Full Screen Mode" in Reader changes to full-screen display, which is ideal for presentations. The Reader application is freely available over the Internet, which means that a presentation in PDF format can be posted online and viewed by anyone with no need for a commercial software package. Slide features, such as font sizes and types, display in a constant way across different computers in PDF. In contrast, it can happen that a slideshow created in PowerPoint on one computer will look different when run on another computer. Some

---

[1] All but two slides in Figures 10.1–10.4 were created using a word processor.

modern word processors can automatically save documents in PDF. There are also some freely available utilities that perform this conversion for older word processors.[2]

Is PowerPoint Evil?

Tufte (2006) described what he referred to as the **cognitive style of PowerPoint,** which works best when information is organized in a strictly hierarchical way that can be presented in a linear, single-path structure using bullet points over multiple slides. However, this cognitive style does not facilitate analytical reasoning with words or numbers (statistical results), given the inherent limitations of the medium of electronic slide shows. This is especially true when it is necessary to understand relations that underlie facts listed in bullet points in order to grasp a bigger picture.

Serious problems can arise when PowerPoint is used as the sole means to communicate about a complex problem. For example, Tufte (2006) claimed that the misuse of PowerPoint may have contributed to the destruction of the Space Shuttle *Columbia* on February 1, 2003, as it reentered the atmosphere over Texas. In a PowerPoint presentation made by engineers for the National Aeronautics and Space Administration (NASA) while *Columbia* was still flying, a critical fact indicating that prelaunch safety standards no longer held was relegated to a small bullet point at the bottom of a complicated text slide. This slide failed to communicate with tragic consequences the potential seriousness of the damage to *Columbia* at launch caused by the impact of a large piece of foam on the leading edge of its wing, which broke apart under the intense friction and heat generated by reentry into the atmosphere.

A handout in a scientific presentation can help mitigate limitations of PowerPoint's cognitive style. Also, the ultimate product in science is a journal article, book chapter, or technical report with full text that was subjected to peer review. For this reason, Tufte (2006) argued that the real presentation computer tool in science and engineering is a word processor, not PowerPoint. In business settings, though, there may be even greater danger that complex information winds up being dumbed-down to fit within the confines of a PowerPoint presentation, especially when there is no corresponding written report. The potential for misuse of PowerPoint in education is also a concern. One example occurs when professors give lectures using PowerPoint presentations created by publishers

---

[2]One I use for Word 2003 is PDF995; *www.pdf995.com/*

for their textbooks. These presentations are usually just chapter content summarized in bullet-point form. No educational value is added if the instructor speaks only from the PowerPoint presentation. Another example is when students learn how to make PowerPoint presentations but not how to write.

The issues just mentioned have led Tufte (2006) and others to ask whether PowerPoint is evil, given its potential for misuse. In the final analysis, PowerPoint is just a tool, and the misuse of a tool is at least partly the fault of its user. Hanft (2003) offered this perspective: PowerPoint may be more a symptom of a deeper societal problem—that of a shortage of reflection and critical thinking—than inherently evil by itself.

Poster Presentations

The first experience as a presenter for many students and young researchers is the scientific poster session. Compared with oral presentations, poster sessions offer a lower-pressure, more intimate forum where the distinction between speaker and audience is blurred. Indeed, it is the ability to interact directly with people who stop by to read the poster that makes these sessions less about data presentation than an exchange of ideas.

A successful experience in a poster session depends in part on good poster design. Posters do not have the same requirements as slides or handouts, and consequently they have a unique format. This is because a poster is intended to be read quickly by people who are moving from one poster stand display to another. Consequently, a poster must be designed to be easily read from a distance of up to several feet away. This means that (1) text should be large and easy to see, (2) illustrations must be simple, and (3) the overall layout makes it clear the order in which the text and illustrations should be viewed. Relatively little text can be included in a poster, so only the most essential points should be included. One way to do so is to list no more than four text bullet points in each section ("Methods," "Results," etc.). Bullet points in posters can be complete sentences, but it must be possible to read all the text within a few minutes. The most common mistake in creating a poster is to include too much text. To enhance readability, use a light background with dark text—the colors white and black, respectively, are just fine—and select a non-serif font in a large size for the text body (e.g., at least 18 points). Posters do not ordinarily have an abstract.

The most common format for scientific posters is column format. That is, the poster is organized as series of vertical lists each with clear labels or numbers that signal the order in which the information is to be read. The number of columns varies most often from two to five, depending on the maximum amount of space available for the poster. For example, posters limited in width to a maximum of 48 in (122 cm) may have two to three columns, and posters with a maximum width of 72–96 in (183–244 cm) may have four to five columns. Posters with more than five columns can be hard to read. Presented in Figure 10.5 are two examples of poster layout. The design in the top part of the figure has

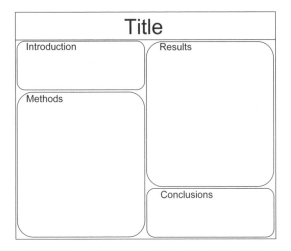

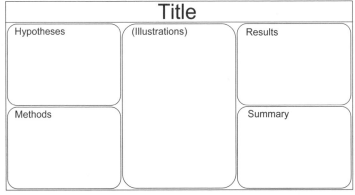

FIGURE 10.5. Examples of two- and three-column layouts for scientific posters.

two columns and could be suitable for a narrower poster width limit. The layout at the bottom of the figure has three columns, which may suit a wider poster width limit. An example of a poster with four columns is presented in Appendix 10.1.

Top-notch posters are created in professional computer programs for graphics, such as Adobe InDesign, QuarkXPress, or LaTeX, and printed on a single, large page with a special printer. However, the cost of using a special printer can be relatively high, especially if part of the poster is in color. PowerPoint can also be used to create posters. There are PowerPoint templates for scientific posters, some freely available over the Internet.[3] Many universities offer free PowerPoint templates for posters with the appropriate logos and color schemes. A disadvantage of using PowerPoint compared with a professional graphics program is that the former may not support larger page widths. For example, PowerPoint 2003 restricted page width to no more than 56 in (142 cm), but some printing services allow the final design to be scaled up in order to be printed on wider pages. Students may not have access to special software or printers, so their posters are most often created in sections and printed on separate pages. For example, the method section may be printed on one page and the results section on another. The final poster is then assembled by putting the individual pages together on the poster board. These "cut-and-paste" posters usually do not look as sophisticated as ones printed on a single sheet, but good content is the most critical factor in poster presentations, too.

Just as for an oral presentation, prepare a handout to distribute during the poster session. The handout could take the same form as one for an oral presentation. An advantage is that the handout gives more detail than can be shown on the poster. Another alternative is to print an image of the poster on a standard sheet of paper.[4] This alternative is not as desirable because it adds no detail beyond that presented in the poster. Include contact information (postal address, e-mail address, etc.) in the handout that accompanies your poster. See Alley (2003, pp. 216–217), M. Davis (2005, pp. 329–333), and Gosling (1999) for more suggestions about poster design and examples.

---

[3]*www.posterpresentations.com*

[4]This assumes that the image in this size is legible. A good poster design should be legible when reproduced as an 8.5 in × 11 in image.

Summary

The single most important thing about an oral presentation is what you say, not what you show. The former requires good ideas expressed in a way that balances breadth and depth in a short presentation time, and the latter should only support what you say and not take center stage. However, the visual aids in too many oral presentations actually distract from the speaker's intended take-home message. This is because too many presenters make electronic slides that are overly complex with too many colors or have superfluous graphical elements or special effects, such as animations or sound clips, that have little to do with presentation content. When planning an oral presentation, spend most of your time organizing what you will say. The best slide design is visually simple so that the background does not overwhelm the foreground (your content). Keep text slides very simple, too, and limit them to no more than three bullet points each with about five words or so. Any potential technical problem—including the total inability to show electronic slides—can be dealt with by preparing a handout as part of your presentation. If all else fails, you could still give the presentation working only from the handout. A handout can also be used to mitigate some of the limitations of oral presentations as a low-bandwidth communication medium by including extra information, such as larger tables, that is difficult to display on the screen. With sufficient practice, you will improve as a public speaker, and your level of anxiety will decline, too, but being nervous is a normal part of giving an oral presentation. In contrast, many people enjoy poster sessions because of the opportunities for more informal contact with those interested in your research. The design for a poster should be simple, too, and a printed handout should be available as part of your poster session.

RECOMMENDED READINGS

The books by Anholt (2006) and M. Davis (2005) are helpful resources for learning about how to give effective oral presentations and poster presentations. Simplicity in visual aids and clarity and substance in spoken content for oral presentations is emphasized in both works. The monograph by Tufte (2006) is a sobering look at the limitations of PowerPoint and related computer tools for communicating complex material that requires analytical reasoning, not just rote memorization. His basic argument is that a mismatch between a communication medium and the information needs in a particular business or scientific context can potentially have disastrous consequences.

Anholt, R. R. H. (2006). *Dazzle 'em with style: The art of oral scientific presentation* (2nd ed.). New York: Elsevier Academic Press.

Davis, M. (2005). *Scientific papers and presentations* (2nd ed.). New York: Academic Press.

Tufte, E. R. (2006). *The cognitive style of PowerPoint: Pitching out corrupts within* (2nd ed.). Cheshire, CT: Graphics Press.

EXERCISES

For your particular research project:

1. Write a three-sentence summary of the essential take-home messages.

2. Write three main points for each of the three sections of a presentation about your research project, the introduction, the methods and results, and the discussion.

3. Convert the nine points you just wrote into drafts of between 10 and 20 text slides for a 20-minute presentation. Each slide can be sketched out using pencil and paper.

4. Evaluate the points you wrote for the previous exercise in terms of whether the essential take-home messages of your presentation are given proper emphasis.

5. Show how to use the technique of zooming in to present the context for the major aims of your study.

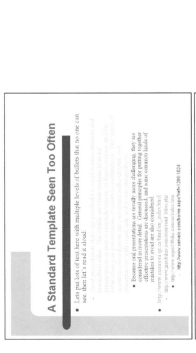

FIGURE 10.1. Examples of bad (top) and better (bottom) text slides.

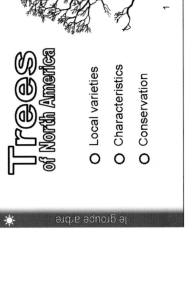

FIGURE 10.2. Examples of bad (top) and better (bottom) title slides.

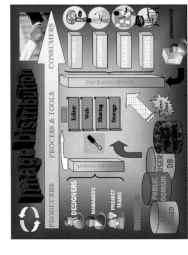

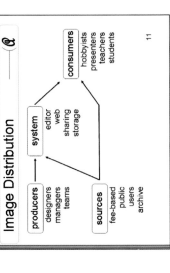

FIGURE 10.4. Examples of bad (top) and better (bottom) slides with illustrations.

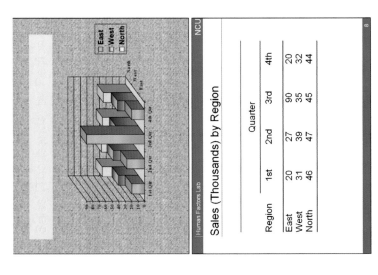

FIGURE 10.3. Examples of bad (top) and better (bottom) slides that convey numerical results.

APPENDIX 10.1

Example Slides,
Handout, and Poster

The slides and handout presented next are for a hypothetical 20-minute presentation based on the classic 1968 study of bystander intervention by Darley and Latané. An example poster based on this article is also presented. The author institutional affiliations and grant support acknowledgments shown in these materials are taken from the original article. Table 1 and Figure 1 in the original article (each on p. 380 in the original work) are adapted here in the example slides, handout, and poster presented next with the permission of John M. Darley (personal communication, September 6, 2007). The copyright for Table 1 and Figure 1 in Darley and Latané is held by the American Psychological Association. Reprinted by permission.

Slides

We can't all be heroes because somebody has to sit on the curb and clap as they go by

Will Rogers

Bystander Intervention in Emergencies: Diffusion of Responsibility[a]

John M. Darley   Bibb Latané
New York University   Columbia University

[a] NSF Grants GS1238, GS1239

1

Attack on Kitty Genovese

- Residential area in NYC
- 38 witnesses
- No one acted

2

Why do bystanders fail to act?

- Urban alienation, anomie
- Fear of harm, police
- Presence of others

3

Presence of others

- Diffusion of responsibility
- Diffusion of blame
- Someone already helped?

4

Hypothesis

More unseen bystanders,

less likely any one will intervene

5

Methods

- $N = 72$ (49 ♂, 13 ♀)
- Mock discussion group
- Others unseen

6

Methods

- Feigned epileptic seizure
- DV: Time to help
- IV: Group (Alone, 1, 4)

7

Group type and response likelihood

Group	n	% Report
Alone	13	85
1 other	26	62
4 others	13	31

Cramer's $V = .55$

8

Cumulative distributions of helping

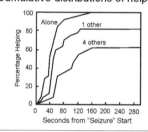

9

Emergency response unrelated to...

- Gender (other, participant)
- Perceived medical skill
- Personality, background

10

Summary

- Group size affects helping
- Non-responders *not* apathic
- But personality not critical

11

Handout

Bystander Intervention in Emergencies:
Diffusion of Responsibility

John M. Darley
New York

Bibb Latané
Columbia University

On March 16, 1964, 28-year-old Catherine "Kitty" Genovese was attacked by a man with a knife as she left her job in Queens, New York. The attack lasted half an hour before Ms. Genovese died. What is especially tragic about this crime is that almost 40 people witnessed or heard the attack, but no one assisted, not even to call the police. Explanations of why so many people failed to intervene include alienation and dehumanization due to the urban environment (Gansberg, 1964; Rosenthal, 1964) and general moral decay.

Another factor may be at work here, the presence of other onlookers. Specifically, when there are several observers, the responsibility to intervene is diffused and does not fall on any one person. The potential blame for not intervening is also diffused (Miller & Dollard, 1941). Consequently, no one may act, even if onlookers are really concerned. This may be especially true when observers cannot directly interact with or even see other observers.

It is hypothesized that the more unseen bystanders to an emergency, the less likely it is that any one observer will try to help. This hypothesis was tested in an experimental setting where (1) a staged but plausible emergency occurred, and (2) each observer was prevented from getting information about the behavior of other observers.

Method

Participants. A total of 72 university students (59 women, 13 men) in introductory psychology classes participated in this study.

Procedure. Each participant was met by a research assistant and led into a small room off a long corridor with other small rooms. It was explained that the participant would take part in a group discussion about with university life. This discussion would be conducted over an intercom system with no face-to-face contact. Only one microphone would be turned on at a time (i.e., they would take turns), and the discussion would be recorded without the experimenter listening in on the conservation while it was taking place.

One of the confederates disclosed that he or she has a seizure disorder. Soon after this confederate

feigned a seizure with choking sounds before the sound was cut off. The experiment was terminated six minutes after a participant failed to seek help.

The dependent variable was the speed of the naïve participant's response (e.g., to leave the room to notify the assistant). The major independent variable is the group size (alone–the victim and participant only; 1–victim, participant, and 1 unseen other; 4–victim, participant, and 4 unseen others). The actual participants also completed a background form and a series of personality tests.

Results

The number of unseen bystanders had a relatively large effect on whether and how quickly participants sought help (Table 1). A clear majority (85%) of the participants left their rooms to seek help when they believed the victim was the only discussant. Fewer sought help when there was one other unseen observer (62%), and even fewer when there were four unseen others (31%). The correlation between group size and the proportion seeking help is .55.

Table 1
Effects of group size on likelihood and speed of response

Group size	n	% reporting[a]	Time (sec.)	Speed score[b]
Alone	13	85	52	.87
1 other	26	62	93	.72
4 others	13	31	166	.51

[a]Cramér's $V = .55$; $\chi^2 (2) = 7.19$, $p = .028$.
[b]$\hat{\eta}^2 = .25$, $F (2, 49) = 7.91$, $p = .002$.

Time for participants to seek help was converted to a speed score (Table 1). In this metric, a speed score of zero means help was never sought. The average speed also clearly differed as a function of group size. Specifically, the proportion of speed variance explained by group size is about .25, and the correlation between group size and response speed is about .50.

Presented in Figure 1 are the cumulative distributions of time to seek help as a function of

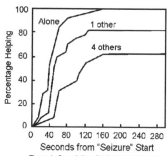

Figure 1. Cumulative distributions of time to help as a function of group size.

group size. Most participants who ever sought help (95%) did so within the first three minutes. Also, no participant who did not seek help within the first three minutes ever did so. These results suggest that few, if any, additional participants would have sought help if the experiment were allowed to continue for a longer time.

We tested several other variations on the three-person condition (participant, victim, 1 unseen other). Some of these involved combinations where the participant thought the unseen other was a man or a women; in another, the unseen other was thought to be a premedical student with emergency room experience or not. These variations had no impact on the results. That is, variations in perceived gender and medical competence of the unseen other had no impact on response speed. Also, men responded to the emergency just as fast as women. Background variables and personality characteristics were also unrelated to response speed across cases in the whole study.

Discussion

Participants seemed to clearly believe that the staged emergency was real, and many genuinely seem confused and distressed about what to do. This included the participants who failed to report the apparent seizure to the assistant. Specifically, these persons did not appear to be apathetic or indifferent to the fate of the confederate with the seizure. Indeed, many seemed upset and nervous.

An obvious question is: Why did these participants not respond? We speculate that they were in a state of indecision or conflict about whether to

respond. This conflict is of the avoidance-avoidance type where guilt and shame about not responding was balanced against the fear of overreacting or looking like a fool. When there were no other observers, this conflict was easily resolved such that most participants responded to the emergency. The conflict was more acute when other unseen observers were present, and resolving this conflict is more difficult as the number of other bystanders is greater.

Other results suggest that personality constructs, such as alienation, dehumanization, or Machiavellianism, may not be as important as once thought as explanations for the failure of bystanders to respond to emergencies. These kinds of explanation imply that those who do not respond are somehow different from the rest of us, and that we would not also fail to help in the same situation. Our results suggest that the explanation may lie more in the response of the bystander to other observers than in apathy, indifference, or personality defects.

Some limitations of these results are noted. The experimental situation in this study where other participants were unable to see or communicate with other observers is unlike some real emergencies, such as a fire, where other observers are close by. The opportunity to communicate with other observers may be sufficient to counteract effects of diffusion or responsibility and blame (Bryan & Test, 1967). However, the conditions of this study are similar to those of the Genovese murder where many witnesses had no direct contact with one another.

References

Bryan, J. H., & Test, M. A. (1967). Models and helping: Naturalistic studies in aiding behavior. *Journal of Personality and Social Psychology, 6,* 400–407.

Gansberg, M. (1964, March 27). 37 who saw murder didn't call the police. *The New York Times,* pp. 1, 38.

Miller, N., & Dollard, J. (1941). *Social learning and imitation.* New Haven, CT: Yale University Press.

Rosenthal, A, M. (1964). *Thirty-eight witnesses.* New York: McGraw-Hill.

Give name of conference, date of presentation, and author contact information somewhere in the handout

Poster

Bystander Intervention in Emergencies: Diffusion of Responsibility

John M. Darley, *New York University*   Bibb Latané, *Columbia University*

Objective

Evaluate whether response to a perceived emergency is affected by the presence of unseen observers

> ### Shocking Queens Murder
>
> March 16, 1964
>
> This morning 28-year-old Catherine Genovese was attacked and killed by a man with a knife in a residential area in New York City. Almost 40 people witnessed the crime, but no one helped, not even to call the police.
>
> *Article, Page A2*

Simulated article, real story

Rationale

- Sometimes bystanders do not act to help victims
- Some explanations refer to alienation, apathy, anomie, or dehumanization

Hypotheses

- The presence of other onlookers may be a factor in bystander non-response
- The responsibility to act is diffused, so is the blame for not helping
- These effects are greater when there are more observers who are unseen

Methods

- $N = 72$ university students
- Participant led to small room
- Asked to take part in anonymous discussion over intercom, then left alone
- Told either alone with confederate, or 1 or 4 additional discussants
- Confederate feigned seizure

Results

- Proportion seeking help and group size:

Group	n	% Report
Alone	13	85
1 other	26	62
4 others	13	31

- Cumulative response time and group size:

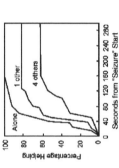

- Response speed unrelated to gender, personality

Discussion

- Participants were not apathetic or indifferent
- However, likelihood of responding is less as there are more unseen observers
- Personality flaws or defects in bystanders does not explain non-response
- Results may not generalize to emergencies where witnesses are close by

Acknowledgments

NSF Grants GS1238, GS1239

Suggested Answers to Exercises

Chapter 3

1. Although internal validity, construct validity, conclusion validity, and external validity are the *main* concerns of, respectively, design, measurement, analysis, and sampling (an aspect of design), they are not the exclusive ones. Some examples: The statistical requirement for score independence is met through a measurement plan that prevents the responses of one case from influencing those of another (e.g., cases are tested separately). The same measurement plan should also reduce the influence of nuisance variables (e.g., the testing method is standardized). In a covariate analysis, the influence of potential confounders as measured by the covariates are controlled when estimating treatment effects. Selection of the sample in a way that restricts the true range of variability may negatively affect statistical conclusion validity by truncating effect sizes. Finally, not all authors agree in the classification of different validity threats under these four categories.

2. There is truth in this comment. One way to maximize internal validity is to study a phenomenon in a laboratory setting where extraneous variables are controlled and precise methods are used. This maximization of precision in one specific setting may reduce the generalizability of the results to other, less controlled situations. Likewise, an attempt to maximize external validity by studying something in real-world settings may introduce so much imprecision that true causal effects are washed out. When resources are limited, researchers must make trade-offs among validity types, including internal versus external validity. Be direct and honest in identifying plausible validity threats when describing your results. Learn from your mistakes, too. This means to plan the next study to deal with an expanded subset of validity threats, given what you learned in previous studies.

3. Construct validity, external validity: Both involve generalization, one from observable scores to hypothetical constructs (construct), the other from a particular study to variations in settings, participants, interventions, or outcomes (external). It is possible to study constructs with no particular hypotheses about cause–effect relations, but it is difficult to separate cause–effect inferences from operationalizations about how presumed causes and effects are to be measured. Conclusion validity, internal validity: Both are concerned with study operations, those involved in the statistical analysis (conclusion) and those involved in manipulating presumed causes while controlling for confounders (internal). Errors in the statistical analysis (e.g., incorrect effect sizes) can lead to errors in causal inference. However, causal reasoning can be flawed even if the analyses were technically correct.

4. No. Probability samples are selected by a chance-based method, such as random selection. This is a sample of convenience because it was available at a local clinic. At best, the sample is a purposive sample in that both men and women patients are included in the sample. However, whether each gender group in the sample is representative is unknown.

5. The 100 students selected for invitation is a probability sample but relative only to the whole class. This group may be representative of the whole class, but it is not guaranteed. Even if so, this group may not be representative of other students outside this particular class. It is unlikely that all those invited will volunteer for the study, and those who do may not be representative of the whole class.

6. Random sampling guarantees representative samples in the long run only. It could happen by chance that individuals with atypical characteristics are included in a particular random sample, and this sample may not be representative. With sufficient replication, though, results averaged across random samples will reflect population characteristics.

7. There are many negative effects of low score reliability: it increases extraneous variance; unreliability in covariate scores reduces accuracy in analyses of covariance; statistical power, observed statistical significance, and effect sizes are all decreased; regression to the mean is greater when there is more measurement error; establishing construct validity is compromised; and the accuracy of causal inferences is comprised.

8. Selection-testing: Exposure to a test affects later scores on the outcome variable for either the treatment group or the control

group. Selection-history: A specific event that takes place concurrently with treatment affects one group or the other. Selection-instrumentation: The nature of measurement is different in one group or the other. All of these threats operate by mimicking a treatment effect.

9. One way to illustrate a case when the predicted mean difference is greater than the observed mean difference in ANCOVA is presented next:

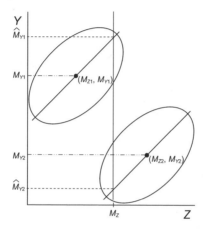

10. Report complete descriptive statistics for all groups in your study (e.g., men, women, and treatment, control). The absence of a profile means that the specific characteristics of the hypothetical population for your study are not known. Therefore, you should be cautious about making claims that your results will generalize to any particular population.

11. The rate of experimentwise Type I error was here correctly calculated:

$$\alpha_{EW} = 1 - (1 - .001)^{50} = .0488 < .05$$

However, this estimate assumes that each of the 50 statistical tests is independent of the others. This is not true when the outcome variables are correlated. Thus, the probability of making a Type I error across the set of 50 correlated tests is actually higher than .05.

12. The group mean difference is $M_1 - M_0 = 13.00 - 11.00 = 2.00$. The source table calculated for these data calculated using the One-Way ANOVA procedure in SPSS appears next:

	Sum of Squares	df	Mean Square	F	Sig.
Between Groups	10.000	1	10.000	1.600	.242
Within Groups	50.000	8	6.250		
Total	60.000	9			

The correlations, regression sums of squares, and regression coefficients calculated for the same data but using the Linear Regression option in SPSS appear next:

Model	R	R Square	Adjusted R Square	Std. Error of the Estimate
1	.408[a]	.167	.062	2.5000

[a]Predictors: (Constant), X

Model		Sum of Squares	df	Mean Square	F	Sig.
1	Regression	10.000	1	10.000	1.600	.242[a]
	Residual	50.000	8	6.250		
	Total	60.000	9			

[a]Predictors: (Constant), X

Model		Unstandardized Coefficients		Standardized Coefficients	t	Sig.
		B	Std. Error	Beta		
1	(Constant)	11.000	1.118		9.839	.000
	X	2.000	1.581	.408	1.265	.242

The source tables across the two sets of analyses are identical. Also, note across these analyses that

$$SS_{Bet}/SS_T = SS_{Reg}/SS_T = R^2 = 10.00/60.00 = .4082 = .167$$

which says that (1) group membership (X) explains about 16.7% of the total variance in Y, and (2) the correlation between the two is about .408. Note also that (1) the unstandardized regression coefficient for X, 2.00, equals the observed mean difference; and (2) the value of t for this effect, 1.265, equals the square root of $F(1, 8) = 1.60$ in both source tables.

Chapter 4

1. Both counterbalancing and crossover control for order effects in designs with a repeated-measures factor. Crossover can be seen as a special form of counterbalancing in designs where two different treatments are evaluated in two different groups. Each group is exposed to every treatment but in a different order. In a crossover design, observations are collected both before and after each treat-

ment. Counterbalancing is a more general way to control order effects, and it can be used in designs where treatment effects are not specifically evaluated.

2. There is a main effect of praise such that the overall mean in the money condition (25.75) is lower than that in the praise condition (28.00). However, there is also an interaction effect in that improvement over trials occurred at different rates for the two groups. Specifically, those rewarded with money showed initial better performance, but the performance of the two groups is similar by the last trial.

3. This conclusion may be unwarranted. Students placed in the program scored at the upper extreme of achievement in grade 1. Due to the regression effect, we expect these children to score at a less extreme (lower) level when retested on a similar measure, which is confounded with any program effect.

4. The particular numerical values you specified are not important if the basic patterns are correct. For example, the cell means in the leftmost 2×2 table presented next indicate main effects only (A, B). However, the cell means in the rightmost table indicate both an interaction effect and just one main effect (AB, A):

	B_1	B_2
A_1	50.00	25.00
A_2	35.00	10.00

	B_1	B_2
A_1	50.00	30.00
A_2	20.00	40.00

5. Two examples are presented next. In the leftmost graphic, cases with extremely high scores on the pretest were assigned to the treatment group (e.g., because they were the sickest patients), and their scores are regressing to the mean over time. In the rightmost graphic, cases in the treatment group had extremely low pretest scores; thus, we expect their scores to regress back up closer to the mean:

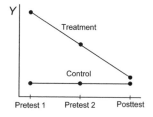
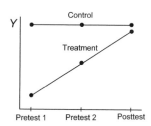

6. It is critical to have a placebo control condition when evaluating a medication. One possible solution is to specify a switching-replications design where the patients who initially receive placebo are later switched to the drug. However, the patients in the drug condition continue to take medication even after the placebo group crosses over to treatment. Presented next is the structural representation for this design:

$$
\begin{array}{ccccccc}
R & O_1 & X & O_2 & X & O_3 \\
R & O_1 &   & O_2 & X & O_3
\end{array}
$$

7. The particular numerical values you specified are unimportant if the basic pattern is correct. For example, the cell means presented next indicate a testing effect for the treatment group only such that the administration of a pretest is associated with higher scores on the posttest. There is also a main effect of pretest and a group × pretest interaction:

	No Pretest	Pretest
Treatment	40.00	50.00
Control	30.00	30.00

8. Level of anxiety is theoretically continuous. Thus, it makes sense in a nonexperimental study to administer an anxiety questionnaire to measure this variable. However, it may be a bad idea to categorize this continuous variable in order to form groups. Instead, use a regression technique to estimate the relation between anxiety and task performance. Examine the scatterplot to determine if there is a nonlinear association. Level of anxiety could be treated as a manipulable variable in an experimental study through the administration of task instructions. For example, tell one group that task performance reflects competency, and another that performance is unrelated to personal characteristics.

9. This problem describes an interrupted time-series design. History is a major threat, especially concerning seasonal effects. For example, there could be greater local pollution at certain times of the year (e.g., pesticide runoff from crops). Thus, results of water quality tests may depend on when samples are taken.

10. One solution is to specify a hybrid of a regression-discontinuity design and a simple randomized design: Students with grade-point averages above the cutoff (> 3.50) are assigned to the program. Stu-

dents with averages in the range 3.00–3.50 are randomly assigned to either the program or not where the proportion of such students placed in the program is determined by resource limitations. Students with averages < 3.00 are not assigned to the program. All groups are administered a posttest. The structural representation for this hybrid design is presented next:

$$O_A \text{ (GPA)}$$

> 3.50	C	X	O_2
3.00–3.50	R	X	O_2
3.00–3.50	R		O_2
< 3.00	C		O_2

11. The observed mean difference in ANOVA is $M_1 - M_0 = 18.00 - 14.00 = 4.00$. The ANOVA source table calculated using the One-Way ANOVA procedure in SPSS appears next:

	Sum of Squares	df	Mean Square	F	Sig.
Between Groups	40.000	1	40.000	4.000	.081
Within Groups	80.000	8	10.000		
Total	120.000	9			

The predicted mean difference calculated using the General Linear Model–Univariate (GLM–U) option in SPSS for the ANCOVA is $\hat{M}_1 - \hat{M}_0 = 19.554 - 12.446 = 7.108$, which is greater than the observed contrast (4.00). Presented next is the ANCOVA source table:

	Type III Sum of Squares	df	Mean Square	F	Sig.
Corrected Model	67.027[a]	2	33.514	4.429	.057
Intercept	60.478	1	60.478	7.992	.026
Z	27.027	1	20.027	3.571	.101
X	66.706	1	66.706	8.815	.021
Error	52.973	7	7.568		
Total	2680.000	10			
Corrected Total	120.00	9			

[a]R Squared = .559 (Adjusted R Squared = .432)

The predicted group mean difference (7.108) is statistically significant in the ANCOVA ($p = .021$), but the observed mean difference (4.00) is not in the ANOVA ($p = .081$). Also note that the error term is smaller in the ANCOVA (7.568) than in the ANOVA (10.000). But what are the other effects listed in the ANCOVA source table, such as "Corrected Model," "Intercept," and "Z"? The GLM–U procedure actually conducts an ANCOVA using multiple regression; this point is elaborated in the next exercise. The homogeneity of regression assumption appears to be reasonable. For example, values of the respective within-group correlations and unstandardized regression coefficients for predicting Y from Z are quite similar (Group 0: $r_{YZ} = .585$, $B_{YZ} = .685$; Group 1: $r_{YZ} = .577$, $B_{YZ} = .667$).

12. The data were analyzed using the Linear Regression option in SPSS. The correlations, regression sums of squares, and coefficients calculated by SPSS are presented next:

Model	R	R Square	Adjusted R Square	Std. Error of the Estimate
1	.747[a]	.559	.432	2.7509

[a]Predictors: (Constant), X, Y

Model		Sum of Squares	df	Mean Square	F	Sig.
1	Regression	67.027	2	33.514	4.429	.057[a]
	Residual	52.973	7	7.568		
	Total	120.000	9			

[a]Predictors: (Constant), X, Z

Model		Unstandardized Coefficients B	Std. Error	Standardized Coefficients Beta	t	Sig.
1	(Constant)	6.162	4.326		1.424	.197
	Z	.676	.358	.653	1.890	.101
	X	7.108	2.394	1.026	2.969	.021

The multiple correlation between the predictors of group membership and the covariate on the one hand and the dependent variable on the other is $R = .747$, and the total proportion of explained variance is $R^2 = .559$, or about 55.9%. The sum of squares for the whole regression is 67.027 and $F(2, 7) = 4.429$ for this effect. Note that the results just mentioned correspond to the respective values for the "Corrected Model" in the ANCOVA source table for the previous exercise. The unstandardized regression coefficient (B) for the group effect (X) is 7.108, which exactly equals the ANCOVA predicted mean difference. For this effect, $t = 2.969$, and $t^2 = 2.969^2 = 8.815$. The latter is the same value as that of the $F(1, 7)$ statistic for the group effect in the ANCOVA source table for the previous exercise. From a regression perspective, this test evaluates the predictive power of group membership when we are controlling for the covariate. Likewise, the results for the covariate Z in the regression analysis concern its predictive power, but now controlling for group membership. In the regression analysis, it is clear that the covariate is a predictor, too. This fact is sometimes overlooked from a traditional ANCOVA perspective.

13. The homogeneity of regression is not tenable (Group 0: $r_{YZ} = -.585$, $B_{YZ} = -.685$; Group 1: $r_{YZ} = .577$, $B_{YZ} = .667$). In the first regression analysis, the total proportion of explained variance estimated using the Linear Regression procedure in SPSS is reported next:

Model	R	R Square	Adjusted R Square	Std. Error of the Estimate
1	.577[a]	.33	.143	3.3806

[a]Predictors: (Constant), X, Z

The proportion of total explained variance is .33 when just group membership (X) and the covariate (Z) are the predictors. However, this analysis is a standard ANCOVA, which assumes homogeneity of regression. Presented next are results for the regression analysis where X, Z, and XZ are all predictors:

Model	R	R Square	Adjusted R Square	Std. Error of the Estimate
1	.747[a]	.559	.432	2.9712

[a]Predictors: (Constant), X, Z, XZ

Model		Sum of Squares	df	Mean Square	F	Sig.
1	Regression	67.027	3	22.334	2.531	.154[a]
	Residual	52.973	6	7.568		
	Total	120.000	9			

[a]Predictors: (Constant), X, Z, XZ

Model		Unstandardized Coefficients B	Std. Error	Standardized Coefficients Beta	t	Sig.
1	(Constant)	21.945	6.515		3.368	.015
	Z	-.685	.550	-.662	-1.246	.259
	XZ	1.352	.772	1.524	1.750	.131
	X	-8.612	7.657	-1.243	-1.125	.304

The proportion of total variance explained in the second regression analysis is .559. This total explanatory power is not statistically significant, but this is expected given the small group size. Presented next is the overall regression equation from this analysis:

$$\hat{Y} = 21.945 - 8.612\,X - .685\,Z + 1.352\,XZ$$

When $X = 0$ and $X = 1$ are plugged into this equation, we get the following separate regression equations for each group:

$$\hat{Y}_0 = 21.945 - 0 - .685\,Z + 0 = 21.945 - .685\,Z$$

$$\hat{Y}_1 = 21.945 - 8.612 - .685\,Z + 1.352\,Z = 13.333 + .667\,Z$$

These separate equations indicate that in the treatment group ($X = 0$), the relation between the covariate Z and the dependent variable Y is negative, but this relation is positive in the control group ($X = 1$). Accordingly, prediction of status on Y depends jointly on whether cases were treated or not and also on their score on the covariate.

14. The observed contrast is $M_1 - M_0 = 11.80 - 3.60 = 8.20$. You must create a new variable for the RD analysis, the difference between the score on the assignment variable and the cutting score for each case (e.g., $DIFF = AS - 8.00$). In a regression analysis, the predictors are X (group membership) and $DIFF$. The data were analyzed using the Linear Regression procedure in SPSS. The results are presented next:

Model	R	R Square	Adjusted R Square	Std. Error of the Estimate
1	.969[a]	.940	.923	1.3681

[a]Predictors: (Constant), DIFF, X

Model		Sum of Squares	df	Mean Square	F	Sig.
1	Regression	204.998	2	102.499	54.762	.000[a]
	Residual	13.102	7	1.872		
	Total	1218.100	9			

[a]Predictors: (Constant), DIFF, X

Model		Unstandardized Coefficients		Standardized Coefficients		
		B	Std. Error	Beta	t	Sig.
1	(Constant)	7.404	1.053		7.003	.000
	X	.782	1.881	.084	.416	.690
	DIFF	.951	.214	.894	4.440	.003

The regression model as a whole explains about 94.0% of the variance in the dependent variable Y. The estimate of the treatment effect is .951, which is the unstandardized regression coefficient for $DIFF$. This value estimates the size of the "break" in the regression line at $AS = 8.00$. This result is smaller than the observed mean difference (8.20), but it takes full account of the assignment variable and its cutting score.

Chapter 5

1. This depends on whether the sampling method is representative. A smaller sample that is representative is better than a larger sample that is not. Also, the characteristic that statistics from large samples tend to be closer on average to the population parameter assumes representative sampling.

2. Both SD and SE_M are standard deviations. The former reflects variability among cases within a group; the latter estimates variability among means from random samples all drawn from the same population and based on the same number of cases. They are related by the expression $SE_M = SD/N^{1/2}$. Thus, the standard error reflects both the variability among cases and the group size. Given $SD > 0$, the value of SE_M decreases as N increases.

3. The standard error of the mean is like an average distance between μ and means from many random samples all based on the same number of cases. Like any average, though, it may not describe any individual observation (e.g., no family has exactly 2.2 children). Also, the statistic SE_M is subject to sampling error, so its value will probably be different in another sample. Without more information, we cannot say just how far $M = 115.00$ is away from μ.

4. False. The value of the mean contrast $M_1 - M_2$ is unrelated to that of its standard error, $SE_{M_1-M_2}$. The latter is determined by the pooled within-group variance and the group sizes.

5. For these data, $M_1 - M_2 = 2.00$, $n_1 = n_2 = 5$, $s_1^2 = 7.50$, $s_2^2 = 5.00$, $s_P^2 = 6.75$, and $SE_{M_1-M_2} = 1.58$. The positive critical value of $t_{\text{two-tail, .05}}(8)$ is 2.306, so the 95% confidence interval for $\mu_1 - \mu_2$ is

$$2.00 \pm 1.58 \ (2.306)$$

or 2.00 ± 3.65, which defines the interval -1.65–5.65. Based on these results, we can say that the population mean difference could be as small as $\mu_1 - \mu_2 = -1.65$ or as large as $\mu_1 - \mu_2 = 5.65$, at the 95% level of confidence. Of course, the real value of $\mu_1 - \mu_2$ could fall outside of this range, too. Remember, a confidence interval is not a guarantee.

6. For these data, $M_1 - M_2 = 2.00$, $n = 5$, $SD_1 = 7.50^{1/2}$, $SD_2 = 5.00^{1/2}$, $r_{12} = .735$, $s_D^2 = 3.50$, and $SE_{M_D} = .837$. The positive critical value of $t_{\text{two-tail}, .05}$ (4) is 2.776, so the 95% confidence interval for μ_D is

$$2.00 \pm .837 \ (2.776)$$

or 2.00 ± 2.32, which defines the interval –.32–4.32. The 95% confidence interval assuming a repeated-measures design (–.32–4.32) is narrower compared with the 95% confidence interval assuming independent samples (–1.65–5.65) for the same scores. This is because the subject effect is relatively strong in the repeated-measures design (e.g., $r_{12} = .735$).

7. Presented next are results for the three group sizes. Increasing n while holding all else constant has no effect on s_P^2, but values of $SE_{M_1 - M_2}$ and $t_{\text{two-tail}, .05}$ become smaller and values of t become larger as the group size increases. The mean difference of 2.00 is not statistically significant at $n = 5$, but it is so for $n = 15$ ($p < .05$) and $n = 30$ ($p < .01$):

	$n = 5$	$n = 15$	$n = 30$
$M_1 - M_2$	2.00	2.00	2.00
s_P^2	6.25	6.25	6.25
SE_{M1-M2}	1.581	.913	.645
t	1.26	2.19	3.10
df	8	28	58
$t_{\text{two-tail}, .05}$	2.306	2.048	2.002
p	> .05	< .05	< .01

8. The observed mean difference is 25 times as large as the estimated standard error of that difference. Both the t test and its p value measure group size and effect size. The value of t can be large and its probability low if the group sizes are large but the magnitude of the mean difference is small.

9. For these data, the grand mean is $M_T = 12.00$. Calculation of MS_A and MS_W using, respectively, Equation 5.14 and Equation 5.15, are demonstrated next for $n = 15$:

$$MS_A = [15 \ (13.00 - 12.00)^2 + 15 \ (11.00 - 12.00)^2$$
$$+ \ 15 \ (12.00 - 12.00)^2]/2 = 15.00$$

$$MS_W = [14 \ (7.50) + 14 \ (5.00) + 14 \ (4.00)]/(45 - 3)$$
$$= (7.50 + 5.00 + 4.00)/3 = 5.50$$

Present next are the ANOVA source tables for the two group sizes. Increasing n but keeping all else constant has no effect on the error term MS_W, but values of MS_A and F become larger as the group size increases:

		Sum of Squares	df	Mean Square	F	Sig.
$n = 15$	Between (A)	30.00	2	15.00	2.73	$p > .05$
	Within	231.00	42	5.50		
	Total	261.00	44			
$n = 30$	Between (A)	60.00	2	30.00	5.45	$p < .01$
	Within	478.50	87	5.50		
	Total	538.50	89			

10. The between-group variance is 200 times larger than the pooled within-group variance. However, the former measures group size plus the squared distances between the group means and the grand mean. Thus, if the group sizes are large, the value of the between-group variance can be large even though the group means are close to the grand mean. Like the t-test, the F-test measures both group size and effect size together.

11. There is no suggested answer for this question because each student may find a different set of examples. For each example, however, you should identify the myth (e.g., odds-against-chance fallacy) and also rewrite the definition so that it is correct.

Chapter 6

1. The t-test expresses the mean difference as the proportion of its standard error, which measures the pooled within-group variability and the group sizes. This explains the sensitivity of t to group size. In contrast, g expresses the mean contrast as a proportion of the pooled within-group standard deviation, which is not affected by group size, holding all else constant, including the ratio n_1/n_2. Hedges's g is the part of t that measures effect size, but not also sample size.

2. To calculate g, we need its denominator, the square root of the pooled within-group variance. The latter is calculated here as

$$s_P^2 = (7.50 + 5.00)/2 = 6.25$$

For all group sizes, $g = 2.00/6.25^{1/2} = .80$. The value of r_{pb} can be calculated for these data using either Equation 6.11 or Equation 6.14. Use of the latter for $n = 5$ is demonstrated next:

$$r_{pb} = .80/[.80^2 + 8 (1/5 + 1/5)]^{1/2} = .41$$

Presented next are results for the three group sizes. Increasing n while holding all else constant has no effect on g, but values of t become larger as the group size increases. The results for r_{pb} show the pattern that sample correlations approach their maximum absolute values in very small samples:

	$n = 5$	$n = 15$	$n = 30$
$M_1 - M_2$	2.00	2.00	2.00
t	1.26	2.19	3.10
df	8	28	58
p	> .05	< .05	< .01
g	.80	.80	.80
r_{pb}	.41	.38	.38

3. An effect size of $g = .50$ implies that the correlation between group membership (treatment vs. control) and outcome is about .24 and that the former explains about $.24^2 = 0.058$, or about 5.8% of the variance in the latter. At the case level, only about one-third of the cases are distinct, that is, they have scores outside the range of the other group ($U_1 = .330$). The rest of the cases, or about 67%, have scores that fall within the region of overlap of two distributions. The median treated case has a score on the outcome variable that exceeds about 70% of the scores among untreated cases ($U_3 = .691$).

4. It seems that the researcher is referring to a T-shirt effect size category based on Cohen's general rule of thumb that $g > .80$ *may* indicate a large effect. However, this guideline is for cases when there is no other convention to differentiate between smaller and larger effects. If data about effect sizes exist, then they should be the standard for describing effect size magnitude; otherwise, be very cautious about using Cohen's guidelines to make absolute statements about whether an effect size is small, medium, or large.

5. The result $g = 0$ means that the two distributions have the same average score. However, the distributions could differ in other ways, including variability, shape, and the relative proportions of scores at the extremes. Depending on the research question, some of these differences may be of interest.

6. In Table 6.5, descriptive statistics on the alcohol problems variable for the depressed group are $M_D = .30$, $SD_D = .90$, and $n_D = 461$, and for the nondepressed group are $M_N = .20$, $SD_N = .60$, and $n_N = 702$. Demonstrated next are the calculations of Hedges's g, its estimated standard error using the first equation in Table 6.4, and the approximate 95% confidence interval for δ using $z_{\text{two-tail}, .05} = 1.96$ as the test statistic:

$$g = (.30 - .20)/\{[460\,(.90^2) + 701\,(.60^2)]/(460 + 701)\}^{1/2}$$
$$= .10/.538^{1/2} = .14$$

$$\text{est. } SE_g = [.14^2/(2 \times 1{,}161) + 1{,}163/(460 \times 701)]^{1/2} = .0601$$

$.14 \pm .0601\,(1.96)$, or $.14 \pm .12$, which defines the interval $.02-.26$.

7. In Table 6.5, descriptive statistics on the substance abuse variable for the depressed group are $p_D = .288$ and $n_D = 461$, and for the nondepressed group are $p_N = .214$ and $n_D = 702$. Demonstrated next are the calculations of OR, its estimated standard error using the last equation in Table 6.4, the approximate 95% confidence interval for ω using $z_{\text{two-tail, }.05} = 1.96$ as the test statistic, and the value of logit d:

$$OR = [.288/(1 - .288)]/[.214/(1 - .214)]$$
$$= (.288/.712)/(.214/.786) = 1.49$$

$$\ln(1.49) = .3988$$

$$\text{est. } SE_{\ln\,(OR)} = \{1/[461 \times .288\,(1 - .288)]$$
$$+ 1/[702 \times .214(1 - .214)]\}^{1/2} = .1391$$

$$.3988 \pm .1391\,(1.96) \text{ or } .3988 \pm .2726$$

which defines the range $.1262-.6714$ in log units;

$$\ln^{-1}(.1262) = e^{.1262} = 1.1345$$

$$\ln^{-1}(.6714) = e^{.6714} = 1.9569$$

which within rounding error defines the interval $1.14-1.95$ in OR units. Logit d is calculated as

$$\text{logit } d = .3988/(\,\text{pi}/3^{1/2}) = .3988/1.8138 = .22$$

8. Presented next are calculations of partial $\hat{\eta}^2$ for each main and interaction effect using the data in Table 6.6. Also reported are values of $\hat{\eta}^2$ for each effect:

$$\text{partial } \hat{\eta}^2_G = .3539/(.3539 + 7.0176) = .048;\ \hat{\eta}^2_G = .045$$

$$\text{partial } \hat{\eta}^2_P = .0393/(.0393 + 7.0176) = .006;\ \hat{\eta}^2_P = .005$$

$$\text{partial } \hat{\eta}^2_{G \times P} = .4943/(.4943 + 7.0176) = .066;\ \hat{\eta}^2_{G \times P} = .063$$

As expected, values of partial $\hat{\eta}^2$ for each effect are greater than the corresponding value of $\hat{\eta}^2$. This is because the former are proportions of explained variance after removing all other sources of systematic variation.

Chapter 7

1. False. One minus a reliability coefficient, or $1 - r_{XX}$, estimates a proportion of error variance. But because a reliability coefficient estimates only a particular type of measurement error, we cannot say that all of the rest of the variance outside the measurement error part is systematic. Here, $\alpha_C = .80$, so we can say that 20% of the variance is due to content sampling error. However, other types of random error, such as time-sampling error, are not measured by α_C. Thus, some of the remaining 80% of the variance may be error variance, too.

2. The Spearman–Brown prophesy formula (Equation 7.4) can be applied here where $k = 2$:

$$\hat{r}_{kk} = [2\,(.35)]/[1 + (2 - 1)\,.35] = .52$$

That is, doubling the length of the test from 10 to 20 items may increase the reliability from .35 to .52, assuming that new items of similar quality are added.

3. In this application of the Spearman–Brown prophesy formula, the desired minimum level of score reliability is represented by $\hat{r}_{kk} = .90$, but k is here unknown. So we need to solve the equation for k:

$$
\begin{aligned}
.90 &= [k\,(.35)]/[1 + (k - 1)\,.35] \\
.90\,[(1 + (k - 1)\,.35] &= .35\,k \\
.90\,[1 + .35\,k - .35] &= .35\,k \\
.90 + .315\,k - .315 &= .35\,k \\
.90 - .315 &= .35\,k - .315\,k \\
.585 &= .035\,k \\
k &= 16.71
\end{aligned}
$$

It is estimated that the expanded test would require a total of 16.17 × 10 items, or about 162 items (i.e., add 152 items to the original test), in order for reliability to be at least .90, given $r_{XX} = .35$ for 10 items and assuming that the new items are of the same quality.

4. This pattern is not unexpected. An odd–even item split for this test, for which items become increasingly difficult, may be optimal. This is because the two halves of the tests should have about the same mix of easier versus harder items, and scores will tend to be consistent across the two halves. In contrast, the internal consistency reliability is the average of all possible split-half reliabilities. Some of these splits will not be optimal, such as a first-half, second-half split of the items. Here, all the easier items are in the first half, and all the harder ones in the second, so the correlation of scores across the two halves may be low. Both results are correct, but the split-half reliability coefficient based on the odd–even split may provide the best information about content sampling error for this test.

5. The Pearson correlation r_{XY} is a measure of linear association for two continuous variables. Equation 7.5 indicates that the maximum absolute value of $\hat{r}_{XY}$ is limited by the reliabilities of both X and Y, or r_{XX} and r_{YY}. The standardized mean difference Hedges's g is related to the point-biserial correlation r_{pb} (see Equation 6.13), which itself is just a Pearson correlation. In a two-group design, measurement error in the dependent variable will limit the absolute value of both r_{pb} and g.

6. Presented next are item and scale descriptive statistics calculated using the Reliability Analysis procedure of SPSS. Note that the means for each item equal p, the proportion of cases with correct scores:

		Mean	Std Dev	Cases
1.	I1	.7500	.4629	8.0
2.	I2	.7500	.4629	8.0
3.	I3	.6250	.5175	8.0
4.	I4	.7500	.4629	8.0
5.	I5	.7500	.4629	8.0

Statistics for Scale	Mean	Variance	Std Dev	Variables
	3.6250	2.2679	1.5059	5

The sum of the item variances and the value of KR-20 are calculated next:

$$\Sigma\ pg = 4\ (.4629^2) + .5175^2 = 1.1249$$

$$\text{KR-20} = [5/(5-1)]\ [1 - (1.1249/2.2679)] = 1.25\ (.5040) = .63$$

We need the interitem correlations in order to use Equation 7.1. These values calculated using SPSS are presented next:

	I1	I2	I3	I4	I5
I1	1.0000				
I2	.3333	1.0000			
I3	.1491	.1491	1.0000		
I4	.3333	.3333	.1491	1.0000	
I5	.3333	.3333	.1491	.3333	1.0000

Presented next are calculations for α_C:

$$\bar{r}_{ij} = [6\,(.3333) + 4\,(.1491)]/10 = .2596$$

$$\alpha_C = [5\,(.2596)]/[1 + (5-1)\,.2596] = 1.2981/2.0385 = .64$$

which within the limits of rounding error is equivalent to the value for KR-20. The value of α_C calculated by SPSS for these data is .6299.

7. The value of α_C for these data calculated using the Reliability Analysis procedure of SPSS is –.1818. There is obviously a problem with these scores. Presented next are the interitem correlations. Observe that the correlations that involve items 3 and 5 are negative, and the value of $\bar{r}_{ij}$ for these items is –.0298. It may be necessary to apply reverse coding to these two items if they are negatively worded compared with the other three items:

	I1	I2	I3	I4	I5
I1	1.0000				
I2	.3333	1.0000			
I3	-.1491	-.1491	1.0000		
I4	.3333	.3333	-.1491	1.0000	
I5	-.3333	-.3333	.1491	-.3333	1.0000

8. Grade 4 teachers or other experts in mathematics instruction should review item content for representativeness (content validity). Scores on the new test should be positively correlated with scores on existing math achievement tests and also with grades in math (concurrent validity, convergent validity). If archival math test scores are available (e.g., from grade 2), then these scores should covary positively with those from the new test (postdictive validity, convergent validity). To assess the degree to which scores on the new math test are affected by reading comprehension, scores from the math test should not correlate too highly with those from a reading skill test (discriminant validity). The new math test should also predict later math skills, such as those measured in grade 6 (predictive validity, convergent validity).

Chapter 8

1. See Figure 8.2 (p. 239).

2. The value of the multiple correlation for the regression equation with both X and X^2 as predictors calculated using the Linear Regression procedure in SPSS is $R = .927$. Values of the regression coefficients are presented next:

Model		Unstandardized Coefficients		Standardized Coefficients		
		B	Std. Error	Beta	t	Sig.
1	(Constant)	29.486	3.714		7.938	.001
	X	-2.714	.494	-5.505	-5.498	.003
	X2	8.319E-02	.015	5.537	5.529	.003

The regression equation for these data

$$\hat{Y} = 29.486 - 2.714\,X + .0832\,X^2$$

describes a curve line with one bend. It is the term X^2 that, when entered into the equation along with X, represents the quadratic component of the relation, and the X represents the linear component, which is slight for these data. Presented next is an adapted version of the scatterplot created using the Curve Estimation procedure of SPSS that shows both the linear and quadratic trends for these data:

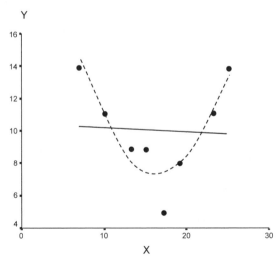

3. See Figure 8.5 (p. 248).

4. Depending on your statistics program, one of the predictors, such as X_2, may be excluded, or the run may end with an error message about multicollinearity. The bivariate correlations among these variables calculated by SPSS are reported next:

	Y	X1	X2	X3
Y	1.000	.648	.236	.617
X1	.648	1.000	-.033	.649
X2	.236	-.033	1.000	.738
X3	.617	.649	.738	1.000

None of these intercorrelations seem excessively high. However, scores on X_3 are the average of the scores on X_1 and X_2 for each case. Just as the sum $X_1 + X_2$ is perfectly collinear with the set X_1 and X_2, so is the ratio $(X_1 + X_2)/2$. Try this analysis: Enter X_1 and X_2 as predictors of X_3 in a new regression analysis. The multiple correlation here is $R = 1.0$.

5. The means are $M_X = 15.500$, $M_Y = 20.125$, and $M_W = 40.375$. Presented next are the correlations calculated in SPSS for these data using each of the three options for handling missing data:

Listwise N = 6

		X	Y	W
X		1.000	.134	.254
Y		.134	1.000	.610
W		.254	.610	1.000

Pairwise

		X	Y	W
X	r	1.000	.134	.112
	N	8	6	7
Y	r	.134	1.000	.645
	N	6	8	7
W	r	.112	.645	1.000
	N	7	7	8

Mean Substitution N = 10

		X	Y	W
X		1.000	.048	.102
Y		.048	1.000	.532
W		.102	.532	1.000

The results change depending on the missing data option used. For example, the correlation between Y and W ranges from .532 to .645 across the three methods. If you do not have a substantive reason for preferring one option for dealing with missing data over others *and* there is an appreciable difference in the results across these alternatives, then it is best to report both sets of results, not just the one that seems the most favorable considering your hypotheses.

References

Abelson, R. P. (1997a). On the surprising longevity of flogged horses: Why there is a case for the significance test. *Psychological Science, 8*, 12–15.

Abelson, R. P. (1997b). A retrospective on the significance test ban of 1999 (If there were no significance tests, they would be invented). In L. L. Harlow, S. A. Mulaik, & J. H. Steiger (Eds.), *What if there were no significance tests?* (pp. 117–141). Mahwah, NJ: Erlbaum.

Agresti, A. (2007). *An introduction to categorical data analysis.* Hoboken, NJ: Wiley.

Aguinis, H. (2004). *Regression analysis for categorical moderators.* New York: Guilford Press.

Aiken, L. S., West, S. G., Sechrest, L., & Reno, R. R. (1990). Measurement in psychology: A survey of PhD programs in North America. *American Psychologist, 45*, 721–734.

Alley, M. (1996). *The craft of scientific writing* (3rd ed.). New York: Springer.

Alley, M. (2003). *The craft of scientific presentations: Critical steps to succeed and critical errors to avoid.* New York: Springer.

Allison, P. D. (2002). *Missing data.* Thousand Oaks, CA: Sage.

American Educational Research Association, American Psychological Association, & National Council on Measurement in Education. (1999). *Standards for educational and psychological testing.* Washington, DC: American Psychological Association.

American Psychological Association. (2005). *Publication manual of the American Psychological Association* (5th ed.). Washington, DC: Author.

Anholt, R. R. H. (2006). *Dazzle 'em with style: The art of oral scientific presentation* (2nd ed.). New York: Elsevier Academic Press.

Armstrong, J. S. (2007a). Significance tests harm progress in forecasting. *International Journal of Forecasting, 23*, 321–327.

Armstrong, J. S. (2007b). Statistical significance tests are unnecessary even when properly done and properly interpreted: Reply to commentaries. *International Journal of Forecasting, 23,* 335–336.

Banasiewicz, A. D. (2005). Marketing pitfalls of statistical significance testing. *Marketing Intelligence and Planning, 23,* 515–528.

Barbour, R. (2007). *Introducing qualitative research: A student's guide to the craft of doing qualitative research.* Thousand Oaks, CA: Sage.

Baron, R. A., Markman, G. D., & Hirsa, A. (2001). Perceptions of men and women as entrepreneurs: Evidence for differential effects of attributional augmenting. *Journal of Applied Psychology, 86,* 923–929.

Belia, S., Fidler, F., Williams, J., & Cumming, G. (2005). Researchers misunderstand confidence intervals and standard error bars. *Psychological Methods, 10,* 389–396.

Berliner, D. C. (2002). Educational research: The hardest science of all. *Educational Researcher, 31*(8), 18–20.

Beutler, L. E., Williams, R. E., Wakefield, P. J., & Entwistle, S. R. (1995). Bridging scientist and practitioner perspectives in clinical psychology. *American Psychologist, 50,* 984–994.

Boice, R. B. (1990). Faculty resistance to writing-intensive courses. *Teaching of Psychology, 17,* 13–17.

Bonate, P. L. (2000). *Analysis of pretest–posttest designs.* Boca Raton, FL: CRC Press.

Bottge, B. A., Rueda, E., LaRoque, P. T., Serlin, R. C., & Kwon, J. (2007). Integrating reform-oriented math instruction in special education settings. *Learning Disabilities Research and Practice, 22,* 96–109.

Breaugh, J. A., & Arnold, J. (2007). Controlling nuisance variables by using a matched-groups design. *Organizational Research Methods, 10,* 523–541.

Buros Institute of Mental Measurements. (n.d.). *Test reviews online!* Retrieved April 13, 2007, from *buros.unl.edu/buros/jsp/search.jsp*

Campbell, D. T., & Erlebacher, A. (1975). How regression artifacts in quasi-experimental evaluations can mistakenly make compensatory education look harmful. In M. Guttentag & E. L. Struening (Eds.), *Handbook of evaluation research* (Vol. 1, pp. 597–617). Beverly Hills: Sage.

Campbell, D. T., & Kenny, D. A. (1999). *Primer on regression artifacts.* New York: Guilford Press.

Campbell, D. T., & Stanley, J. C. (1963). *Experimental and quasi-experimental designs for research.* Chicago: Rand McNally.

Campbell, N. R. (1920). *Physics, the elements.* Cambridge, UK: Cambridge University Press.

Campbell, T. C. (2005). An introduction to clinical significance: An alternative index of intervention effect for group experimental studies. *Journal of Early Intervention, 27,* 210–227.

Carlson, M. (2002). *Winning grants step by step: The complete workbook for plan-*

ning, developing and writing successful grant proposals. San Francisco: Jossey-Bass.

Carver, R. P. (1978). The case against significance testing. *Harvard Educational Review, 48,* 378–399.

Chambers, E. A. (2004). An introduction to meta-analysis with articles from the *Journal of Educational Research* (1992–2002). *Journal of Educational Research, 98,* 35–45.

Chambless, D. L. (1993). *Task Force on Promotion and Dissemination of Psychological Procedures*. Retrieved August 27, 2007, from *www.apa.org/divisions/div12/est/chamble2.pdf*

Chatfield, C. (2004). *The analysis of time series: An introduction* (6th ed.). Boca Raton, FL: CRC Press.

Chow, S. L. (1998). *Statistical significance*. Thousand Oaks, CA: Sage.

Ciarleglio, M. M., & Makuch, R. W. (2007). Hierarchical linear modeling: An overview. *Child Abuse and Neglect, 31,* 91–98.

Cohen, J. (1968). Multiple regression as a general data-analytic system. *Psychological Bulletin, 70,* 426–443.

Cohen, J. (1988). *Statistical power analysis for the behavioral sciences* (2nd ed.). New York: Academic Press.

Cohen, J. (1994). The earth is round ($p < .05$). *American Psychologist, 49,* 997–1003.

Cohen, J., Cohen, P., West, S. G., & Aiken, L. S. (2003). *Applied multiple regression/correlation analysis for the behavioral sciences* (3rd ed.). Mahwah, NJ: Erlbaum.

Cole, J. R., & Cole, S. (1972). The Ortega Hypothesis: Citation analysis suggests that only a few scientists contribute to scientific progress. *Science, 178,* 368–375.

Cone, J. D., & Foster, S. L. (2006). *Dissertations and theses from start to finish: Psychology and related fields* (2nd ed.). Washington, DC: American Psychological Association.

Conley, R. R., Ascher-Svanum, A., Zhu, B., Faries, D. E., & Kinon, B. J. (2007). The burden of depressive symptoms in the long-term treatment of patients with schizophrenia. *Schizophrenia Research, 90,* 186–197.

Conners, F. A., Mccown, S. M., & Roskos-Ewoldson, B. (1998). Unique challenges in teaching undergraduates statistics. *Teaching of Psychology, 25,* 40–42.

Cook, T. D., & Campbell, D. T. (1979). *Quasi-experimentation: Design and analysis issues for field settings*. Chicago: Rand McNally.

Costello, E. J., Erkanli, A., & Angold, A. (2006). Is there an epidemic of child or adolescent depression? *Journal of Child Psychology and Psychiatry, 47,* 1263–1271.

Creswell, J. W. (2003). *Research design: Qualitative, quantitative, and mixed methods approaches* (2nd ed.). Thousand Oaks, CA: Sage.

Cumming, G. (2005). Understanding the average probability of replication: Comment on Killeen (2005). *Psychological Science, 16,* 1002–1004.

Cumming, G., & Maillardet, R. (2006). Confidence intervals and replication: Where will the next mean fall? *Psychological Methods, 11,* 217–227.

Darley, J. M., & Latané, B. (1968). Bystander intervention in emergencies: Diffusion of responsibility. *Journal of Personality and Social Psychology, 8,* 377–383.

Davis, C. M., Yarber, W. L., Bauserman, R., Schreer, G. E., & Davis, S. L. (Eds.). (1998). *Handbook of sexuality-related measures* (2nd ed.). Thousand Oaks, CA: Sage.

Davis, M. (2005). *Scientific papers and presentations* (2nd ed.). New York: Academic Press.

Dawes, R. M. (1994). *House of cards.* New York: Free Press.

Dawes, R. M. (2001). *Everyday irrationality: How pseudo-scientists, lunatics, and the rest of us systematically fail to think rationally.* Cambridge, MA: Westview Press.

Demakis, G. J. (2006). Meta-analysis in neuropsychology: An introduction. *Clinical Neuropsychologist, 20,* 5–9.

DeRubeis, R. J., Hollon, S. D., Amsterdam, J. D., Shelton, R. C., Young, P. R., Salomon, R. M., et al. (2005). Cognitive therapy vs. medications in the treatment of moderate to severe depression. *Archives of General Psychiatry, 62,* 409–416.

Dixon, P. M., & O'Reilly, T. (1999). Scientific versus statistical inference. *Canadian Journal of Experimental Psychology, 53,* 133–149.

Dombrowski, S. C., Kamphaus, R. W., & Reynolds, C. R. (2004). After the demise of the discrepancy: Proposed learning disabilities diagnostic criteria. *Professional Psychology: Research and Practice, 35,* 364–372.

Dong, P., Loh, M., & Mondry, A. (2005). The "impact factor" revisited. *Biomedical Digital Libraries, 2*(7). Retrieved August 14, 2007, from *www.bio-diglib. com/content/pdf/1742-5581-2-7.pdf*

Dunleavy, E. M., Barr, C. D., Glenn, D. M., & Miller, K. R. (2006). Effect size reporting in applied psychology: How are we doing? *The Industrial–Organizational Psychologist, 43*(4), 29–37.

Dybå, T., Kampenes, V. B., & Sjøberg, D. I. K. (2006). A systematic review of statistical power in software engineering experiments. *Information and Software Technology, 48,* 745–755.

Educational Testing Service. (2007). *Test Link overview.* Retrieved April 13, 2007, from *www.ets.org/testcoll/*

Elefteriades, J. A. (2002). Twelve tips on writing a good scientific paper. *International Journal of Angiology, 11,* 53–55.

Elliot, A. J., Maier, M. A., Moller, A. C., Friedman, R., & Meinhardt, J. (2007). Color and psychological functioning: The effect of red on performance attainment. *Journal of Experimental Psychology: General, 136,* 154–168.

Ellis, M. V. (1999). Repeated measures designs. *Counseling Psychologist, 27,* 552–578.

Embretson, S. E., & Reise, S. P. (2000). *Item response theory for psychologists.* Mahwah, NJ: Erlbaum.

Evanschitzky, H., Baumgarth, C., Hubbard, R., & Armstrong, J. S. (2007). Replication research's disturbing trend. *Journal of Business Research, 60,* 411–415.

Fidler, F. (2002). The fifth edition of the APA *Publication Manual:* Why its statistics recommendations are so controversial. *Educational and Psychological Measurement, 62,* 749–770.

Fox, J. (1991). *Regression diagnostics: An introduction.* Newbury Park, CA: Sage.

Frederich, J., Buday, E., & Kerr, D. (2000). Statistical training in psychology: A national survey and commentary on undergraduate programs. *Teaching of Psychology, 27,* 248–257.

Gad-el-Hak, M. (2004). Publish or perish—An ailing enterprise. *Physics Today, 57,* 61–62.

Gescheider, G. A. (1998). *Psychophysics: The fundamentals* (3rd ed.). Mahwah, NJ: Erlbaum.

Gibbs, W. W. (2005). Obesity: An overblown epidemic? *Scientific American, 292* (6), 70–77.

Gigerenzer, G. (1993). The superego, the ego, and the id in statistical reasoning. In G. Keren & C. Lewis (Eds.), *A handbook for data analysis in the behavioral sciences: Vol. 1. Methodological issues* (pp. 311–339). Hillsdale, NJ: Erlbaum.

Goldman, B. A., & Mitchell, D. F. (2002). *Directory of unpublished experimental mental measures* (Vol. 8). Washington, DC: American Psychological Association.

Gorard, S. (2006). Towards a judgment-based statistical analysis. *British Journal of Sociology of Education, 27,* 67–80.

Gosling, P. J. (1999). *Scientist's guide to poster presentations.* New York: Springer.

Gould, S. J. (1996). *Full house: The spread of excellence from Plato to Darwin.* New York: Three Rivers Press.

Greene, J. P. (2005). *Education myths: What special interest groups want you to believe about our schools—and why it isn't so.* Lanham, MD: Rowman & Littlefield.

Greenwald, A. G., Gonzalez, R., Harris, R. J., & Guthrie, D. (1996). Effect sizes and *p* values: What should be reported and what should be replicated? *Psychophysiology, 33,* 175–183.

Grissom, R. J., & Kim, J. J. (2005). *Effect sizes for research: A broad practical approach.* Mahwah, NJ: Erlbaum.

Grocer, S., & Kohout, J. (1997). *The 1995 APA survey of 1992 psychology baccalaureate recipients.* Retrieved August 22, 2007, from *research.apa.org/95survey/homepage.html*

Haller, H., & Krauss, S. (2002). Misinterpretations of significance: A problem students share with their teachers? *Methods of Psychological Research Online*, 7 (1), Article 1. Retrieved July 3, 2007, from *www.mpr-online.de/issue16/art1/article.html*

Hamilton, D. P. (1990). Publishing by—and for?—the numbers. *Science, 250*, 1331–1332.

Hamilton, D. P. (1991). Research papers: Who's uncited now? *Science, 251*, 25.

Hanft, A. (2003, August). Grist: More power than point. *Inc Magazine*. Retrieved February 10, 2007, from *www.inc.com/magazine/20030801/ahanft.html*

Harris, R. J. (1997). Significance tests have their place. *Psychological Science, 8*, 8–11.

Hartwig, F., & Dearing, B. E. (1979). *Exploratory data analysis*. Newberry Park, CA: Sage.

Hedges, L. V. (1987). How hard is hard science, how soft is soft science? *American Psychologist, 42*, 443–455.

Heiberger, M. M., & Vick, J. M. (2001). *The academic job search handbook* (3rd ed.). Philadelphia: University of Pennsylvania Press.

Heinrichs, R. W. (2000). *In search of madness: Schizophrenia and neuroscience*. New York: Oxford University Press.

Henke, R. R., & Perry, K. (2007). *To teach or not to teach? Teaching experience and preparation among 1992–93 bachelor's degree recipients 10 years after college: Statistical analysis report* [Electronic version] (Rep. No. NCES 2007-163). Retrieved August 22, 2007, from *nces.ed.gov/pubs2007/2007163.pdf*

Henson, R. K. (2006). Effect-size measures and meta-analytic thinking in counseling psychology research. *Counseling Psychologist, 34*, 601–629.

Hill, L. G., & Betz, D. L. (2005). Revisiting the retrospective pretest. *American Journal of Evaluation, 26*, 501–517.

Honnef, K. (2000). *Warhol* (rev. ed.). (C. Fahy & I. Burns, Trans.). Cologne, Germany: Taschen. (Original work published 1989)

Horowitz, J. A., & Walker, B. E. (2005). *What can you do with a major in education: Real people. Real jobs. Real rewards*. Hoboken, NJ: Wiley.

Huberty, C. J. (2002). A history of effect size indices. *Educational and Psychological Measurement, 62*, 227–240.

Huberty, C. J., & Morris, J. D. (1988). A single contrast test procedure. *Educational and Psychological Measurement, 48*, 567–578.

Huck, S. W. (1992). Group heterogeneity and Pearson's r. *Educational and Psychological Measurement, 52*, 253–260.

Hunter, J., Schmidt, F., & Jackson, G. (1982). *Meta-analysis: Cumulating research findings across studies*. Beverly Hills, CA: Sage.

International Committee of Medical Journal Editors. (2006). *Uniform requirements for manuscripts submitted to biomedical journals: Writing and editing for biomedical publication*. Retrieved July 18, 2007, from *www.icmje.org/icmje.pdf*

James, L., Mulaik, B., & Brett, J. (1982). *Causal analysis: Assumptions, models, and data*. Beverly Hills, CA: Sage.

Johnston, S. J. (2007). Excel's 65535 problem. *PC World, 25*(12), 68.

Joint Committee on Testing Practices. (2004). *Code of Fair Testing Practices in Education*. Retrieved April 21, 2007, from *www.apa.org/science/fairtestcode.html*

Jones, B., & Kenward, M. G. (2003). *Design and analysis of cross-over trials* (2nd ed.). Boca Raton, FL: Chapman & Hall/CRC.

Justice, L. M., Meier, J., & Walpole, S. (2005). Learning new words from storybooks: An efficacy study with at-risk kindergartners. *Language, Speech, and Hearing Services in Schools, 36*, 17–32.

Kawasaki, G. (2005, December 30). *The 10/20/30 rule of PowerPoint*. Retrieved February 3, 2007, from *blog.guykawasaki.com/2005/12/the_102030_rule.html*

Kehle, T. J., Bray, M. A., Chafouleas, S. M., & Kawano, T. (2007). Lack of statistical significance. *Psychology in the Schools, 44*, 417–422.

Keller, J. (2003, January 5). Killing me Microsoftly with PowerPoint. *Chicago Tribune Magazine*, pp. 8–12, 28–29.

Keppel, G., & Wickens, T. D. (2004). *Design and analysis: A researcher's handbook* (4th ed). Upper Saddle River, NJ: Prentice Hall.

Keppel, G., & Zedeck, S. (1989). *Data analysis for research designs*. New York: Freeman.

Keselman, H. J., Algina, J., & Kowalchuk, R. K. (2001). The analysis of repeated measures designs: A review. *British Journal of Mathematical and Statistical Psychology, 54*, 1–20.

Keselman, H. J., Huberty, C. J., Lix, L. M., Olejnik, S., Cribbie, R. A., Donahue, B., et al. (1998). Statistical practices of education researchers: An analysis of the ANOVA, MANOVA, and ANCOVA analyses. *Review of Educational Research, 68*, 350–368.

Keselman, H. J., Rogan, J. C., Mendoza, J. L., & Breen, L. J. (1980). Testing the validity conditions of repeated measures *F* tests. *Psychological Bulletin, 87*, 479–481.

Kessler, R.C., Demler, O., Frank, R. G., Olfson, M., Pincus, H. A., Walters, E. E., et al. (2005). Prevalence and treatment of mental disorders, 1990 to 2003. *New England Journal of Medicine, 352*, 2515–2523.

Killeen, P. R. (2005). An alternative to null-hypothesis significance tests. *Psychological Science, 15*, 345–353.

Kirk, R. (1996). Practical significance: A concept whose time has come. *Educational and Psychological Measurement, 56*, 746–759.

Kline, R. B. (2004). *Beyond scientific testing: Reforming data analysis methods in behavioral research*. Washington, DC: American Psychological Association.

Kline, R. B. (2005). *Principles and practice of structural equation modeling* (2nd ed.). New York: Guilford Press.

Kmetz, J. L. (2002). *The skeptic's handbook: Consumer guidelines and a critical assessment of business and management research* (rev. ed.). Retrieved August 29, 2007, from *papers.ssrn.com/sol3/papers.cfm?abstract_id=334180*

Kraemer, H. C., & Kupfer, D. J. (2005). Size of treatment effects and their importance to clinical research and practice. *Biological Psychiatry, 59,* 990–996.

Krantz, D. H. (1999). The null hypothesis testing controversy in psychology. *Journal of the American Statistical Association, 44,* 1372–1381.

Kuder, G. F., & Richardson, M. W. (1937). The theory of the estimation of test reliability. *Psychometrika, 2,* 151–160.

Kulczycki, A., Kim, D.-J., Duerr, A., Jamieson, D. J., & Macaluso, M. (2004). The acceptability of the female and male condom: A randomized crossover trial. *Perspectives on Sexual and Reproductive Health, 36,* 114–119.

Laband, D. N., & Tollison, R. D. (2003). Dry holes in economic research. *Kyklos, 56,* 161–174.

Lesik, S. A. (2006). Applying the regression-discontinuity design to infer causality with non-random assignment. *The Review of Higher Education, 30,* 1–19.

Lesiuk, T. (2005). The effect of music listening on work performance. *Psychology of Music, 33,* 173–191.

Linden, A., & Adams, J. L. (2007). Determining if disease management saves money: An introduction to meta-analysis. *Journal of Evaluation in Clinical Practice, 13,* 400–407.

Luellen, J. K., Shadish, W. R., & Clark, M. H. (2005). Propensity scores: An introduction and experimental test. *Evaluation Review, 29,* 530–558.

Lykken, D. T. (1991). What's wrong with psychology, anyway? In D. Cicchetti & W. Grove (Eds.), *Thinking clearly about psychology* (Vol. 1, pp. 3–39). Minneapolis: University of Minnesota Press.

Lynam, D. R., Moffitt, T., & Stouthamer-Loeber, M. (1993). Explaining the relation between IQ and delinquency: Class, race, test motivation, or self-control? *Journal of Abnormal Psychology, 102,* 187–196.

Lyon, G. R., Shaywitz, S. E., Shaywitz, B. A., & Chhabra, V. (2005). Evidence-based reading policy in the United States: How scientific research informs instructional practices. In D. Ravitch (Ed.), *Brookings papers on education policy 2005* (pp. 209–250). Washington, DC: Brookings Institute.

Mabe, M. (2003). The growth and number of journals. *Serials, 16,* 191–197.

MacCallum, R. C., Zhang, S., Preacher, K. J., & Rucker, D. O. (2002). On the practice of dichotomization of quantitative variables. *Psychological Methods, 7,* 19–40.

Maddox, T. (2003). *Tests: A comprehensive reference for assessments in psychology, education, and business* (5th ed.). Austin, TX: PRO-ED.

Marek, R. J. (2004). *Opportunities in social science careers.* New York: McGraw-Hill.

Marsh, H. W., & Hattie, J. (2002). The relation between research productivity and teaching effectiveness: Complementary, antagonistic, or independent constructs? *Journal of Higher Education, 73,* 603–641.

Martella, R. C., Nelson, R., & Marchand-Martella, N. C. (1999). *Research methods: Learning to become a critical consumer.* New York: Allyn & Bacon.

Maxwell, S. E., Delaney, H. D., & Dill, C. A. (1984). Another look at ANCOVA versus blocking. *Psychological Bulletin, 95,* 136–147.

Mayer, R. E. (2001). *Multimedia learning.* New York: Cambridge University Press.

McCartney, K., & Rosenthal, R. (2000). Effect size, practical importance, and social policy for children. *Child Development, 71,* 173–180.

McEwan, M. J., & Anicich, V. G. (2007). Titan's ion chemistry: A laboratory perspective. *Mass Spectrometry Reviews, 26,* 281–319.

McKnight, P. E., McKnight, K. M., Sidani, S., & Figueredo, A. J. (2007). *Missing data: A gentle introduction.* New York: Guilford Press.

Meehl, P. E. (1978). Theoretical risks and tabular asterisks: Sir Karl, Sir Ronald, and the slow progress of soft psychology. *Journal of Consulting and Clinical Psychology, 46,* 806–834.

Meehl, P. (1990). Why summaries of research on psychological theories are often uninterpretable. *Psychological Reports, 66*(Suppl. 1), 195–244.

Menard, S. (Ed.). (2007). *Handbook of longitudinal research: Design, measurement, and analysis across the social sciences.* San Diego: Academic Press.

Messick, S. (1995). Validation of inferences from persons' responses and performances as scientific inquiry into score meaning. *American Psychologist, 50,* 741–749.

Miller, D. W. (1999, August 6). The black hole of education research: Why do academic studies play such a minimal role in efforts to improve the schools? *Chronicle of Higher Education, 45*(48), A17–A18.

Morgan, G. A., Gliner, J. A., & Harmon, R. J. (2000). Quasi-experimental designs. *Journal of the American Academy of Child and Adolescent Psychiatry, 39,* 794–796.

Morris, S. B. (2000). Distribution of standardized mean change effect sizes for meta-analysis on repeated measures. *British Journal of Mathematical and Statistical Psychology, 53,* 17–29.

Mulaik, S. A., Raju, N. S., & Harshman, R. A. (1997). There is a time and place for significance testing. In L. L. Harlow, S. A. Mulaik, & J. H. Steiger (Eds.), *What if there were no significance tests?* (pp. 65–115). Mahwah, NJ: Erlbaum.

Murphy, L. L., Spies, R. A., & Plake, B. S. (Eds). (2006). *Tests in print VII.* Lincoln: Buros Institute of Mental Measurements, University of Nebraska–Lincoln.

Nickerson, R. S. (2000). Null hypothesis significance testing: A review of an old and continuing controversy. *Psychological Methods, 5,* 241–301.

Northey, M., & Tepperman, L. (2007). *Making sense: A student's guide to research and writing in the social sciences* (3rd ed.). New York: Oxford University Press.

Nunnally, J. C., & Bernstein, I. H. (1994). *Psychometric theory* (3rd ed.). New York: McGraw-Hill.

Oakes, M. (1986). *Statistical inference: A commentary for the social and behavioral sciences.* New York: Wiley.

Odom, S. L., Brantlinger, E., Gersten, R., Horner, R. H., Thompson, B., & Harris, K. R. (2005). Research in special education: Scientific methods and evidence-based practices. *Exceptional Children, 71,* 137–148.

Olejnik, S., & Algina, J. (2000). Measures of effect size for comparative studies: Applications, interpretations, and limitations. *Contemporary Educational Psychology, 25,* 241–286.

Ostrow, A. C. (Ed.). (2002). *Directory of psychological tests in the sport and exercise sciences* (2nd ed.). Morgantown, WV: Fitness Information Technology, Western Virginia University.

Pagani, L., Larocque, D., Tremblay, R. E., & Lapointe, P. (2003). The impact of Junior Kindergarten on behaviour in elementary school children. *International Journal of Behavioral Development, 27,* 423–427.

Pallant, J. (2007). *SPSS survival manual: A step-by-step guide to data analysis* (3rd ed.). Maidenhead, Berkshire, UK: Open University Press.

Paradi, D. (2003). *Summary of the annoying PowerPoint survey.* Retrieved January 20, 2007, from *www.communicateusingtechnology.com/pptresults.htm*

Paradi, D. (2005). *What annoys audiences about PowerPoint presentations?* Retrieved January 20, 2007, from *www.thinkoutsidetheslide.com/pptresults2005. htm*

Park, R. L. (2003). The seven warning signs of bogus science. *Chronicle of Higher Education, 49*(21), B20.

Pearl, J. (2000). *Causality: Models, reasoning, and inference.* New York: Cambridge University Press.

Pedhazur, E. J., & Schmelkin, L. P. (1991). *Measurement, design, and analysis: An integrated approach.* Hillsdale, NJ: Erlbaum.

Prentice, D. A., & Miller, D. T. (1992). When small effects are impressive. *Psychological Bulletin, 112,* 160–164.

Rausch, J. R., Maxwell, S. E., & Kelly, K. (2003). Analytic methods for questions pertaining to a randomized pretest, posttest, follow-up design. *Journal of Clinical Child and Adolescent Psychology, 32,* 467–486.

Retsas, A. (2000). Barriers to using research evidence in nursing practice. *Journal of Advanced Nursing, 31,* 599–606.

Richards, J. C., & Miller, S. K. (2005). *Doing academic writing in education: Connecting the personal and the professional.* Mahwah, NJ: Erlbaum.

Robinson, D., & Levin, J. (1997). Reflections on statistical and substantive significance, with a slice of replication. *Educational Researcher, 26*(5), 21–26.

Robinson, D. H., Levin, J. R., Thomas, G. D., Pituch, K. A., & Vaughn, S. (2007). The incidence of "causal" statements in teaching-and-learning research journals. *American Educational Research Journal, 44*, 400–413.

Rogers, J. L., Howard, K. I., & Vessey, J. T. (1993). Using significance tests to evaluate equivalence between two experimental groups. *Psychological Bulletin, 113*, 553–565.

Rosenthal, R., Rosnow, R. L., & Rubin, D. B. (2000). *Contrasts and effect sizes in behavioral research.* New York: Cambridge University Press.

Rossi, J. S. (1987). How often are our statistics wrong? *Teaching of Psychology, 14*, 98–101.

Roth, P. L. (1994). Missing data: A conceptual review for applied psychologists. *Personnel Psychology, 47*, 537–560.

Rutledge, T., & Loh, C. (2004). Effect sizes and statistical testing in the determination of clinical significance in behavioral medicine research. *Annals of Behavioral Medicine, 27*, 138–145.

Sagan, C. (1996). *The demon-haunted world: Science as a candle in the dark.* New York: Random House.

Sanderson, P. M., Wee, A., & Lacherez, P. (2006). Learnability and discriminability of melodic medical equipment alarms. *Anaesthesia, 61*, 142–147.

Scheier, L. M., & Dewey, W. L. (Eds.) (2007). *The complete writing guide to NIH behavioral science grants.* New York: Oxford University Press.

Schmidt, F. L., & Hunter, J. E. (1997). Eight common but false objections to the discontinuation of significance testing in the analysis of research data. In L. L. Harlow, S. A. Mulaik, & J. H. Steiger (Eds.), *What if there were no significance tests?* (pp. 37–64). Mahwah, NJ: Erlbaum.

Schneeweiss, S., Maclure, M., Soumerai, S. B., Walker, A. M., & Glynn, R. J. (2002). Quasi-experimental longitudinal designs to evaluate drug benefit policy changes with low policy compliance. *Journal of Clinical Epidemiology, 55*, 833–841.

Schwarz, N., Knäuper, B., Hippler, H.-J., Noelle-Neumann, E., & Clark, L. (1991). Rating scales: Numeric values may change the meaning of scale labels. *Public Opinion Quarterly, 55*, 570–582.

Sedlmeier, P., & Gigerenzer, G. (1989). Do studies of statistical power have an effect on power of studies? *Psychological Bulletin, 105*, 309–315.

Shadish, W. R. (2002). Revisiting field experimentation: Field notes for the future. *Psychological Methods, 7*, 3–18.

Shadish, W. R., Cook, T. D., & Campbell, D. T. (2001). *Experimental and quasi-experimental designs for generalized causal inference.* New York: Houghton Mifflin.

Simon, H. A. (1988). The science of design: Creating the artificial. *Design Issues, 4* (1/2), 67–82.

Simons, T. (2004, April 7). *Does PowerPoint make you stupid?* Retrieved January 21, 2007, from *www.presentations.com/msg/search/article_display.jsp?vnu_content_id= 1000482464*

Smith, M. L., & Glass, G. V. (1977). Meta-analysis of psychotherapy outcome studies. *American Psychologist, 32*, 752–760.

Smithson, M. J. (2001). *Workshop on: Noncentral confidence intervals and power analysis.* Retrieved July 26, 2007, from *psychology.anu.edu.au/people/smithson/details/CIstuff/Noncoht2.pdf*

Spies, R. A., & Plake, B. S. (Eds.). (2005). *The Sixteenth Mental Measurements Yearbook.* Lincoln: Buros Institute of Mental Measurements, University of Nebraska–Lincoln.

Starbuck, W. H. (2005). How much better are the most prestigious journals?: The statistics of academic publication. *Organization Science, 16*, 180–200.

Steel, P. (2007). The nature of procrastination: A meta-analytic and theoretical review of quintessential self-regulatory failure. *Psychological Bulletin, 133*, 65–94.

Steiger, J. H. (2001). Driving fast in reverse: The relationship between software development, theory, and education in structural equation modeling. *Journal of the American Statistical Association, 96*, 331–338.

Strunk, W., & White, E. B. (2000). *The elements of style* (4th ed.). New York: Longman.

Stuss, D. T., Robertson I. H., Craik, F. I. M., Levine, B., Alexander, M. P., Black, S., et al. (2007). Cognitive rehabilitation in the elderly: A randomized trial to evaluate a new protocol. *Journal of the International Neuropsychological Society, 13*, 120–131.

Swerdlow, N. R., Stephany, N., Wasserman, L. C., Talledo, J., Sharp, S., Minassian, A., et al. (2005). Intact visual latent inhibition in schizophrenia patients in a within-subject paradigm. *Schizophrenia Research, 72*, 169–183.

Tabachnick, B. G., & Fidell, L. S. (2007). *Using multivariate statistics* (5th ed.). Boston: Allyn & Bacon.

Thompson, B. (2001). Significance, effect sizes, stepwise methods, and other issues: Strong arguments move the field. *Journal of Experimental Education, 70*, 80–93.

Thompson, B. (2002). What future quantitative social science research could look like: Confidence intervals for effect sizes. *Educational Researcher, 31*, 25–32.

Thompson, B. (Ed.). (2003). *Score reliability.* Thousand Oaks, CA: Sage.

Thompson, B. (2006). *Foundations of behavioral statistics: An insight-based approach.* New York: Guilford Press.

Thompson, B., & Vacha-Haase, T. (2000). Psychometrics *is* datametrics: The test is not reliable. *Education and Psychological Measurement, 60*, 174–195.

Thorndike, R. M. (2005). *Measurement and evaluation in psychology and education* (7th ed.). Upper Saddle River, NJ: Prentice Hall.

Touliatos, J., Perlmutter, B. F., Straus, M. A., & Holden, G. W. (Eds.). (2001). *Handbook of family measurement techniques* (Vols. 1–3). Thousand Oaks, CA: Sage.

Trochim, W. M. K., Cappelleri, J. C., & Reichardt, C. S. (1991). Random measurement error does not bias the treatment effect estimate in the regression-discontinuity design: II. When an interaction effect is present. *Evaluation Review, 10,* 571–604.

Trochim, W., & Donnelly, J. P. (2007). *The research methods knowledge base* (3rd ed.). Mason, OH: Atomic Dog.

Trochim, W., & Land, D. (1982). Designing designs for research. *The Researcher, 1,* 1–6.

Trujillo, C. A. (2007). Building internal strength, sustainable self-esteem, and inner motivation as a researcher. *Journal of Research Practice, 3*(1), Article M8. Retrieved November 12, 2007, from *jrp.icaap.org/index.php/jrp/article/view/62/88*

Trusty, J., Thompson, B., & Petrocelli, J. V. (2004). Practical guide to implementing the requirement of reporting effect size in quantitative research in the *Journal of Counseling and Development. Journal of Counseling and Development, 82,* 107–110.

Tufte, E. R. (2001). *The visual display of quantitative information* (2nd ed.). Cheshire, CT: Graphics Press.

Tufte, E. R. (2006). *The cognitive style of PowerPoint: Pitching out corrupts within* (2nd ed.). Cheshire, CT: Graphics Press.

Ulmer, R. G., & Northrup, V. S. (2005). *Evaluation of the repeal of the all-rider motorcycle helmet law in Florida* [Electronic version] (Rep. No. DOT HS 809 849). Retrieved June 28, 2007, from *www.nhtsa.dot.gov/people/injury/pedbimot/motorcycle/FlaMCReport/pages/Index.htm*

Vacha-Haase, T., Kogan, L. R., & Thompson, T. (2000). Sample composition and variabilities in published versus those in test manuals: Validity of score reliability inductions. *Educational and Psychological Measurement, 60,* 509–522.

Vacha-Haase, T., Ness, C., Nilsson, J., & Reetz, D. (1999). Practices regarding reporting of reliability coefficients: A review of three journals. *Journal of Experimental Education, 67,* 335–341.

van Dalen, H. P., & Klamer, A. (2005). Is science a case of wasteful competition? *Kyklos, 58,* 395–414.

van den Akker, J., Gravemeijer, K., McKenney, S., & Nieveen, N. (Eds.). (2006). *Educational design research.* New York: Routledge.

Van de Vijver, F., & Hambleton, R. K. (1996). Translating tests: Some practical guidelines. *European Psychologist, 1,* 89–99.

van Sluijs, E., van Poppel, M., Twisk, J., & van Mechelen, W. (2006). Physical activity measurements affected participants' behavior in a randomized controlled trial. *Journal of Clinical Epidemiology, 59,* 404–411.

Wayne, J. H., Riordan, C. M., & Thomas, K. M. (2001). Is all sexual harassment viewed the same?: Mock juror decisions in same- and cross-gender cases. *Journal of Applied Psychology, 86,* 179–187.

Webb, E. J., Campbell, D. T., Schwartz, R. D., & Sechrest, L. (1966). *Unobtrusive measures: Nonreactive research in the social sciences.* Chicago: Rand McNally.

Wilcox, R. R. (1998). How many discoveries have been lost by ignoring modern statistical methods? *American Psychologist, 53,* 300–314.

Wilkinson, L., & the Task Force on Statistical Inference. (1999). Statistical methods in psychology journals: Guidelines and explanations. *American Psychologist, 54,* 594–604.

Wood, J. M., Nezworski, M. T., Lilienfeld, S. O., & Garb, H. N. (2003). *What's wrong with the Rorschach: Science confronts the controversial inkblot test.* San Francisco: Jossey-Bass.

Woody, S. R., Weisz, J., & McLean, C. (2005). Empirically supported treatments: 10 years later. *Clinical Psychologist, 58,* 5–11.

Wuensch, K. L. (2006). *Using SPSS to obtain a confidence interval for Cohen's d.* Retrieved July 23, 2007, from *core.ecu.edu/psyc/wuenschk/SPSS/CI-d-SPSS. doc*

Ziliak, S. T., & McCloskey, D. N. (2008). *The cult of statistical significance: How the standard error costs us jobs, justice, and lives.* Ann Arbor: University of Michigan Press.

Zuckerman, I. H., Lee, E., Wutoh, A. K., Xue, Z., & Stuart, B. (2006). Application of regression-discontinuity analysis in pharmaceutical health services research. *Health Services Research, 41,* 550–563.

Author Index

Abelson, R. P., 135, 207
Adams, J. L., 19
Agresti, A., 48
Aguinis, H., 113
Aiken, L. S., 5, 193, 194
Algina, J., 83, 167
Alley, M., 279, 284, 290, 295, 304
Allison, P. D., 245
Angold, A., 262
Anholt, R. R. H., 290, 291, 295, 299, 305, 306
Anicich, V. G., 264, 266
Armstrong, J. S., 117, 120, 134
Arnold, J., 113
Ascher-Svanum, A., 180, 181
Asimov, I., 236

B

Banasiewicz, A. D., 124
Barbour, R., 74
Baron, R. A., 182, 183
Barr, C. D., 154
Baumgarth, C., 134
Bauserman, R., 204
Belia, S., 148
Berliner, D. C., 31, 32
Bernstein, I. H., 195, 196, 197, 199, 200, 221
Betz, D. L., 85
Beutler, L. E., 26
Boice, R. B., 256
Bonate, P. L., 113
Bottge, B. A., 102
Bray, M. A., 120

Breaugh, J. A., 113
Breen, L. J., 83
Brett, J., 45
Buday, E., 5

C

Campbell, D. T., 42, 45, 62, 63, 71, 96, 97, 107
Campbell, N. R., 193
Campbell, T. C., 175
Cappelleri, J. C., 105
Carlson, M., 278
Carver, R. P., 124
Chafouleas, S. M., 120
Chambers, E. A., 19
Chambless, D. L., 17
Chatfield, C., 113
Chhabra, V., 25
Chow, S. L., 135
Ciarleglio, M. M., 113
Clark, L., 198
Clark, M. H., 113
Cohen, J., 50, 120, 138, 156, 164, 172, 173
Cole, J. R., 23
Cole, S., 23
Condron, M., 45
Cone, J. D., 277
Conley, R. R., 180, 181, 182
Conners, F. A., 119
Cook, T. D., 42, 45, 71, 96
Costello, E. J., 262
Creswell, J. W., 74
Cumming, G., 128, 145, 187

D

Darley, J. M., 10, 289, 290, 307
Davis, C. M., 204
Davis, M., 253, 255, 279, 288, 296, 299, 304, 305, 306
Davis, S. L., 204
Dawes, R. M., 17, 131
Dearing, B. E., 241, 249
Delaney, H. D., 85, 113
Delany, H. D., 113
Demakis, G. J., 19
DeRubeis, R. J., 79
Dewey, W. L., 278
Dill, C. A., 85, 113
Dixon, P. M., 130
Dombrowski, S. C., 24
Dong, P., 20
Donnelly, J. P., 60, 62, 71, 74
Duerr, A., 90
Dunleavy, E. M., 154
Dybå, T., 132, 133

E

Elefteriades, J. A., 261, 262
Elliot, A. J., 266
Ellis, M. V., 113
Embretson, S. E., 218
Entwistle, S. R., 26
Erkanli, A., 262
Erlebacher, A., 97
Evanschitzky, H., 134

F

Faries, D. E., 180, 181
Fidell, L. S., 234
Fidler, F., 148, 154
Figueredo, A. J., 241
Fischer, M. H., 39–40
Foster, S. L., 277
Fox, J., 247
Frederich, J., 5, 119, 193
Friedman, R., 266

G

Gad-el-Hak, M., 33
Garb, H. N., 25
Gescheider, G. A., 192
Gibbs, W. W., 263
Gigerenzer, G., 132, 133, 136
Glasbergen, R., 286
Glass, G. V., 17–18
Glenn, D. M., 154
Gliner, J. A., 92
Glynn, R. J., 93
Goldman, B. A., 203
Gonzalez, R., 127
Gorard, S., 174
Gosling, P. J., 304
Gould, S. J., 15
Gravemeijer, K., 71
Greene, J. P., 17
Greenwald, A. G., 127
Grissom, R. J., 184, 185
Grocer, S., 16
Guthrie, D., 127

H

Haller, H., 120, 124, 125
Hambleton, R. K., 204
Hamilton, D. P., 22
Hanft, A., 302
Harmon, R. J., 92
Harris, R. J., 127, 135
Harshman, R. A., 128
Hartwig, F., 241, 249
Hattie, J., 34
Hedges, L. V., 28
Heiberger, M. M., 13
Heinrichs, R. W., 179–180
Henke, R. R., 16
Henson, R. K., 153, 154, 184, 185
Hill, L. G., 85
Hippler, H. -J., 198
Hirsa, A., 182, 183
Holden, G. W., 204
Honnef, K., 3
Horowitz, J. A., 13
Howard, K. I., 129
Hubbard, R., 134
Huberty, C. J., 48, 155, 166

Huck, S. W., 65
Hunter, J., 18, 132, 133
Hunter, J. E., 138, 139

J

Jackson, G., 18
James, L., 45
Jamieson, D. J., 90
Johnston, S. J., 228
Jones, B., 113
Justice, L. M., 86

K

Kampenes, V. B., 132, 133
Kamphaus, R. W., 24
Kawano, T., 120
Kawasaki, G., 295
Kehle, T. J., 120
Keller, J., 283
Kelly, K., 86, 114
Kenny, D. A., 62
Kenward, M. G., 113
Keppel, G., 51, 54
Kerr, D., 5
Keselman, H. J., 83, 134
Kessler, R. C., 263
Killeen, P. R., 127
Kim, D. -J., 90
Kim, J. J., 184, 185
Kinon, B. J., 180, 181
Kirk, R., 121, 154, 174
Klamer, A., 12, 19, 22, 23
Kline, R. B., 5, 19, 29, 113, 121, 124,
    127, 136, 137, 138, 140, 155, 158,
    159, 163, 166, 169, 172, 174, 184,
    185, 186, 187, 188, 203, 214, 233
Kmetz, 29
Knäuper, B., 198
Kogan, L. R., 206
Kohout, J., 16
Kowalchuk, R. K., 83
Kraemer, H. C., 154
Krantz, D. H., 135
Krauss, S., 120, 124, 125
Kuder, G. F., 209
Kulczycki, A., 90

Kupfer, D. J., 154
Kwon, J., 102

L

Laband, D. N., 22
Lacherez, P., 83
Land, D., 43, 57
Lapointe, P., 100–101
Larocque, D., 100–101
LaRoque, P. T., 102
Latané, B., 10, 289, 290, 307
Lee, E., 106
Lenth, R., 132
Lesik, S. A., 105
Lesiuk, T., 108
Levin, J., 134
Levin, J. R., 272
Lilienfeld, S. O., 25
Linden, A., 19
Loh, C., 157
Loh, M., 20
Luellen, J. K., 113
Lykken, D. T., 22, 27, 28, 29, 30, 31,
    34, 35
Lynam, D. R., 57
Lyon, G. R., 25

M

Mabe, M., 19
Macaluso, M., 90
MacCallum, R. C., 49, 50
Maclure, M., 93
Maddox, T., 203
Maier, M. A., 266
Maillardet, R., 145
Makuch, R. W., 113
Marchand-Martella, N. C., 69
Marek, R. J., 13
Markman, G. D., 182, 183
Marsh, H. W., 34
Martella, R. C., 69
Maxwell, S. E., 85, 86, 113, 114
Mayer, R. E., 299
McCartney, K., 154
McCloskey, D. N., 120
Mccown, S. M., 119

McEwan, M. J., 264, 266
McKenney, S., 71
McKnight, K. M., 241
McKnight, P. E., 241
McLean, C., 25
Meehl, P. E., 28, 130
Meier, J., 86
Meinhardt, J., 266
Menard, S., 113
Mendoza, J. L., 83
Messick, S., 215–216
Miller, D. T., 174
Miller, D. W., 34, 35
Miller, K. R., 154
Miller, S. K., 256
Mitchell, D. F., 203
Moffitt, T., 57
Moller, A. C., 266
Mondry, A., 20
Morgan, G. A., 92
Morris, J. D., 48, 159
Morris, S. B., 159
Mulaik, B., 45, 128
Mulaik, S. A., 128
Murphy, L. L., 203

N

Nelson, R., 69
Nezworski, M. T., 25
Nickerson, R. S., 138, 139
Nieveen, N., 71
Nighswander, L., 283
Noelle, Neumann, E., 198
Northey, M., 256
Northrup, V. S., 109, 110
Nunnally, J. C., 195, 196, 197, 199,
    200, 221

O

Oakes, M., 120, 124, 125
Odom, S. L., 17
Olejnik, S., 167
O'Reilly, T., 130
Ostrow, A. C., 204

P

Pagani, L., 100–101
Pallant, J., 249, 250
Paradi, D., 285, 287, 288
Parisi, M., 197
Park, R. L., 128
Pearl, J., 45
Pedhazur, E. J., 26, 31, 42, 46, 57,
    68–69, 119, 191
Perlmutter, B. F., 204
Perry, K., 16
Petrocelli, J. V., 154
Pituch, K. A., 272
Plake, B. S., 202, 203
Preacher, K. J., 49
Prentice, D. A., 174

R

Raju, N. S., 128
Rausch, J. R., 86, 114
Reichardt, C. S., 105
Reise, S. P., 218
Retsas, A., 26
Reynolds, C. R., 24
Richards, J. C., 256
Richardson, M. W., 209
Riordan, C. M., 280, 281
Robinson, D., 134
Robinson, D. H., 272
Rogan, J. C., 83
Rogers, J. L., 129
Rosenthal, R., 154, 155
Roskos-Ewoldson, B., 119
Rosnow, R. L., 155
Rossi, J. S., 26
Roth, P. L., 249, 250, 269
Rubin, D. B., 155
Rucker, D. O., 49
Rueda, E., 102
Rutledge, T., 157

S

Sagan, C., 47
Sanderson, P. M., 83

Schmelkin, L. P., 26, 31, 42, 46, 57, 68–69, 119, 191
Schmidt, F., 18, 132, 133
Schmidt, F. L., 138, 139
Schneeweiss, S., 93
Schreer, G. E., 204
Schwartz, R. D., 63
Schwarz, N., 198
Sechrest, L., 63
Sedlmeier, P., 132, 133
Serlin, R. C., 102
Shadish, W. R., 42, 44, 48, 55, 56, 60, 61, 67, 68, 69, 71, 92, 94, 100, 108, 110, 113, 114
Shaywitz, B. A., 25
Shaywitz, S. E., 25
Sheier, L. M., 278
Sidani, S., 241
Simon, H. A., 73
Simons, T., 285
Sjøberg, D. I. K., 132, 133
Smith, M. L., 17–18, 259
Smithson, M. J., 187–188
Soumerai, S. B., 93
Spearman, C. E., 192
Spies, R. A., 202, 203
Stanley, J. C., 107
Starbuck, W. H., 20, 22
Steel, P., 290
Steiger, J. H., 229
Stein, G., 255
Sternberg, R. J., 13
Stouthamer-Loeber, M., 57
Straus, M. A., 204
Strunk, W., 256
Stuart, B., 106
Stuss, D. T., 89
Swerdlow, N. R., 264

T

Tabachnick, B. G., 234
Tagore, R., 119
Tepperman, L., 256
Thomas, G. D., 272
Thomas, K. M., 280, 281
Thompson, B., 18, 50, 51, 65, 113, 140, 148, 154, 173, 193, 205, 206, 207, 220, 221, 263
Thompson, T., 206

Thorndike, R. M., 194, 196, 199, 205, 221
Tollison, R. D., 22
Touliatos, J., 204
Tremblay, R. E., 100–101
Trochim, W., 41, 43, 57, 60, 62, 71, 74
Trochim, W. M. K., 105
Trujillo, C. A., 262
Trusty, J., 154
Tufte, E. R., 271, 275, 279, 285, 301, 302, 305, 306
Twisk, J., 87
Tzu, C., 16

U

Ulmer, R. G., 109, 110

V

Vacha-Haase, T., 193, 205, 206
van Dalen, H. P., 12, 19, 22, 23
Van de Vijver, F., 204
van den Akker, J., 71
van Mechelen, W., 87
van Poppel, M., 87
van Sluijs, E., 87, 88
Vaughn, S., 272
Vessey, J. T., 129
Vick, J. M., 13

W

Wakefield, P. J., 26
Walker, A. M., 93
Walker, B. E., 13
Walpole, S., 86
Warhol, A., 3
Wayne, J. H., 280, 281
Webb, E. J., 63
Wee, A., 83
Weisz, J., 25
Wells, H. G., 45
White, E. B., 256
Wickens, T. D., 51
Wilcox, R. R., 51
Wilkinson, L, 51, 112, 132, 150, 225, 226–228, 234, 267, 269, 270, 272

Williams, J., 148
Williams, R. E., 26
Wood, J. M., 25
Woody, S. R., 25
Wuensch, K. L., 187, 188
Wutoh, A. K., 106

X

Xue, Z., 106

Y

Yarber, W. L., 204

Z

Zedeck, S., 54
Zhang, S., 49
Zhu, B., 180, 181
Ziliak, S. T., 120
Zuckerman, I. H., 106

Subject Index

f following a page number indicates a figure;
t following a page number indicates a table.

A priori level of statistical significance, 122
A priori power analysis
    effect size and, 154–155
    overview, 132
    recommendations regarding, 137, 137*t*
A × subject (S) interaction, 150
Abstracts, 263–264, 264*t*
Academic career path
    overview, 11–12
    "publish or perish" and, 33–34
Academic integrity, 253–254
Accidental sampling, 68
Active voice, 258
Ad hoc samples, 68
Adobe Portable Document Format (PDF) in oral presentations, 300–301
Alternate-forms reliability, 208
Ambiguous temporal precedence threat to internal validity, 58, 58*t*
American Educational Research Association, 192–193
American Psychological Association (APA)
    Code of Fair Testing Practices in Education and, 193
    Standards for Educational and Psychological Testing and, 192–193
American Psychological Association (APA) style, 7, 9, 255–256
Analysis of covariance (ANCOVA)
    design and, 113
    experimental design and, 82

overview, 51–54, 53*f*, 319–320
predicted mean difference and, 315
pretest–posttest design and, 96–99, 98*f*
proxy pretest in, 85–86
Analysis of data. *see also* Design; Statistics
    goals of, 47–54, 53*f*
    overview, 9, 47–54, 53*f*, 138
    problems students may have with, 5–6
    recommendations regarding, 136–138, 137*t*
    research trinity and, 40*f*
    threats to inference accuracy and, 8
Analysis of variance (ANOVA)
    batch mode processing and, 232
    design and, 78–81
    effect size and, 157, 158
    effect size estimation and, 166–168
    experimental design and, 82
    generalizability theory and, 220
    moderator effects and, 92
    overview, 44, 49–54, 315–316, 319–320
    proxy pretest in, 85–86
    results section of an empirical study and, 269–271
    simplicity and, 227
Anthropomorphism, 259
APA style, 7, 9, 255–256
Approximate truth, 40–41, 40*f*
Assignment variable, 93
Association, 45
Assumptions problem, 134
Asymptotic standard error, 175

Attention control group, 77
Attrition threat to internal validity, 58*t*, 59
Autoregressive integrative moving average (ARIMA) model, 109
Available-case methods, 242

B

Balanced design, 79, 80*t*
Basic randomized experiment, 76–79, 79–84, 80*t*
Basic type of experimental design, 77*t*
Batch mode processing, 230–231
Bayesian statistics, 127
Behavioral scientist career path, 10–12
Between-subject factorial design, 79
Bias, adapting or translating tests and, 205
Big Five false beliefs about *p* values, 124–128, 125*t*
Binet–Simon scales of mental ability, 192
Bivariate regression, 50–51
Bivariate relations, 245–249, 246*f*, 247*f*, 248*f*
Blocking factor, 81–82
Box plot, 238–239, 239*f*
Box-and-whisker plot, 238–239, 239*f*
Build sequence, 288
Burnout, 19–20
Buros Institute of Mental Measurements, *Mental Measurements Yearbook* (MMY) and, 203

C

Capitalization on chance, 158
Career paths, 10–12
Case-control designs, 110–111
Case-history design, 110–111
Case-level indexes
    overview, 163–165, 164*f*, 165*t*
    relation of group-level indexes to, 165–166, 165*t*
Case-referent design. *see* Case-control designs
Categorical data analysis, 48
Causal effects, path analysis and, 111

Causal questions
    overview, 75–76
    validity and, 314
Causality fallacy, 128, 129*t*
Cause–effect relations, 42, 314
Cause-probing designs, 42
Cell mean, 80
Central *t*-distribution, 143
Chartjunk, 275, 276*f*, 298
Chi-square statistic, homogeneity of covariance and, 83
Circularity. *see* Homogeneity of covariance
Citation half-lives, 20–21
Citations
    impact factor (IF) and, 20–21
    uncited works, 22
Classical test (measurement) theory
    multi-item measurement and, 197
    overview, 192, 220–221
    recent developments in, 217–220, 219*f*
    score reliability and, 213–214
Clinical significance, 175
Cluster sampling, 67
Code of Fair Testing Practices in Education, 193
Coefficient alpha
    overview, 208–209
    score reliability and, 212
Cognitive style of PowerPoint, 301
Coherence principle, 299–300
Commercial test measures, finding measures and, 200–204, 202*t*
Common method variance, 62–63
Comparative studies, 74
Compensatory equalization of treatment threat to internal validity, 58*t*, 60
Compensatory rivalry threat to internal validity, 58*t*, 60
Completely between-subject factorial design, 79
Completely within-subject factorial design, 82
Computer technology. *see* Technology
Conclusion validity
    analysis and, 48
    overview, 40, 40*f*, 64–66, 64*t*, 313
Concurrent validity, 215, 330
Conduct statistical tests, 48

Confidence interval, 47, 175–178, 177*t*
Confidence interval for μ, 143,
     145–146, 323
Confidence intervals for means,
     143–146
Confidence-level misconception, 145
Confounders. *see* Confounding variables
Confounding variables, 44
Consequential aspect of validity, 216
Construct bias, adapting or translating
     tests and, 205
Construct confounding threat to construct validity, 62, 63*t*
Construct validity
     measurement and, 46
     overview, 40, 40*f*, 62–64, 63*t*, 221,
          313, 314
     threats to, 62–64, 63*t*
Content aspect of validity, 215
Content error, 220–221
Content sampling error, 208
Content validity, 214
Context effects, problems associated
     with soft research and, 31
Contrast comparison, 78
Contribution to knowledge, lack of in
     published articles, 27–28
Control groups
     designs without, 107–108
     overview, 318
Controlled quasi-experimental designs,
     92–94, 95*t*
Convenience samples, 68
Convergent validity, 215, 330
Correlation ratio, 157
Correlational designs. *see* Nonexperimental design
Counterbalanced within-subject design,
     82, 316–317
Covariance. *see also* Analysis of covariance (ANCOVA)
     analysis and, 47, 51–53, 53*f*
     research hypotheses and, 43
Covariance structures, 91
Covariate, 51–52
Criterion-related validity, 214
Critical ratio, 147
Cronbach's alpha
     overview, 208–209
     score reliability and, 212

Crossed design, 79
Crossover type of experimental design,
     77*t*, 89–90, 316–317
Cumulative knowledge, lack of in published articles, 28–29
Cumulativeness, theoretical. *see* Theoretical cumulativeness

D

Data analysis. *see also* Analysis of data
     data screening and, 233–249, 234*t*,
          238*f*, 239*f*, 246*f*, 247*f*, 248*f*
     managing complex analyses,
          229–233, 232*t*
     overview, 225–229, 249
Data screening, 233–249, 234*t*, 238*f*,
     239*f*, 246*f*, 247*f*, 248*f*
Decision study. *see* D-study
Descriptive questions, 74–75
Design. *see also* Experimental design;
          Quasi-experimental designs
     complex designs and, 166–168
     connecting to research questions,
          74–76
     controlled quasi-experimental designs, 92–94, 95*t*
     effect size estimation and, 166–168
     five structural elements of, 42–43
     nonequivalent-group designs,
          94–103, 98*f*, 102*f*
     nonexperimental design, 57,
          111–112
     overview, 41–46, 74, 112–113, 113*t*
     problems associated with soft research and, 31
     regression-discontinuity designs,
          93–94, 103–106, 104*f*, 107*f*
     research trinity and, 40*f*
     threats to inference accuracy and, 8
Dichotomization
     analysis and, 49–50
     effect size and, 169–172, 169*t*
     experimental design and, 82
     simplicity and, 227
Difference score, 142
Differential attrition, case-control designs and, 110–111
Differential item functioning, adapting
     or translating tests and, 205

Direct manipulation, 55
Discriminant validity, 215
Discussion section of an empirical
    study, 271–273
Dissertations, writing skills and,
    276–278
Distribution shape, data analysis and,
    236–241, 238*f*, 239*f*
Double-pretest design
    overview, 101
    results from, 102*f*
D-study, 220

E

Ecological validity, 67
Education research, education policy
    and, 24
Educational Testing Service (ETS),
    203–204
Effect size. *see also* Effect size estima-
    tion
    data analysis and, 226
    dichotomous outcomes and,
        169–172, 169*t*
    noncentrality interval estimation
        for, 186–189, 187*f*
    overview, 326
    score reliability and, 213
    statistical tests and, 151
Effect size estimation. *see also* Effect
    size
    complex designs and, 166–168
    confidence intervals and, 175–178,
        177*t*
    contexts for, 154–155
    examples of, 178–184, 181*t*, 183*t*
    measures of association and,
        166–168
    noncentrality interval estimation
        for, 186–189, 187*f*
    overview, 47, 153, 184
    parametric effect sizes and, 155–
        158
    t-shirt sizes example, 172–175, 174*t*
    when comparing two samples,
        158–166, 164*f*, 165*f*
80/20 rule, 23
Elimination of an extraneous variable,
    56

Empirical studies, writing sections of,
    263–273, 264*t*, 266*t*
Empirically validated methods, basing
    practice on, 17
Entrepreneur research, example of ef-
    fect size estimation and, 182–184,
    183*t*
Equivalence fallacy, 129, 129*t*
Equivalent model, 111–112
Error bars, 47
Error term, 149
Estimated eta-squared, 157
Estimated omega-squared, 158
Estimation of effect size. *see* Effect size
    estimation
Evaluation apprehension threat to con-
    struct validity, 63, 63*t*
Exact level of statistical significance, 122
Expectancy control group, 77
Expectation–maximization method,
    244–245
Experimental design
    analysis and, 47
    overview, 41–42, 76–92, 77*t*, 80*t*
Experimentwise (familywise) rate of
    Type I error, 66
Exploratory Software for Confidence
    Intervals (ECSI), 186–187
External aspect of validity, 216
External validity
    overview, 40, 40*f*, 67–70, 70*t*, 313,
        314
    replication and, 133–134
    threats to, 69–70, 70*t*
Extraneous variables, 43–44

F

Facets, generalizability theory and,
    219–220
Factorial repeated-measures design, 82
Factorial type of experimental design,
    77*t*
Failure fallacy, 129, 129*t*
Failure of randomization, 56
Familywise rate of Type I error, 66
Fishing, 66
Fishing and inflation of Type I error
    rate threat to conclusion validity,
    64*t*, 66

Fixed-effects factor, 51
Focused comparison, 78
Fourfold table, 169, 169t
Freewriting, 255
Frequentist approach to probability,
  144–145
F-test
  homogeneity of covariance and, 83
  overview, 148–151

G

G-coefficient, 220
Geisser–Greenhouse correction, 83
General linear model, 50, 231
Generalizability aspect of validity, 216
Generalizability coefficient, 220
Generalizability theory, 219–220
Generalization of results
  purposive sampling and, 68–69
  replication and, 133–134
  validity and, 314
Glass's delta, 160
Goal of research, data analysis and,
  225–229
Graduate thesis, writing skills and,
  276–278
Grand mean, 80
Grant proposals, writing sections of,
  277–278
Graphical displays, 273–276, 275f, 276t
Graphical user interface (GUI),
  229–230
Group differences indexes, 155
Group matching, 78
Group mean difference, 315–316
Group overlap indexes, 155
Group-level indexes
  overview, 159–163
  relation of to case-level indexes,
    165–166, 165t
Group-mean substitution, 242–243
G-theory, 219–220

H

Handouts in oral presentations,
  293–294, 301–302
Hawthorne effect, 61

Hedges's g, 159–160, 180, 326–327
Heterogeneity of variance, 51
Heteroscedasticity, 246
Hidden bias, 100
Hierarchical (nested) data structures,
  91
Hierarchical linear modeling (HLM),
  91
History threat to internal validity
  overview, 58–59, 58t
  reducing, 61–62
Homogeneity of covariance, 82–83
Homogeneity of regression
  overview, 53–54, 321
  pretest–posttest design and, 98
Homogeneity of variance, 51
Homoscedasticity, 246
Huynh–Feldt correction, 83
Hypotheses, research, 43, 47–48
Hypothetical constructs
  measurement process and, 194–195
  validity and, 314

I

Idiographic factors, problems associ-
  ated with soft research and, 31
IF (impact factor), 20–21
Illusory correlation, 131
Imitation threat to internal validity,
  58t, 60
Impact factor (IF), 20–21
Inaccurate effect size estimation threat
  to conclusion validity, 64t, 65
Inclusion of an extraneous variable, 56
Independence of observations
  analysis and, 51
  overview, 44
Indirect citation, 273
Individual differences principle, 300
Individual-differences assessment, 192
Inference, statistical
  analysis and, 48
  statistical tests and, 136
  threats to, 8
Inflated diction, 258
Information explosion, 19
Information fatigue (burnout), 19–20
Institute for Scientific Information
  (ISI), 20–21

Instrumentation threat to internal validity
  overview, 58*t*, 59
  reducing, 61–62
Interaction effect, 80, 92
Internal consistency reliability, 208
Internal validity
  case-control designs and, 110–111
  double-pretest design and, 101
  nonequivalent-group designs, 101–103
  overview, 40, 40*f*, 54–62, 58*f*, 313
  pretest–posttest design and, 95
  threats to, 58–61, 58*t*
Interrater reliability, 208
Interrupted time-series designs, 108–109, 110*f*, 318
Interval estimation, 47
Introduction of an empirical study, 264–266, 266*t*
Inverse probability error
  overview, 126–127
  statistical significance and, 125*t*
IQ scores, education policy and, 24
Isolation, 45
Item bias, adapting or translating tests and, 205
Item response theory (IRT), 217–219, 219*f*
Item-characteristic curve (ICC), 218
Item–total correlations, 209

J

Joint Committee on Testing Practices, 192–193

K

KR-20 internal consistency reliability, 209
Kurtosis, 237–240, 238*f*

L

Latent growth model, 91
Latent-trait theory. *see* Item response theory (IRT)

Least publishable unit (LPU), 33
Leptokurtic, 237–240
Likert scale, 197–198
Linear Regression option in SPSS, 331
Listwise deletion, 242
Literature reviews, 264–266, 266*t*
Local Type I error fallacy, 125*t*
Locally available samples, 68
Logistic regression, 100
Logit, 171
Longitudinal type of experimental design, 77*t*, 90–92
Low power threat to conclusion validity, 64*t*, 65–66
Lower asymptote, 218
Lower hinge, 239
Lurking variables. *see* Confounding variables

M

Magnitude fallacy, 128, 129*t*
Main effect, 80
Margin bound, 162
Marginal mean, 80
Marker, 179
Maturation threat to internal validity
  overview, 58*t*, 59
  reducing, 61–62
Mauchly's test, 83
Mean
  experimental design and, 80
  statistical tests for comparing, 146–151
Mean split, 49
Mean structures, 91
Mean substitution, 242
Meaningfulness fallacy, 128, 129*t*
Measurement
  adapting or translating tests, 204–205
  checklist for evaluation measures, 216, 217*t*
  evaluation of score reliability and validity and, 205–216
  finding measures, 200–204, 202*t*
  overview, 46, 191–193, 220–221
  process overview, 194–200
  recent developments in test theory and, 217–220, 219*f*

research trinity and, 40*f*
role of, 5–6, 193–194
threats to inference accuracy and,
    8–9
Measurement error interaction effects,
    220
Measurement issues, problems associat-
    ed with soft research and, 31–32
Measurement scale, 196–200
Measurement theory, instruction of, 5
Measures of association, 155, 156–158
Median split, 49
Mediator effect, 91–92
Mediator variable, 92
Mental Measurements Yearbook (MMY),
    202–203
Meta-analysis, 17–19
Meta-analytic thinking, 17–19
Method bias, adapting or translating
    tests and, 205
Methodology, role of, 5–6
Methods section of an empirical study,
    266–268
Metric, 196–200
Microsoft PowerPoint. *see* PowerPoint
    presentations
Minimally sufficient analysis, 226–227
Missing data
    data analysis and, 241–245
    results section of an empirical study
    and, 269
Mixed design. *see* Mixed within-subject
    factorial design
Mixed within-subject factorial design,
    82
Modality principle, 300
Model-based imputation methods, 244
Moderated multiple regression, 99
Moderator effect, 80, 92
Moments about the mean, 239–240
Monomethod bias threat to construct
    validity, 62, 63*t*
Mono-operation bias threat to con-
    struct validity, 63, 63*t*
Monotonic transformation, 199–200
Multicollinearity, 245
Multi-item measurement, 196–200
Multiple regression
    batch mode processing and, 232
    data screening and, 245–249, 246*f*,
    247*f*, 248*f*

overview, 50–51
simplicity and, 227
Multiple treatment interference threat
    to external validity, 69, 70*t*
Multivariate analysis of variance
    (MANOVA), 227–228, 231

N

Negative kurtosis, 237–240, 238*f*
Negative skew, 237–240, 238*f*
Newman–Keuls procedure, *F*-test and, 150
Nill hypothesis, 134–135
No-attention control group, 77
Nomothetic factors, problems associ-
    ated with soft research and, 31
Noncentral *t*-distribution, 143
Noncentrality interval estimation, 176,
    186–189, 187*f*
Noncentrality parameter, 186
Noncommercial test measures, finding
    measures and, 202*t*
Nonequivalent dependent variables,
    86–87
Nonequivalent-group design, 93,
    94–103, 98*f*, 102*f*
Nonexperimental design
    internal validity and, 57
    overview, 42, 111–112
Nonprobability sampling
    overview, 68
    purposive sampling and, 69
Normal probability plot, 246
Novelty and disruption effects threat
    to internal validity, 58*t*, 61
Nuisance (noise) variables, 43–44
Null hypothesis
    myths regarding statistical signifi-
    cance and, 130–131
    null hypothesis problem, 134–135
    overview, 135
    statistical significance and, 118*t*,
    121–124, 125
    statistical tests and, 136

O

Objectivity fallacy, 129*t*, 130
Observations, independence of. *see* In-
    dependence of observations

Odds ratio
  confidence intervals and, 175–178
  overview, 170–171
Odds-against-chance fallacy, 124–125,
  125*t*
Omnibus comparison, 78
One-group pretest–posttest design,
  107–108
One-shot case study, 107
One-to-one matching, 78
Online availability of articles, 20–21
Open-access journals, 19
Operational definition, 195
Oral presentations
  creating effective presentations with
    PowerPoint and, 289–299
  issues with PowerPoint and, 300–302
  overview, 9–10, 283–288, 287*t*, 305
  poster presentations, 302–304, 303*f*
  principles of multimedia presenta-
    tions and, 299–300
  problems students may have with,
    6–7
Order effects, 82
Outcome interaction threat to external
  validity, 69, 70*t*
Outliers, 235–236
Out-of-range scores, 235
Overreliance on statistical tests threat
  to conclusion validity, 64*t*, 65

P

Pairwise deletion, 242
Paradigm
  overview, 23
  problems associated with soft re-
    search and, 32
Parametric effect sizes, 155–158
Partial eta-squared, 167
Passive observational designs. *see* Non-
  experimental design
Passive voice, 258
Path analysis, 111
Pattern matching, 244
PDF format in oral presentations,
  300–301
Pearson correlation, 329
Performance anxiety in oral presenta-
  tions, 284

Phi coefficient, 171
Placebo control group, 76–77, 318
Plagiarism, 253–254
Platykurtic, 237–240
Point estimate, 47
Point-biserial correlation, 161
Policy, gap between research and,
  24–25
Poor construct definition threat to con-
  struct validity, 62, 63*t*
Population validity, 67, 323
Positive bias, 51
Positive kurtosis, 237–240, 238*f*
Positive skew, 237–240, 238*f*
Postdictive validity, 215
Poster presentations, 302–304, 303*f*
Posttest-only design, 94, 319
Power
  overview, 65–66
  statistical significance and, 132–
    133
Power Analysis module of STATIS-
  TICA
  overview, 187
  reliability and, 211
  simplicity and, 228
PowerPoint presentations
  creating effective presentations
    with, 289–299
  issues with, 300–302
  oral presentations, 283–288
  overview, 9–10, 283, 287*t*, 305
  principles of, 299–300
  problems with, 6–7, 286–288, 287*t*
Practice, gap between research and,
  24–26
Predicted means
  analysis of covariance (ANCOVA)
    and, 52–53, 53*f*
  overview, 52, 315, 319–320
Predictions
  moderated multiple regression and,
    99
  research hypotheses and, 43
Predictive validity, 215, 330
Presentations
  creating effective presentations with
    PowerPoint and, 289–299
  examples of slides, handouts and
    posters, 307–312
  issues with PowerPoint and, 300–302

oral presentations, 283–299, 287*t*
overview, 283, 305
poster presentations, 302–304,
    303*f*
principles of multimedia presenta-
    tions and, 299–300
Presumed causes and effects, design
    and, 42
Pretest–posttest type of experimental
    design
    one-group pretest–posttest design,
        107–108
    overview, 77*t*, 84–87, 94–101, 98*f*,
        318
    results from, 102*f*
    switching replications type of ex-
        perimental design and, 89
Pretest–posttest–follow-up (PPF) de-
    sign, 86
Prewriting activities, 254–255
Primary studies, meta-analysis and, 18
Principle of proximal similarity, 67
Probabilistic revolution, 136
Probability sampling
    overview, 67, 314
    purposive sampling and, 68–69
Propensity score analysis (PSA),
    99–100
Propensity scores, 99–100
Proxy pretest, 84, 85
Psychometrics, instruction of, 5
Publication Manual of the APA (2005),
    7, 255–256. *see also* American
    Psychological Association (APA)
    style
"Publish or perish," 33–34
Purposive sampling, 68–69

Q

Qualitative research, 74
Quality fallacy, 128, 129*t*
Quantitative research, 74
Quasi-experimental designs
    analysis and, 47
    overview, 41–42, 107–111, 110*f*
    problems associated with soft re-
        search and, 31
Questionnaires, finding measures and,
    200–204

R

Random hot-deck imputation, 244
Random irrelevancies in study setting
    threat to conclusion validity,
    64–65, 64*t*
Random sampling, 67–68, 314
Random within-group heterogeneity
    threat to conclusion validity, 64*t*,
    65
Random-effects factor, 50–51
Randomization
    internal validity and, 61
    missing data and, 243
    overview, 41, 55–56
    probability sampling and, 314
    random sampling and, 67–68
Randomized blocks design, 81–82
Randomized clinical trials, 41–42
Randomized control trials, 41–42
Randomized experiments, 41–42
Randomized factorial design, 76–79,
    79–84, 80*t*
Randomized longitudinal designs,
    90–92
Randomized pretest–posttest design,
    84–87
Range restriction threat to conclusion
    validity, 64*t*, 65
Rater drift, 59
Reactive self-report changes threat to
    construct validity, 63, 63*t*
Redundancy principle, 300
Reference sections of empirical stud-
    ies, 273
Regression equation
    Linear Regression option in SPSS,
        320–323
    overview, 98–99, 331
    pretest–posttest design and, 98, 98*f*
Regression threat to internal validity
    overview, 58*t*, 59
    reducing, 62
Regression-based imputation, 243
Regression-based substitution, 243
Regression-discontinuity designs,
    93–94, 103–106, 104*f*, 107*f*,
    318–319
Reification fallacy, 129, 129*t*
Rejection of manuscripts, 22
Relation between variables, 43

Relational questions, 75
Relationship indexes, 155
Reliability
    adapting or translating tests and,
        204–205
    classical test theory and, 192
    empirical studies and, 268
    evaluation of, 205–216
    measurement and, 46
    overview, 220–221, 314
Reliability Analysis procedure of SPSS,
    329–330
Reliability coefficients, 207–208,
    220–221, 328
Reliability induction, 206
Removed-treatment design, 108
Repeated pretest, 84–85
Repeated-treatment design, 108,
    316–317
Replicability fallacy
    overview, 127
    statistical significance and, 125t
Replication
    lack of in published articles, 29–30
    statistical significance and, 133–134
Representative samples
    overview, 323, 330
    randomization and, 314
Research hypotheses, 43, 47–48
Research question, connecting to a
    possible design, 74–76
Research trinity
    analysis, 47–54, 53f
    conclusion validity, 64–66, 64t
    construct validity, 62–64, 63t
    design, 41–46
    external validity, 67–70, 70t
    internal validity, 54–62, 58f
    measurement, 46
    overview, 39–41, 40f, 70–71
    role of measurement in, 193
Researcher expectancies threat to con-
    struct validity, 63–64, 63t
Resentful demoralization threat to in-
    ternal validity, 58t, 60–61
Residuals, 246
Results section of an empirical study
    example of, 280–282, 281t, 282f
    overview, 268–271
Retrospective (post hoc) power analy-
    sis, 132

Retrospective design, 110–111
Retrospective interpretation, meta-
    analytic thinking and, 18
Retrospective pretest, 85
Reversal design, 77t, 89–90, 316–317
Reverse coding, 209–210
Reverse scoring, 209–210
Risk difference
    confidence intervals and, 175–178
    overview, 169–171
Risk ratio
    confidence intervals and, 175–178
    overview, 170–171
Rorschach inkblot test, gap between
    research and the use of, 25

S

Sample size, power and, 133
Sampling, 67–70, 70t, 314, 323
Sampling distribution, 140
Sampling error
    confidence-level misconception and,
        145
    overview, 140, 220–221
    replication and, 134
    statistical significance and, 122–123
Sanctification fallacy, 129, 129t
SAS/STAT
    batch mode processing and, 231
    simplicity and, 228
Scaling measurement, 196–200
Scheffé procedure, F-test and, 150
Schizophrenia research, 179–182,
    181t
Score imputation, 242
Score reliability
    classical test theory and, 192
    empirical studies and, 268
    evaluation of, 205–216
    factors that influence, 212–213
    measurement and, 46
    overview, 220–221, 314
    types of, 208–211
Score validity
    classical test theory and, 192
    empirical studies and, 268
    evaluation of, 205–216
    overview, 221
    types of, 214–216

Secondary analysis, meta-analysis as a type of, 18
Selection bias
    case-control designs and, 110–111
    overview, 59–60
Selection maturation, pretest–posttest design and, 95
Selection process, 93–94, 314–315
Selection threat to internal validity, 58*t*, 59–60
Selection-attrition threat to internal validity, 60
Selection-maturation threat to internal validity, 60
Selection-regression threat to internal validity
    double-pretest design and, 101
    overview, 60
Self-archiving research repositories, 19
SEM. *see* Structural equation modeling (SEM)
Setting interaction threat to external validity, 69, 70*t*
Signed correlation, 161
Simple random sampling, 67
Simple randomized design. *see* Basic randomized experiment
Simplicity in research, data analysis and, 225–229
Single-item measure, 198–199
Skew, 237–240, 238*f*
Skewness problem, 22–23
Slow reveal, 288
Social interaction threats to internal validity, 60
Soft science, problems associated with research in, 30–32
Soft social science model, 29
Solomon Four-Group Design
    internal validity and, 61
    overview, 77*t*, 87–88
Spatial continuity principle, 299
Spearman–Brown prophesy formula, 212–213, 328
Sphericity. *see* Homogeneity of covariance
Split-half reliability, 210–211
Split-plot design. *see* Mixed within-subject factorial design
Spontaneous remission, 77

SPSS
    batch mode processing and, 231, 232–233, 232*t*
    Linear Regression option in, 320–323, 331
    Reliability Analysis procedure of, 329–330
    simplicity and, 228
Stage fright in oral presentations, 284
Standard error, 140
Standard error bars, 144
Standard error of the mean, 140–143, 323
Standardized mean differences
    comparing two samples and, 159–166, 164*f*, 165*t*
    overview, 155–156
Standards for Educational and Psychological Testing, 192–193
STATISTICA
    overview, 187
    reliability and, 211
    simplicity and, 228
Statistical conclusion validity, 40–41, 40*f*
Statistical control, 56
Statistical inference
    analysis and, 48
    statistical tests and, 136
    threats to, 8
Statistical results, incorrect, 26–27
Statistical significance
    drawbacks of statistical tests and, 132–135
    misinterpretation of, 124–130, 125*t*, 129*t*
    myths regarding, 130–131
    overview, 118*t*, 121–124
Statistical software, 211
Statistical tests
    for comparing means, 146–151
    defense of, 135–136
    drawbacks of, 132–135
    effect size and, 151
    overreliance on, 32–33
    overview, 119–121
    recommendations regarding, 136–138, 137*t*
Statistician's two step, 68
Statistics
    analysis and, 47–48
    managing complex analyses, 229–233, 232*t*

Statistics *(continued)*
 myths regarding, 130–131
 overview, 8–9, 117–121, 138
 recommendations regarding,
  136–138, 137*t*
 review of the fundamentals of,
  140–151
 role of, 5
 simplicity and, 226–227
 validity and, 314
Statistics reform, 5
Stem-and-leaf plot, 237–238, 238*f*, 239*f*
Stratified sampling, 67
Structural aspect of validity, 215–216
Structural elements of design, 42–43.
 see also Design
Structural equation modeling (SEM)
 nonexperimental design and,
  111–112
 overview, 91, 92
 results section of an empirical study
  and, 270–271
 simplicity and, 228
Style guides for writing, 255–256
Subject effect, 142
Substantive aspect of validity, 215
Success fallacy, 128, 129*t*
Switchback design. *see* Crossover type
 of experimental design
Switching replications type of experimental design, 77*t*, 88–90

T

Tailored testing, 218
Task Force on Promotion and Dissemination of Psychological Procedures of the Clinical Psychology
 division of the APA, 17
Technical style guide, 255–256
Technology. *see also* PowerPoint presentations
 information explosion and, 19
 managing complex analyses,
  229–233, 232*t*
 noncentrality interval estimation
  and, 186–188
 oral presentations and, 6–7
 poster presentations, 304
 presentations and, 285

simplicity and, 228
statistical significance and, 122–123
statistical software reliability and,
 211
Templates in PowerPoint, 296–297
Temporal contiguity principle, 299
Temporal precedence, 45
10, 20, 30, 3 × 5 rule of PowerPoint
 presentations, 295
Test Link database, 203–204
Test theory. *see* Classical test (measure-
 ment) theory
Test user qualifications, 201
Testing threat to internal validity
 overview, 58*t*, 59
 reducing, 61–62
Test–retest reliability, 208
The Elements of Style (200), 256
Theoretical cumulativeness
 overview, 28
 problems associated with soft re-
  search and, 32
Thesis research projects, components
 of, 6
Three-parameter IRT model, 218
Title of an empirical study, 263–264
Transformations, 236, 240–241
Treatment diffusion threat to internal
 validity, 58*t*, 60
Treatment effect, regression-disconti-
 nuity designs and, 103–106, 104*f*,
 107*f*
Treatment interaction threat to exter-
 nal validity, 69, 70*t*
Treatment × outcome interaction
 threat to external validity, 69, 70*t*
Treatment × setting interaction threat
 to external validity, 69, 70*t*
Treatment × treatment interaction
 threat to external validity, 69, 70*t*
Treatment × unit interaction threat to
 external validity, 69, 70*t*
Trinity, research. *see* Research trinity
t-tests, 146–148, 325
Two-parameter IRT model, 218
Type I errors
 experimentwise rate of, 66
 F-test and, 150
 null hypothesis and, 135
 overview, 135, 315
 statistical significance and, 118*t*, 124

Type II errors
homogeneity of covariance and, 83
null hypothesis and, 135
overview, 135

U

Unbalanced design, 79
Uncited published works, 22
Unit interaction threat to external va-
lidity, 69, 70*t*
Univariate data screening, basic steps
of, 234*t*
Unreliability of treatment implementa-
tion threat to conclusion validity,
64, 64*t*
Unreliable scores threat to conclusion
validity, 64*t*
Unreliable scores threat to construct
validity, 63*t*
Unsigned correlation, 161
Upper asymptote, 218
Upper hinge, 239

V

Validity. *see also* Conclusion validity;
Construct validity; External validity; Internal validity
adapting or translating tests and,
204–205
case-control designs and, 110–111
classical test theory and, 192
empirical studies and, 268
evaluation of, 205–216
measurement and, 46
overview, 313, 314, 330
research trinity and, 40–41, 40*f*
threats to, 58–61, 58*t*, 69–70, 70*t*

Validity fallacy
overview, 128
statistical significance and, 125*t*
Variance-accounted-for effect size, 157
Violated assumptions of statistical tests
threat to conclusion validity, 64*t*, 65

W

Wait-list control group, 77
Washout period, 90
Waste problem, 22–23
Within-subject factorial design, 82
Word processor use in oral presentations, 301–302
Writing skills
example results section, 280–282,
281*t*, 282*f*
getting started and, 254–255
graphical displays and, 273–276,
275*f*, 276*t*
at a higher level, 276–278
learning and, 254
overview, 253, 278–279
plagiarism and, 253–254
principles of, 256–263, 260*t*
"publish or perish" and, 12
role of style guides in, 255–256
scientific writing, 261–263
writing sections of empirical studies, 263–273, 264*t*, 266*t*
Writing style guide, 256
Written presentations, problems students may have with, 6

Z

Zero fallacy, 129, 129*t*
Zooming in method, 291

About the Author

Rex B. Kline, PhD, is Associate Professor of Psychology at Concordia University in Montréal. Since earning a doctorate in psychology, his areas of research and writing have included the psychometric evaluation of cognitive abilities in children, child clinical assessment, structural equation modeling, statistics reform, and usability engineering in computer science. Dr. Kline has published four books, several chapters, and more than 40 articles in research journals.